Surveillance as S

Surveillance happens to us all, every day, as we walk beneath street cameras, swipe cards, surf the Net. Agencies are using increasingly sophisticated computer systems – especially searchable databases – to keep tabs on us at home, work, and play. Once the word surveillance was reserved for police activities and intelligence gathering; now it is an unavoidable feature of everyday life.

Surveillance as Social Sorting proposes that surveillance is not simply a contemporary threat to individual freedoms, but that, more insidiously, it is a powerful means of creating and reinforcing long-term social differences. As practiced today, it is actually a form of social sorting – a means of verifying identities but also of assessing risks and assigning worth. Questions of how categories are constructed therefore become significant ethical and political questions.

Bringing together contributions from North America and Europe, *Surveillance as Social Sorting* offers an innovative approach to the interaction between societies and their technologies. It looks at a number of examples in depth and will be an appropriate source of reference for a wide variety of courses.

David Lyon is Professor of Sociology at Queen's University, Kingston, Ontario.

Surveillance as Social Sorting

Privacy, risk, and digital discrimination

Edited by David Lyon

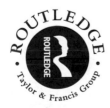

London and New York

First published 2003
by Routledge
11 New Fetter Lane, London EC4P 4EE

Simultaneously published in the USA and Canada
by Routledge
29 West 35th Street, New York, NY 10001

Routledge is an imprint of the Taylor & Francis Group

© 2003 David Lyon

Typeset in Times by
Keystroke, Jacaranda Lodge, Wolverhampton
Printed and bound in Great Britain by
TJ International Ltd, Padstow, Cornwall

British Library Cataloguing in Publication Data
A catalogue record for this book is available from the British Library

Library of Congress Cataloging in Publication Data
A catalog record for this book has been requested

ISBN 0–415–27873–2 (pbk)
ISBN 0–415–27872–4 (hbk)

Contents

Contributors

Lori Andrews is Distinguished Professor, Chicago-Kent College of Law, and Director, Institute for Science, Law, and Technology at the Illinois Institute of Technology.

Kirstie Ball is Lecturer in Organizational Management, Department of Commerce, University of Birmingham. She is the author of a number of theoretical and empirical papers on surveillance in organizations including those published in *Organization Studies*, and *Ethics and Information Technology*, and is joint editor (with David Lyon, Clive Norris, Steven Graham, and David Wood) of *Surveillance in Society*, an on-line journal and web-based study resource. She has spoken nationally and internationally on surveillance practice at work, and has appeared in the national media in relation to this issue. She also writes on new managerialism (with Damian Hodgson and Chris Carter); discourse and the body in organizations (with Damian Hodgson); and human resource information systems.

Colin Bennett received his Bachelor's and Master's degrees from the University of Wales, and his Ph.D. from the University of Illinois at Urbana-Champaign. Since 1986 he has taught in the Department of Political Science at the University of Victoria, where he is now Professor. From 1999 to 2000, he was a fellow with the Harvard Information Infrastructure Project, Kennedy School of Government, Harvard University. His research interests have focused on the comparative analysis of information privacy protection policies at the domestic and international levels. He has published *Regulating Privacy: Data Protection and Public Policy in Europe and the United States* (1992); *Visions of Privacy: Policy Choices for the Digital Age* (1999); and multiple articles in a variety of international journals. He is currently involved in an interdisciplinary and international research project (funded by the National Science Foundation) which examines the relation of emergent geographic information technologies to changing patterns of individual identification.

Michael Curry is a Professor of Geography at the University of California, Los Angeles. His areas of interest are the social and cultural implications of the development of geographic information technologies, such as geographic information systems, and the geographical implications of the development of information technologies. He is the author of two books, *The Work in the World: Geographical Practice and the Written Word* (1996) and *Digital Places: Living with Geographic Information Technologies* (1998), and a number of articles and book chapters. His current work concerns the relationship between conceptualizations of place and of privacy. E-mail: curry@geog.ucla.edu. Website: http://baja.sscnet.ucla.edu/~curry/.

David Lyon is Professor of Sociology at Queen's University, Kingston, Ontario, where he is also Director of the Surveillance Project (http://qsilver.queensu.ca/sociology/Surveillance/intro.htm). He works in the sociology of technology, of religion, and social theory. His books include *The Electronic Eye: The Rise of Surveillance Society* (1994), *Surveillance Society: Monitoring Everyday Life* (2001) and, co-edited with Elia Zureik, *Computers, Surveillance and Privacy* (1996).

Greg Marquis obtained his Ph.D. from Queen's University in 1987 and teaches Canadian and criminal justice history at the University of New Brunswick Saint John. Author of *Policing Canada's Century: A History of the Canadian Association of Chiefs of Police* (1993) and *In Armageddon's Shadow: The Civil War and Canada's Maritime Provinces* (1998, 2000), his work has appeared in *Acadiensis*, the *Journal of the Canadian Historical Association*, *Histoire sociale/Social History*, the *Canadian Journal of Criminology*, *Criminal Justice History* and the *Journal of Imperial and Commonwealth History*. His current research is twentieth-century Canadian alcohol policy. E-mail: gmarquis@unbsj.ca

Dorothy Nelkin holds a University Professorship at New York University, teaching in the Department of Sociology and the School of Law. Her research in science studies focuses on the relationship between science and the public as expressed in disputes, the media and popular culture, public attitudes, and institutional responses to scientific information. Formerly on the faculty of Cornell University, she has had visiting appointments at University College in London, the École Polytechnique in Paris, and MIT. Her books include: *Controversy: Politics of Technical Decisions* (1992), *The Creation Controversy* (1982), *Workers at Risk* (1984), *Selling Science* (1995), *Dangerous Diagnostics* (with L. Tancredi) (1989, 1994), *The DNA Mystique* (with S. Lindee) (1995), and *Body Bazaar: The Market for Human Tissue in the Biotechnology Age* (with L. Andrews) (2001).

Clive Norris is Professor of Sociology at the University of Sheffield. He has written extensively on the sociology of policing and surveillance. In 1998 he completed another, two-year, ESRC-funded study entitled *CCTV and Social Control*. He is joint editor with Gary Armstrong and Jade Moran of *Surveillance, Closed Circuit Television and Social Control* (1998), and co-author with Gary Armstrong of *The Maximum Surveillance Society: The Rise of CCTV* (1999). His most recent book, with Clive Coleman, is *Introducing Criminology* (2000). He is currently working on a three-year European Commission funded project, entitled *Urbaneye*, comparing the use of CCTV in seven European countries.

David Phillips is Assistant Professor of Radio-Television-Film at the University of Texas-Austin. He studies the political economy and social shaping of information and communication technologies, especially technologies of privacy, identification, and surveillance. He is the author, most recently, of "Negotiating the Digital Closet: Online Pseudonymity and the Politics of Sexual Identity" (forthcoming in *Information, Communication, and Society*) as well as numerous conference papers exploring the relations among policy, economics, ideology, culture, and technology.

Jennifer Poudrier is Assistant Professor of Sociology at the University of Saskatchewan, Saskatoon. Her research focuses on the social, cultural, and political implications of new genetic science and deals with issues that lie at the intersections of Aboriginal studies, medical sociology and science studies. She is currently completing her doctoral dissertation entitled "The 'Genetic Revolution,' Aboriginal Health and the 'Thrifty Gene' Theory: Cautionary Facts from DNA Fiction."

Charles Raab is Professor of Government at the University of Edinburgh. He has taught and published extensively in the field of public policy, including information policy. His current interests lie in regulatory policies and regimes for privacy protection, public access to information, and electronic government and democracy, with regard to information and communications systems and technologies. Funding sources for his research include the Economic and Social Research Council (UK), the European Commission, and the National Science Foundation (USA). He has advised the UK Government's Cabinet Office on privacy and data-sharing, and is on the editorial board of *Information, Communication, and Society*. E-mail: c.d.raab@ed.ac.uk Website: http://www. pol.ed. ac.uk/people.html#raab.

Priscilla Regan is an Associate Professor in the Department of Public and International Affairs at George Mason University. Prior to joining that faculty in 1989, she was a Senior Analyst in the Congressional Office of Technology Assessment (1984–89) and an Assistant Professor of Politics and Government at the University of Puget Sound (1979–84). Since the mid-1970s, Dr Regan's primary research interest has been the analysis of the social, policy, and legal implications of organizational use of new information and communications technologies. Dr Regan has published over twenty articles or book chapters, as well as *Legislating Privacy: Technology, Social Values, and Public Policy* (1995). As a recognized researcher in this area, Dr Regan has testified before Congress and participated in meetings held by the Department of Commerce, Federal Trade Commission, Social Security Administration, and Census Bureau. Dr Regan received her Ph.D. in Government from Cornell University in 1981 and her BA from Mount Holyoke College in 1972.

Felix Stalder is interested in the social dynamics created with new technologies, particularly in the areas of electronic money, digital identity and open-source approaches to software and other forms of digital content. He holds a Ph.D. from the University of Toronto, is a post-doctoral fellow with the Surveillance Project at Queen's University and a director of Openflows, an open source media company. He has published extensively in academic and non-academic journals. Much of his writing is accessible at http: //felix.openflows.org.

Irma van der Ploeg (Ph.D.) is a research fellow for the Netherlands Organization for Scientific Research at the Institute for Health Policy and Management of Erasmus University, Rotterdam. She has written on philosophical, political, and normative aspects of medical reproductive technologies, information technology, and biometrics. E-mail: vanderploeg@bmg.eur.nl.

Dwayne Winseck is Associate Professor at the School of Journalism and Communication, Carleton University, Ottawa, Canada. Before arriving in Ottawa in 1998, he lived and taught in Britain, the People's Republic of China, the Turkish Republic of Northern Cyprus and the United States. His research focuses on the political economy of communication, media history, communication policy, theories of democracy, and global communication. He has authored and co-edited three books on these topics, *Reconvergence: A Political Economy of Telecommunications in Canada* (1998); *Democratizing Communication: Comparative Perspectives on Information and Power* (1997); and *Media in Global Context* (1997). He has also published numerous book chapters as well as journal articles in the *Canadian Journal of Communication, Gazette, Javnost/the Public, New Media and Society*, the *European Journal of Communication, Media, Culture and Society*, and elsewhere.

Elia Zureik is a Professor of Sociology at Queen's University. His research interests focus on work and the new technology. He is currently researching the use of surveillance and monitoring technologies in the workplace. He can be reached at zureike@post.queensu.ca.

Preface and acknowledgements

Most of the chapters of this book were originally papers presented at an international research workshop at Queen's University, Kingston, Ontario, Canada, in May 2001. It was a highly collegial and intellectually exciting event, which we hope comes across in the book too. The workshop was organized by the Surveillance Project, a cross-disciplinary initiative based in the Sociology Department at Queen's, and funded in its first three years by a grant from the Social Sciences and Humanities Research Council of Canada. The workshop was also supported by the fact that several participants have a National Science Foundation grant for their research on Intelligent Transportations Systems. Details of the Surveillance Project may be found at: http://qsilver.queensu.ca/sociology/Surveillance/intro.htm. The Project is also a founding partner in the on-line journal and resource center, *Surveillance and Society* (surveillance-and-society.org).

As editor I am deeply grateful for the help of all authors in preparing their chapters for publication, and to the team in the Surveillance Project for providing such a stimulating context in which this work was done. My graduate students, Jason Pridmore, Tamy Superle, and Joran Weiner were particularly helpful in making the workshop work well. A big thank you is due to Anna Dekker, my editorial assistant, for her tireless and cheerful work on the details, and I am also grateful to Edwina Welham for her help at Routledge. I'm always aware of the loving support of Sue, but it's been more apparent than ever during the preparation of this book, because a fracturing fall on hidden ice in the last months of editorial work put me first in hospital, then on crutches. sdg

Thanks to Blackwell Publishing for permission to reprint the (now revised and updated) article by Dorothy Nelkin and Lori Andrews as Chapter 5 of this book.

David Lyon, Kingston, Ontario

Introduction

David Lyon

Once, the word "surveillance" was reserved for highly specific scrutiny of suspects, for police wiretapping or for foreign intelligence. No more. Surveillance – the garnering of personal data for detailed analysis – now occurs routinely, locally and globally, as an unavoidable feature of everyday life in contemporary societies. Organizations of all kinds engage in surveillance and citizens, consumers, and employees generally comply with that surveillance (with some noteworthy exceptions). Surveillance is frequently, but not exclusively, carried out using networked computer systems, which vastly increase its capacities and scope.

Once, concerns about surveillance were couched primarily in the language of privacy and, possibly, freedom. There is something sacrosanct, so the argument goes, about the "private" realm where I am "free to be myself" and where I need not fear the prying eyes of snoops and spies. There are some things I feel it inappropriate to reveal promiscuously to others, let alone to be revealed about me without my knowledge or consent. While these issues are still significant, it is becoming increasingly clear to many that they do not tell the whole story. For surveillance today sorts people into categories, assigning worth or risk, in ways that have real effects on their life-chances. Deep discrimination occurs, thus making surveillance not merely a matter of personal privacy but of social justice.

"Surveillance as social sorting" indicates a new departure for surveillance studies. Not entirely new, of course, especially if one thinks of the work of Oscar Gandy (1993) on the "panoptic sort." Gandy shows how consumer surveillance using database marketing produces discriminatory practices that cream off some and cut off others. Data about transactions is used both to target persons for further advertising and to dismiss consumers who are of little value to companies. What Gandy demonstrates in the consumer realm can be explored in other areas as well. That further exploration across a range of social terrains, undertaken here, suggests some new directions for surveillance studies.

To consider surveillance as social sorting is to focus on the social and economic categories and the computer codes by which personal data is organized with a view to influencing and managing people and populations. To take a prominent example, after the "terrorist" attacks of 11 September 2001, many feared that persons with "Arab" or "Muslim" backgrounds would be profiled at airport or border checkpoints. Such categories would carry consequences (Lyon 2001). More generally, though, in everyday life our life-chances are continually checked or enabled and our choices are channeled using various means of surveillance. The so-called digital divide is not merely a matter of access to information. Information itself can be the means of creating divisions.

This is the theme traversed in the first chapter, focusing in particular on the relation between technological and social change. Everyday surveillance, whether in the form of facial recognition systems using cameras in the street, loyalty clubs in the supermarket, or on-board criminal record checks in police cruisers, all use remote searchable databases. The fact that personal data can be sorted at a distance, and checked for matches, is a key feature of surveillance today. But this is no mere technological achievement – these very systems are themselves the product of the restless search for better ways of coping with increasingly mobile, independent populations. Surveillance is not itself sinister any more than discrimination is itself damaging. However, I argue that there are dangers inherent in surveillance systems whose crucial coding mechanisms involve categories derived from stereotypical or preju-dicial sources. Given that surveillance now touches all of us who live in technologically "advanced" societies in the routine activities of everyday life, on the move as well as in fixed locations, the risks presented go well beyond anything that quests for "privacy" or "data protection" can cope with on their own.

The second chapter continues in an analytical and theoretical vein, this time with the workplace as the focus. Despite the claims made by some that new technologies in work situations contribute to more "horizontal" manage-ment and more involvement of workers, Elia Zureik argues that some of the most significant debates about the expansion of contemporary surveillance may be illustrated in this sphere. After helpfully exploring the concept of surveillance – and concluding, among other things, that it is ubiquitous, and increasingly based on networked control technologies – Zureik surveys the major contributions to surveillance studies in the workplace.

To understand what is happening, he insists, more than one theoretical perspective is required (and Kirstie Ball, in a later chapter, concurs). While the greater involvement of workers has reduced the crude dualisms of "scientific management," what this actually means depends on the context. Empowerment and disempowerment, skilling and deskilling, control and autonomy can coexist, depending on technological deployment, gender, and authority structures. Zureik notes that gender relations in the workplace are particularly significant for understanding surveillance during the present economic and technological restructuring, in which the incorporation of women's labor has been vital. As Manuel Castells observes, the "organization man" is on the way out; the "flexible woman" on her way in (2001: 95). How consent is obtained, and whether or not workers resist surveillance, is an empirical matter, not one that can be judged in advance using vulgar assumptions about panopticism or the negative effects of technology.

One important feature of surveillance discussed by Zureik is that it raises questions about human subjects and bodies, a theme that is elaborated further by Irma van der Ploeg in her consideration of "biometrics and the body as information." She takes issue with the hype surrounding information dependence in today's societies, dismissing the idea that the world has moved towards a more disembodied and virtual existence. But rather than simply stressing embodiment, van der Ploeg asks how far the very distinction between the embodied person and information about that person can be maintained. In a day when body data – biometrics – are increasingly sought for surveillance purposes, could it be that such information is not merely "about" the body but part of what the body is? Illustrating her case with examples such as fingerprinting, iris scans, and facial recognition systems common to today's high-tech social sorting practices – she concludes that our normative approaches, or ethics, require rethinking. What happens to personal data is a deeply serious question if that data in part actually constitutes who the person is.

Questions of identity are central to surveillance, and this is both a question of data from embodied persons and of the larger systems within which those data circulate. But verifying identities is only the beginning. In Chapter 4 Felix Stalder and I examine the specific case of electronic identity cards, which are rapidly becoming a key means of social as well as individual classification. A spate of proposals for new and enhanced national ID card systems followed the attacks of 11 September 2001. Most involve the use of a biometric and an embedded programmable chip, commonly known as "smart cards." This represents quite a shift from conventional paper-based documents that have characterized the history of identification papers for the past two centuries. We note the technical advantages and difficulties associated with such "smart IDs," but emphasize the fact that the social questions are more significant. After all, someone will always appear to offer technological enhancements, but the social cannot so simply be fixed. The central social question is again that of social sorting and classification, a process that is facilitated, for better and for worse, by the use of smart cards.

Staying with the question of the integrity of body data and its surveillant use in social sorting, Dorothy Nelkin and Lori Andrews shift the focus once again to genetic data. Twenty years ago, genetic data was used for the first time in a non-medical context, to identify a rapist, and today such practices are commonplace. Not only criminal cases, but in military and employment situations, the use of DNA samples is growing rapidly.

As Nelkin and Andrews note, DNA samples offer more than a means of identification. When they reveal things about health and predisposition, they can expose persons to workplace or health discrimination, creating "at risk" categories, some of which reinforce racial and ethnic stereotypes. Only ten years after the first legal use of genetic data, the USA set up the means of establishing DNA databanks, a process that has also occurred in varying ways in other countries. While Nelkin and Andrews acknowledge the legitimate and socially beneficial aspects of this, they also insist that the dangers of "surveillance creep" be kept prominently in mind.

While Nelkin and Andrews draw most of their illustrations from the military, Jennifer Poudrier takes a close look at a specific case of genetic surveillance, involving Canadian First Nations people in Ontario. Again, van der Ploeg's concerns about the constitutive power of "body data" become evident here – diabetes diagnoses are associated with "racial" types, in ways that could be quite prejudicial to aboriginal health. Poudrier shows how the kinds of ethnic stereotyping feared by Nelkin and Andrews actually emerge from a combination of dubious theory – the "thrifty gene" – and a regrettable reductionism in epidemiological models of propensity to disease. The latter tend to elevate the significance of genetic data, such that other competing and complementary factors are downplayed or ignored in the quest to isolate the causes of high rates of diabetes. Again, Poudrier does not deny legitimate and worthy aspects of this quest. But stereotypes may all too easily be reinforced by such means, in ways that exacerbate rather than ameliorate the chances of those who are deemed to be "at risk."

Each of the matters discussed so far – workplaces, DNA checks, ID cards, and so on – could refer to relatively fixed geographical environments, and they often do. However, part of the reason why ID cards are needed is the high mobility characterizing many countries in today's world. Not all employment situations are literally work*places*; many employees are on the move as part of their work. And given international travel, employment, and health concerns, even genetic data migrate across borders too. High-speed transport and communication make mobility a pervasive feature of today's world, which some even see as a new defining category for sociology (Urry 2000). Regulating these mobilities yields new roles for surveillance.

Just as surveillance practices have emerged to keep tabs on people in fixed locations, so parallel practices now keep track of persons on the move. The truck driver's tachometer that records speeds, stops, and other data has now been supplemented by an array of GPS (Global Positioning Satellite) devices that locate and monitor not only long-distance truckers but persons using cell phones, renting cars, or just driving their own cars on toll highways. Add to this the increasingly intensive surveillance of the virtual travelers who "surf the net," "visiting" non-place "sites," and a whole new dimension of social sorting opens up.

As with other topics, this is not a mere "technological" phenomenon, nor is it necessarily negative, socially speaking. But in the case of what David Phillips and Michael Curry call the "phenetic urge," it does become a matter for serious social and political analysis. "Phenetics" is classification based on measurable similarities and differences (as opposed, for example, to genetic ones) and they apply this to the changing uses of geodemographic systems. As noted earlier, marketers use transactional data for determining whom to target, but they also combine this with knowledge about neighborhood characteristics, normally based on zip codes and postal codes. Phillips and Curry show how the assumption that "you are where you live" clusters consumers according to – somewhat stereotypical – categories such as "pools and patios" or "bohemian mix," but does little to reveal how cities alter their composition night and day. This has encouraged more fluid approaches, based on the reality that urban areas may be better conceived of as "flows" (Castells 2000) in which work, home and entertainment occur in different places; hence the growth of "location-based systems" for consumer surveillance.

Thus the same kinds of technologies that facilitate high levels of mobility – the "flows" – also provide platforms for surveillance of persons on the move. When many cell phones are in use, for example, their owners may readily be traced, a fact that is advertised as a benefit – especially since cell phones have been used to find victims in emergency situations. Any problems that cell phone users may have with this tend to be addressed by reference to "privacy" policies which, as Phillips and Curry say, put the emphasis on "personally identifiable information" rather than the fact that groups or regions may be categorized and characterized in particular ways. Something very similar may be said about other kinds of locational devices discussed by Colin Bennett, Charles Raab, and Priscilla Regan in the following chapter that deals with "intelligent transportation systems." They too take very seriously the privacy problems associated with, in this case, automated toll highways, but also note that the capacity and the incentive to amass categorical data on road users increases all the time.

For Bennett, Raab, and Regan, who carefully compare and contrast three road toll systems in Canada, the USA, and the UK, the jury is still out on how far such systems represent much more than an efficient cash-free means of easing traffic flows. Even when offered an anonymous means of paying tolls on Toronto's highway 407, for instance, few drivers avail themselves of it. Yet as these authors also observe, the trends all point towards growing marketing interest in capturing more classifiable driver data, and towards the growth of GIS (Geographical Information Systems) and other technological means of collecting and analyzing it. Not satisfied with older notions that "we are where we live," marketers may add the idea that "we are what we drive."

This phenetic urge spreads into other areas too, such as Internet use, even if they do not involve physical travel. Extending the previous thought, we could describe this as "we are where we surf." The Internet has become a major means of classifying and categorizing its users, through an array of increasingly sophisticated devices that began with "cookies." These small pieces of software code are deposited on users' hard drives when they log onto a site, where they remain, sending data back to their originating company. The association of "webs" with traps is thus not entirely misplaced (Elmer 1997; Lyon 1998). However, as with the workplace, or geodemographic marketing, there is a bigger context to be considered. Surveillance, as Zureik notes, is a feature of large-scale organization, and thus invites a political-economy approach as well as discursive, constructivist, and ethnographic ones.

Dwayne Winseck provides such a context in his chapter on "netscapes of power," in which he explores how media monopolies have extended themselves into the "Internet era." In particular, Winseck elaborates the notion that risk management has become an axial principle of social organization within media companies, and that this encourages the drive to regulate behavior through network architecture, cyberlaw, and, of course, surveillance. This last involves, for example, more and more detailed clickstream monitoring geared to "knowing the audience" for web sites of all kinds. He agrees with Gandy and with Rohan Samarajiva's (1997) conclusions that these attempts to manage consumption heighten surveillance and augment advertisers' ability to discriminate between audiences they value and those they do not. The Internet thus comes to resemble, in uncanny ways, the social situations in which it is embedded as a "form of life" (Bennett 2001: 207–8).

Winseck makes the important point that "privacy" is treated ambiguously in these contexts. Because of the huge pressure within corporations to obtain valuable personal data, especially in the form of user profiles, some systems are deliberately created with only minimal levels of "privacy" protection. At the same time, privacy enhancing technologies (PETs) may be offered to offset such trends. While they are often effective, however, PETs also fall back on technocratic solutions and personal choices. Instead of seeing cyberspace as a genuinely social space that is publicly protected, the onus is thus placed on the person to know about and to buy any necessary protection.

Another division emerges, based this time on awareness and, in some cases, ability to pay.

In Part IV of the book, "Targeting trouble: social divisions," the power of categorizing surveillance is seen in three unfolding contexts, each of which highlights some important and emerging features. Kirstie Ball looks at computer-based performance monitoring (CBPM) in a rapidly growing sector – the call center. She shows how categories are created through surveillance and why this raises questions of distributive and procedural justice. Greg Marquis takes the rise of private policing – another expanding phenomenon – as another key site of surveillance, showing how it builds on a long history of "typing" suspect populations, which is accentuated by the use of new technologies. Clive Norris also examines a growth sector – closed circuit television (CCTV) surveillance in public places – demonstrating decisively how categories of suspicion are constructed.

Ball shows how electronic surveillance is used extensively in call centers as a key management tool. Statistics of worker performance, often including voice recordings, are used to classify workers and to evaluate them against company criteria. Ball argues that such situations cannot be properly understood by one analytic method alone and shows the value of complementary approaches. She shows that the management line (relating to "empowerment") actually appropriates to its advantage some workers' orientations to "life-in-work" in the surveillance setting. Ball questions the value of some "best practice" approaches common in call center management styles, suggesting that much more attention be paid to how workers actually negotiate their place within the organization, and how access to justice in monitored situations might really be achieved.

One area that one might expect "best practice" to entail criteria of "justice" is policing. But no one can visit a shopping mall, an airport, or sports facility today without noticing that they are policed by security personnel paid by or contracted to the company. Private police increasingly operate alongside municipal and regional police forces to deter, detect, and deal with infractions of the law and undesirable behaviors. Surveillance is central to both agencies. The old distinction made between police work – maintaining order and enforcing criminal law – and security work – preventing economic loss – is, as Marquis shows, less plausible today. "Public" police, too, use criteria deriving from risk management relating to economic loss (Ericson and Haggerty 1997). Whether in public places such as bus stations, or in semi-private locations such as workplaces, private police often work on the same guidelines as public police, and may use the same databases to deal with different "orders" of "troublemakers."

To take this further, it is worth noting that a key case of public police learning from private is in the deployment of CCTV. Cameras currently sprout like spring flowers (if that analogy is not too innocent) from roofs and pole-mountings in almost every major city in North America, Europe, and Asia. But they do not merely "watch." Clive Norris takes up this theme in a finely nuanced final chapter, showing how some explanations of CCTV are deficient precisely because they underplay the classificatory power – the phenetic urge – of these systems. While many theorists have drawn upon Michel Foucault's rendition of the panopticon as a model for modern surveillance, Norris shows that the case for CCTV as an "unseen observer" is less obvious than it might at first seem.

Norris traces the trend towards more automated and algorithmic systems, and he argues that this marks a distinct shift away from the negotiable space available in earlier forms of social control. As he notes, "Access is either accepted or denied; identity is either confirmed or rejected; behavior is either legitimate or illegitimate." Without downplaying the discriminatory practices of face-to-face or human-operated CCTV systems, Norris nonetheless insists that the new, neatly classifying methods of digital surveillance may not be particularly fair either. Those whose behaviors do not fall in with the "entrepreneurial mission" of the shopping mall, for instance, are targeted for exclusion. Classification and categorization for inclusion or exclusion is of the essence in such surveillance systems. Which is what not only this chapter, but this book, is all about.

Surveillance is thus seen, in a many-faceted series of chapters, as a means of social sorting. It classifies and categorizes relentlessly, on the basis of various – clear or occluded – criteria. It is often, but not always, accomplished by means of remote networked databases whose algorithms enable digital discrimination to take place. Risk management, we are reminded, is an increasingly important spur to surveillance. But its categories are constructed in socio-technical systems by human agents and software protocols and are subject to revision, or even removal. And their operation depends in part on the ways that surveillance is accepted, negotiated, or resisted by those whose data is being processed. While fears for personal privacy are still a significant aspect of this fluid and fluctuating process, the following chapters also demonstrate that voices questioning the social justice of surveillance are also starting to be heard.

Bibliography

Bennett, C. (2001) "Cookies, Web-bugs, Webcams, and Cue-cats: Patterns of Surveillance on the World Wide Web," *Ethics and Information Technology*, 3(3): 197–210.

Castells, M. (2000) *The Rise of Network Society*, Oxford and Malden, MA: Blackwell.

—— (2001) *The Internet Galaxy: Reflections on the Internet, Business, and Society*, Oxford and New York: Oxford University Press.

Elmer, G. (1997) "Spaces of Surveillance: Indexicality and Solicitation on the Internet," *Critical Studies in Mass Communication*, 14(2).

Ericson, R. and Haggerty, K. (1997) *Policing the Risk Society*, Toronto: University of Toronto Press.

Gandy, O. (1993) *The Panoptic Sort: A Political Economy of Personal Information*, Boulder, CO: Westview Press.

Lyon, D. (1998) "The World-Wide-Web of Surveillance: The Internet and Off-World Power Flows," *Information, Communication, and Society*, 1(1).

Lyon, D. (2001) "Surveillance after September 11," *Sociological Research Online*, 6(3). Online. Available HTTP: <http://www.socresonline.org.uk/6/3/lyon.html> (accessed 28 February 2002).

Samarajiva, R. (1997) "Telecom Regulation in the Information Age," in W. Melody (ed.) *Telecommunication Reform*, Lyngby: Technical University of Denmark.

Urry, J. (2000) *Sociology Beyond Societies: Mobilities for the Twenty-First Century*, London: Routledge.

Part I
Orientations

1 Surveillance as social sorting

Computer codes and mobile bodies

David Lyon

This first chapter explores some of the key themes involved in "surveillance as social sorting." The first four paragraphs state the argument in brief, before I suggest a number of ways in which social sorting has become central to surveillance. In what follows I look at some implications of surveillance as a routine occurrence of everyday life; focus on the emergent "coding" and "mobile" aspects of surveillance; and conclude by suggesting some fresh directions for surveillance studies in the early twenty-first century.[1]

Surveillance has spilled out of its old nation-state containers to become a feature of everyday life, at work, at home, at play, on the move. So far from the single all-seeing eye of Big Brother, myriad agencies now trace and track mundane activities for a plethora of purposes. Abstract data, now including video, biometric, and genetic as well as computerized administrative files, are manipulated to produce profiles and risk categories in a liquid, networked system. The point is to plan, predict, and prevent by classifying and assessing those profiles and risks.

"Social sorting" highlights the classifying drive of contemporary surveillance. It also defuses some of the more supposedly sinister aspects of surveillance processes (it's not a conspiracy of evil intentions or a relentless and inexorable process). Surveillance is always ambiguous (Lyon 1994: 219; Newburn and Hayman 2002: 167–8). At the same time social sorting places the matter firmly in the social and not just the individual realm – which "privacy" concerns all too often tend to do. Human life would be unthinkable without social and personal categorization, yet today surveillance not only rationalizes but also automates the process. How is this achieved?

Codes, usually processed by computers, sort out transactions, interactions, visits, calls, and other activities; they are the invisible doors that permit access to or exclude from participation in a multitude of events, experiences, and processes. The resulting classifications are designed to influence and to manage populations and persons thus directly and indirectly affecting the choices and chances of data subjects. The gates and barriers that contain, channel, and sort populations and persons have become virtual.

But not only does doing things at a distance require more and more surveillance. In addition, the social sorting process occurs, as it were, on the move. Surveillance now deals in speed and mobility. In the race to arrive first, surveillance is simulated to precede the event. In the desire to keep track, surveillance ebbs and flows through space. But the process is not one-way. Socio-technical surveillance systems are also affected by people complying with, negotiating, or resisting surveillance. Now let me spell this out, a little less breathlessly.

A key trend of today's surveillance is the use of searchable databases to process personal data for various purposes. This key is not "technological," as if searchable databases could be thought of as separate from the social, economic, and political purposes in which they are embedded. Rather, the use of searchable databases is seen as a future goal, even if, at present, the hardware and software may not all be readily available or sufficiently sophisticated. The point is that access to improved speed of handling and richer sources of information about individuals and populations is believed to be the best way to check and monitor behavior, to influence persons and populations, and to anticipate and pre-empt risks.

One of the most obvious examples of using searchable databases for surveillance purposes occurs in current marketing practices. Over the past two decades a huge industry has mushroomed, clustering populations according to geodemographic type. Canada, for instance, is organized by Compusearch into groups – from U1, Urban Elite to R2, Rural Downscale – which are then subdivided into clusters. U1 includes "The Affluentials" cluster: "Very affluent and middle-aged executive and professional families. Expensive, large, lightly-mortgaged houses in very stable, older, exclusive sections of large cities. Older children and teenagers" (TETRAD 2001). U6, Big City Stress is rather different: "Inner city urban neighbourhoods with the second lowest average household income. Probably the most disadvantaged areas of the country . . . Household types include singles, couple, and lone parent families. A significant but mixed 'ethnic' presence. Unemployment levels are very high" (TETRAD 2001).

Using such clusters in conjunction with postal codes – zip codes in the USA – marketers sift and sort populations according to their spending patterns, then treat different clusters accordingly. Groups likely to be valuable to marketers get special attention, special deals, and efficient after-sales service, while others, not among the creamed-off categories, must make do with less information, and inferior service. Web-based tools have broadened these processes to include other kinds of data, relating not only to geodemographics but to other indicators of worth as well. In processes known variously as "digital redlining" (Perri 6 2001) or "weblining" (Stepanek 2000), customers are classified according to their relative worth. So much for the sovereign consumer! The salesperson may now know not only where you live, but details such as your ethnic background (Stepanek notes that in the USA Acxiom matches names against demographic data to yield "B" for black, "J" for Jewish, "N" for Nipponese-Japanese and so on).

Already one may see how off-line and on-line data-gathering may be matched or merged. As the Internet has become more important as a marketing device, so efforts have increased to combine the power of off-line (mainly geodemographic) with on-line (mainly surfing patterns and traces) databases. This was behind the purchase of Abacus (off-line) by Doubleclick (on-line) in 1999, that resulted in a lengthy court case following an outcry. When marketers merge individually identifiable information pertaining to postal or zip code characteristics with evidence of purchasing habits or interests gleaned by tracking Internet use into a searchable database, they create a closer relationship with relevant customers. In a striking case, an American physician was recently offered a list of all her perimenopausal patients not on some estrogen replacement therapy (Hafner 2001). On-line and off-line data may be combined to produce fine-tuned sales.

Another field in which searchable databases have become more important for surveillance is policing. During 2001, Toronto, Ontario, Canada police introduced upgrades in their patrol vehicles that extended the scope of information-based activities. The e-Cops – Enterprise Case and Occurrence Processing System – was adopted, which uses wireless data communications to connect police officers using laptops in their cruisers to Web-based tools for crime detection and prevention (Marron 2001). Not only can officers now connect directly with Toronto Police Service files as well as the Ontario Ministry of Transport drivers' license records and suspect lists held at the Canadian Police Information Centre (CPIC), but also with an IBM database and business-intelligence software.

This initiative, like database marketing, makes use of geodemographic information. In this case, it identifies geographical patterns of crimes with a view not only to detection but to pre-empting crime by indicating where a particular offender may strike next. The new systems automate tasks that previously required clerical staff as information-processing intermediaries, and connect tools that used to be used in relative isolation. Thus, the system is more fully integrated, and, it is argued, more cost-effective. Background information on suspects is now instantly available and retrievable by officers at their car seat laptops. And the searchable database may be used to indicate whether the suspect is likely to be a serial offender, on a "crime spree" or a novice.

As with database marketing, the policing systems are symptomatic of broader trends. In this case the trend is towards attempted prediction and pre-emption of behaviors, and of a shift to what is called "actuarial justice" in which communication of knowledge about probabilities plays a greatly increased role in assessments of risk (Ericson and Haggerty 1997). How certain territories are mapped socially becomes central to police work that is dependent on information infrastructures. But such mapping also depends on stereotypes, whether to do with territory – "hot spots" – or social characteristics such as race, socio-economic class or gender. As Ericson and Haggerty observe, these categories cannot be impartial because they are produced by risk institutions that already put different value on young and old, rich and poor, black and white, men and women (Ericson and Haggerty 1997: 256).

The two examples, from marketing and from policing, clearly indicate how searchable databases have become central to surveillance. If surveillance is understood as a systematic attention to personal details, with a view to managing or influencing the persons and groups concerned, then the searchable database may be seen as an ideal in other emerging areas as well. Risk management and insurance assessment in particular tend to encourage the quest for greater accuracy of identification and faster communication of the risk, preferably before the risk is realized. New technologies, such as biometrics, using fingerprints, handprints, iris scans, or DNA samples, are harnessed for accuracy of identification (see Nelkin and Andrews in this volume), and the networking of these to increase speed of communication are thus part of an increasingly common pattern.

Two further developments also illustrate these surveillance shifts. One refers to the rapid proliferation of Closed Circuit Television (CCTV) or "video surveillance" and the other to a growing range of locational devices that not only situate data subjects in fixed space, but also while on the move. Again, these are not merely technological innovations with social impacts. They are technologies that are actively sought and developed because they answer to particular political-economic pressures. The political pull factors have to do with neo-conservative governments wishing to contract out services and to cut costs, especially labor costs. In so doing, they are also attempting to reduce public fear of crime and create spaces for "safe" consumption in the city. Pull factors on the commercial side include narrowing profit margins and the desire to capture markets through relationships with customers. The push factors, on the other hand, relate to the drive to sell (companies) and to adopt (agencies, organizations, governments) new technologies.

The UK is the currently unrivalled world capital for video surveillance in public places, but other countries are rapidly following the British example. Major cities in North America, Europe and Asia are using CCTV as a means to control crime and to maintain social order. For example, Sudbury was the first city in Ontario to install public video cameras in 1996, in a move inspired directly by the example of Glasgow, Scotland. Sudbury police obtained help from rotary clubs and Canadian Pacific Rail to put up their first cameras which, it is now claimed, have led to significant reductions in crime rates – which are falling faster than those in other Canadian cities (Tomas 2000). In most cases, searchable databases are not yet used in conjunction with CCTV, though the aim of creating categories of suspicion within which to situate unusual or deviant behaviors is firmly present (see Norris in this volume).

In some cases, however, searchable databases are already in use in public and private situations, to try to connect facial images of persons in the sight of the cameras with others that have been digitally stored. In Newham, London, CCTV is thus enhanced by intelligent systems capable of facial recognition (Norris and Armstrong 1999). In a celebrated case in 2000, the turnstiles at the annual Superbowl events in Florida were watched by such a CCTV system, that compared the 100,000 plus images of those entering the stadium against stored images of the faces of known offenders (19 matches were made). This was a test-run by a camera system company, to demonstrate the capabilities of the machines, which at least suggests the nature of technology push factors in this case (Slevin 2001).

Much more commonplace than street-level facial recognition systems – at least before 11 September 2001 – are the facial recognition technologies used at casinos to catch cheats. As with the turnstiles, the casino entrances offer the opportunity to capture relatively clear images. These may then be matched with database images and used to apprehend known offenders (CNN 2001). The increasing use of digital security cameras is likely to encourage this trend (Black 2001). Since 11 September 2001, however, widespread interest has been expressed in many cities for facial recognition CCTV systems to reduce the likelihood of "terrorist" attacks. The new political will and public willingness to countenance the spread of such systems in public places has been more than matched by confident "expert" announcements about available technology, even though their capacity actually to perform as required is unproven (Rosen 2001).

Sophisticated CCTV systems, such as those in Newham, London, may be used to follow people from street to street if they are of interest to the operators. Thus not only fixed sites, but moving targets may also be subject to surveillance. Cameras, however, are not the most common kinds of devices used for keeping track of persons on the move. Other locational technologies that use Global Positioning Satellites (GPS) and Geographic Information Systems (GIS) in conjunction with wireless telephony provide much more powerful surveillance potential. There is already a popular market for such mobile phone and satellite technologies among parents wishing to keep track of their children, but broader commercial interest is found among car rental companies, emergency, and security services.

Selected new cars from Ford offer the On-Star service that enables, for example, hotels or restaurants to alert users when they are near by. This is a predictable extension of electronic business. Following a federal ruling in the USA, cell phones will carry wireless tracking technology to permit the pinpointing of persons making emergency calls (Romero 2001). This, too, is predictable, and the benefit to persons in trouble, palpable. But such systems also permit other agencies – insurance companies, employers – to discover the whereabouts of individuals and it is only a matter of time before they will develop the means of profiling them too (see Bennett, Raab, and Regan in this volume). In the UK, recent legislation, the Regulation of Investigatory Powers Act, allows police unparalleled access to new-generation cell phones ("mobile" phones in the UK or Australia) for tracing the location of callers (Barnett 2000). Along with Intelligent Transportation Sytems (ITS), these mushrooming technologies permit surveillance to shift decisively into the realm of movement through space.

Explaining everyday surveillance

There is a sense in which new technologies are employed to compensate for losses incurred through the deployment of other technologies. New information, and especially communication technologies and improved transportation, have enabled many things to be done at a distance in the past half century. An unprecedented stretch in relationships allows parties to engage in dispersed production – of everything from automobiles to music – administration, interpersonal communication, commerce, entertainment, and, of course, war. Relationships no longer depend on embodied persons being co-present with each other. Abstract data and images stand in for the live population of many exchanges and communications today. Some of those abstract data and images are deliberately intercepted or captured in order to keep track of the now invisible persons who are nonetheless in an immense web of connections. Thus the disappearing body is made to reappear for management and administrative purposes by more or less the same technologies that helped it to vanish in the first place (Lyon 2001b).

Understood thus, surveillance appears much less sinister. The older metaphors of Big Brother or the panopticon, redolent of heavy-handed social control, seem somehow less relevant to an everyday world of telephone transactions, Internet surfing, street-level security, work monitoring, and so on. And indeed, it seems appropriate to think of such surveillance as in some ways positive and beneficial, permitting new levels of efficiency, productivity, convenience, and comfort that many in the technologically advanced societies take for granted. At the same time, the apparently innocent embeddedness of surveillance in everyday life does raise some important

questions for sociological analysis. The surface-level associations of surveillance with the containment of risk may at times obscure the ways that
expanding surveillance may actually contribute to as well as curtail risks.

It is no accident that interest in privacy has grown by leaps and bounds in
the past decade. This shift maps exactly onto the increased levels and
pervasiveness of surveillance in commercial as well as in governmental
and workplace settings. By the same token, it also relates to increased surveillance of middle-class and male populations. Lower socio-economic
groups and women have long been accustomed to the gaze of various
surveillants. As well, growth of privacy concerns has to be seen in the
context of increasing individualized societies (Bauman 2001), and above
all on the individualizing of risk, as social safety nets deteriorate one by
one. Information privacy, based almost everywhere on "fair information
practices," relates to communicative control, that is, how far data subjects
have a say over how their personal data are collected, processed, and used.
Such privacy policies are now enshrined in law and in voluntary self-
regulation in many countries and contexts.

But privacy is both contested, and confined in its scope. Culturally and
historically relative, privacy has limited relevance in some contexts. As we
shall see in a moment, everyday surveillance is implicated in contemporary
modes of social reproduction – it is a vital means of sorting populations for
discriminatory treatment – and as such it is unclear that it is appropriate to
invoke more privacy as a possible solution. Of course, fair information
practices do go some way to addressing the potential inequalities generated,
or at least facilitated, by surveillance as social sorting. But this latter process
appears to be a social structural one which, however strenuous the claims to
privacy as a common or public good (see Regan 1995), seem to call for
different or at least additional policy instruments and political initiatives.

Another sociological issue is that mapping surveillance is no longer a
merely regional matter. Once, sociology could confidently assume that social
relations were in some ways isomorphic with territories – and of course,
ironically, this assumption is precisely what lies behind the geodemographic
clustering activities of database marketers. But the development of different
kinds of networking relationships challenges this simple assumption. Social
relationships have became more fluid, more liquid (Bauman 2000) and
surveillance data, correspondingly, are more networked, and must be seen
in terms of flows (Urry 2000). It is not merely *where* people are when
they use cell phones, e-mail, or surf the Internet. It is *with whom* they are
connected and how that interaction may be logged, monitored, or traced that
also counts.

A third sociological question raised by everyday surveillance has to
do with the processes of surveilling and being surveilled. It is often implied

that the one can be read off the other – that some mode of surveillance, say, street-level CCTV, simply works to reduce crime, or that a person's paranoid fears of a Big Brother welfare department are fully justified. In fact, many surveillance situations have received little sociological attention, with the result that it is easy to fall back on the perspectives of technological determinism or legal responses in the attempt to understand what is happening. In fact, at least three stages of the process should be isolated for analytical purposes. The creation of codes by data-users is one stage, revealing both the political economy of technology and the implications of certain technical capacities. The extent to which data subjects comply is a second stage; this explores the circumstances under which the surveilled simply go along with their surveillance, how far they negotiate with surveillance, and when they actually resist it. This leads to a third question: what does it take for opposition to surveillance to be mobilized politically in an organized fashion – whether *ad hoc* or long-term – and what are the pragmatic or ethical grounds for so doing?

Social sorting

Everyday surveillance depends increasingly on searchable databases. Even where this is not yet or not fully the case – such as with the predominantly human-operated CCTV systems – a central aim is social sorting. The surveillance system obtains personal and group data in order to classify people and populations according to varying criteria, to determine who should be targeted for special treatment, suspicion, eligibility, inclusion, access, and so on. What, in relation to database marketing, Oscar Gandy calls the "panoptic sort" is, in short, a discriminatory technology, whether or not it is fully automated in every case (Gandy 1993, 1995, 1996). It sieves and sorts for the purpose of assessment, of judgement. It thus affects people's lifestyle choices – if you won't accept the cookie that reports your surfing habits to the parent company, don't expect that information or access will be available – and their life-chances – details about the neighborhood in which you live affect items such as your insurance premiums, what sorts of services are available (Graham and Marvin 2001), how the area is policed, and what advertising you receive.

If surveillance as social sorting is growing, this is not merely because some new devices have become available. Rather, the devices are sought because of the increasing number of perceived and actual risks and the desire more completely to manage populations – whether those populations are citizens, employees, or consumers. The dismantling of state welfare, for instance, that has been occurring systematically in all the advanced societies since its zenith in the 1960s, has the effect of individualizing risks. Whereas the very concept of state welfare involves a social sharing of risks, the converse occurs when that state welfare goes into decline. What are the results of this?

For those still in dire need, because of unemployment, illness, single parenthood, or poverty otherwise generated, surveillance is tightened as a means of discipline. Cases of fraud are more actively sought through data-matching and other means – Ontario residents who cross the USA border when on unemployment benefit may have their details cross-checked by Canada Customs with a view to sniffing out double-dipping – and the criteria of eligibility become more strictly means-tested. In Ohio, the human services department warns its clients that "your social security number may be used to check your income and/or employment information with past or present employers, financial resources through IRS, employment compensation, disability benefits [.]" The document continues: the "number as well as other information will be used in computer matching and program reviews or audits to make sure your household is eligible for food stamps . . . school lunch, ADC and Medicaid" (cf. Gilliom 2001: 18). For those whose risks have become primarily a personal or family responsibility, insurance companies will employ increasingly intrusive means to verify the health, employment, and other risks associated with each application. Personal data are constantly sought for such exchanges, which require surveillance knowledge to be communicated.

The individualization of risk thus fosters ever-spiralling levels of surveillance, implying that automated categorization occurs with increasing frequency. Now, as we noted above, categorization is endemic and vital to human life, especially to social life. The processes of institutional categorization, however, received a major boost from modernity, with its analytical, rationalizing thrust. All modern social institutions, for example, depend upon differentiation, to discover who counts as a citizen, which citizens may vote, who may hold property, which persons may marry, who has graduated from which school, with what qualifications, who is employed by whom, and so on. Many of these matters were less scrupulously checked before the coming of modernity, and there was a certain vagueness and (what might now be seen as) blurring of boundaries.

The growth of modern institutions – above all the nation-state and the capitalist enterprise – meant that those who were citizens, employees, and, in time, consumers found themselves with institutional or organizational identities that had to be calibrated with their self-identities. This does not imply that no group or clan identities existed before modern times, or that self-identity is somehow a pre-social endowment of the person. Rather, it is a reminder that organizational identities have proliferated during modern times, and that they have become increasingly significant factors in the determination of life-chances. With the concomitant rise of modern understandings of the self, traffic between organizational and self identities has become more and more busy and more complex.

What happens when computers are brought into the picture? In short, the social power of information is reinforced. For one thing, the records of those organizational identities, long ago relegated to filing cabinets, seldom disturbed, are now on the move. Data doubles – various concatenations of personal data that, like it or not, represent "you" within the bureaucracy or the network – now start to flow as electrical impulses, and are vulnerable to alteration, addition, merging, and loss as they travel. For another, the ongoing life of the data doubles now depends upon complex information infrastructures. This may help to democratize the information; it may equally lead to tyrannies. As John Bowker and Leigh Star say:

> Some are the tyrannies of inertia – red tape – rather than explicit public policies. Others are the quiet victories of infrastructure builders inscribing their politics into the systems. Still others are almost accidental – systems that become so complex that no one person and no organization can predict or administer good policy.
>
> (Bowker and Star 1999: 50)

For all that modernity may have helped to spawn organizational identities, and now data doubles, within complex information infrastructures, it has not ensured that the identities and data doubles are classified free from stereotypes or other prejudicial typing. As we have seen, marketers use geodemographic and customer-behavior data – which themselves may be misleading – to create their categories, and they may also add highly questionable criteria such as racial and ethnic monikers to the mix. High-tech policing may involve wireless web-based data searches, but it has not moved beyond notions such as city "hotspots" to pinpoint areas requiring special police attention, where "annoying behavior" may occur, or where it is important that certain social elements, above all the poor, be cleaned away for tourism. And the more policing also comes to rely on CCTV surveillance, the more other kinds of prejudicial categories will come into play. In Britain, being young, male and black ensures a higher rate of scrutiny by the street-mounted cameras (Norris and Armstrong 1999).

Computer codes

Although computers are not necessarily used for all kinds of surveillance – some is still face to face and some, like most CCTV systems, still require human operators – most surveillance apparatuses in the wealthier, technological societies depend upon computers. Searchable databases have become especially significant, along with remote networking capacities. The current use of computers is extending from fixed usage to mobile, allowing either the surveillants or the surveilled – or both – to be on the move. As in other areas, it is not merely information processing that is important, but communication.

But what information is processed and communicated? The assessments and judgements made on data subjects depend on coded criteria, and it is these codes that make surveillance processes work in particular ways. They are the switches that place one person in, say, the Affluentials category, and the next in Big City Stress, one person as having health risks, the next as having good prospects. As Bowker and Star note, "values, opinions, and rhetoric are frozen into codes." They extend Marx to suggest that " . . . software is frozen organizational and policy discourse" (Bowker and Star 1999: 135). For one thing, different stakeholders help to determine the coding. As Ericson and Haggerty show, insurance companies play an increasingly large role in determining policing categories (Ericson and Haggerty 1997: 23; see also Ericson, Barry and Doyle 2000). And human resources managers opposed to labor union organization may help to code e-mail or Internet monitoring devices.

Computer codes are thus extremely important for the ways that surveillance works. In a strong sense, surveillance systems are what are in the codes. They regulate the system – as Lawrence Lessig says with regard to cyberspace, '*Code is law*' (Lessig 1999: 6). Lessig also observes that it seems to have come as a surprise to some that cyberspace is necessarily regulated. Indeed, the very term "cyberspace" has obvious affinities with "cybernetics," the science of remote control, connected from the outset with a vision of perfect regulation. Paradoxically, Lessig argues, the commercialization of cyberspace is constructing an architecture that perfects control. In this way it simply perpetuates what James R. Beniger explained about information technology in general – it contributes to a "control revolution" (Beniger 1986). What is true of the Internet is also true of other forms of computer coding. And that is why it is so important that codes be analyzed and assessed in surveillance settings.

Without themselves being involved in the kinds of sociology of technology that is required fully to understand these codes, certain French theorists – notably Paul Virilio and Gilles Deleuze – have observed that the processes of social ordering have been undergoing change over the past decade or two. They argue that today's surveillance goes beyond that of Michel Foucault's disciplinary society, where persons are "normalized" by their categorical locations, to what Deleuze calls the "society of control" where similarities and difference are reduced to code (Deleuze 1992). The coding is crucial, because the codes are supposed to contain the means of prediction, of anticipating events (like crimes), conditions (like AIDS), and behaviors (like consumer choices) that have yet to occur (see also Bogard 1996). The codes form sets of protocols that help to alter the everyday experience of surveillance. As Virilio says, physical obstacles and temporal distances become less relevant in a world of information flows. The old world of surveillance, that depended on the layout of the city (dating back to times of city walls and gates), is now supplanted – or, I would argue, supplemented – by newer surveillance that depends rather on what Virilio calls "audio-visual protocols" (Virilio 1994). Virilio refers to this kind of surveillance *"pros*pection" because the codes promise advance vision, perceiving future events (Virilio 1989).

These computer codes become more significant for surveillance each time it becomes possible to add some further dimension to the data collected and processed. The information infrastructure handles more and more different kinds of codes, and, as it does so, the surveillance capacities of other, once relatively separate and distinct, areas are upgraded. The codes of dataveillance (see Clarke 1988) have been augmented not only by Virilio's audio-visual protocols but also by biometric, genetic, and locational ones. These too carry with them the baggage of their origins and of their stakeholders' values, opinions, and rhetoric. Thus, for example, the "coded body" of a person who attempts to cross a national border may find that she is already welcome or already excluded on the basis of an identity that is established (not merely determined, see van der Ploeg 1999) by the codes.

It hardly needs saying that asylum seekers are among the most vulnerable to such coding – or that this may be a politically acceptable level on which to set up new systems of codes involving biometrics. It was reported in May 2001, for instance, that the Canadian Department of Immigration intends to introduce a smart card that may contain identifiers such as eye scans or thumbprints (Walters 2001). After the attacks of 11 September 2001, the climate of political acceptability altered quite radically, and smart-card national identifiers became one of the most mooted technical defences against "terrorism" (see Stalder and Lyon in this volume). These have the capacity to be coded for several different purposes.

Mobile bodies

Of course, in the twenty-first century more and more people do want to cross borders. Not only asylum seekers and other refugees, but the flows of travellers also includes business people, tourists, sports players, entertainers, students, and so on. If globalization is rightly thought of as the process in which the world becomes one place, then it is only to be expected that borders will become increasingly porous. Mobility, both physical and virtual, is a mark of the information and communication age. Equally predictable, in an increasingly mobile world, is that surveillance practices would evolve in parallel ways. But there are different aspects of this shift.

First, the networked forms of surveillance are as powerful as ever, and are best seen in the activities of major corporations – such as Doubleclick or Disney – on the one hand, or policing and government administration on the other. There are also potential and actual links between surveillance taking place in public and private organizations. Pharmaceutical companies, for instance, may on occasion gain access to the databases of government-run health care schemes and vice versa (Hafner 2001). But, second, this shades into another kind of surveillance organization, or, as Gilles Deleuze and Félix Guattari have it, "assemblage" (Deleuze and Guattari 1987; see also Haggerty and Ericson 2000). This surveillance is not limited to the corporation or government department, but grows and expands rhizomically, like those creeping plants in the suburban lawn or vegetable garden. Some CCTV systems seem to "creep" in this way, moving according to an unpredictable, networking logic that Norris and Armstrong call "expandable mutability" (1999; see also Nelkin and Andrews in this volume).

A third aspect of surveillance in a world of mobilities is that numerous new devices are available for pinpointing the location of data subjects. These represent a specific development in the computing and telecommunications industries, and are based on wireless telephony, video, newly available GPS data, and, of course, searchable databases. Some are Intelligent Transportation Systems (ITS) such as automated road-tolling technologies, or on-board navigational or monitoring devices. Others connect GPS and GIS capabilities with cell phones to enable the location of callers – especially in emergency situations – to be easily traced to within a few metres. These technologies represent an emerging area but there is enough evidence of their use already – both in fixed highway tolling systems and in emergency cell phone call locating – to suggest that it is no passing trend.

One way or another, surveillance seems perfectly capable of keeping up with social trends towards greater mobility. After all, surveillance depends increasingly upon the very same technologies that enable mobility to expand in the first place. Old notions of order, pattern, and regularity seem less salient to a world of mobilities, rendering plausible Urry's view that emergent regimes have more to do with "regulating mobilities" (Urry 2000: 186) rather like a gamekeeper regulates stock that otherwise cross boundaries at will. This does not mean that national states will lose their power to regulate (globalization, after all, implies a concurrent localization), or that more hierarchical organizations (corporations, police departments) will wither away. Rather it suggests that surveillance information – along with those from whom the data are abstracted – will simply be among the fluids that circulate and flow within and beyond what were once taken for granted as "societies."

Conclusions

Sociologies of surveillance as social sorting are underdeveloped. Such studies have tended either to fall back on the theoretical resources of liberal, Orwell-inspired ideas, and of poststructuralist, panoptic schemes (Boyne 2000), or to start with the commonest policy responses – data protection and privacy – and work back to analysis from there (Gilliom 2001: 8). The foregoing account has suggested some limitations of such approaches which, whatever their strengths, do not really deal with questions of disappearing bodies, coding, categorization, and mobilities. Much research is called for, of an ethnographic, explanatory, and an ethical kind. The ethnographic would help us understand processes of coding and of experiencing surveillance in everyday life. The explanatory would develop theories of social sorting and the social power of information in surveillance settings. The ethical would give a critical cutting edge to studies that clearly touch on issues of fairness and dignity.

The grammar of the codes offers rich veins for social research. Exploring from the perspectives of the sociology of technology and of political economy how codes are made up and modified would yield clues about "switching power" (Castells 1996) in contemporary societies. What are the desires that drive the coding processes enacted by data seekers and users? Possible candidates include control, governance, security, safety, and profit. How do different stakeholders bring their interests to bear on the coding processes? Which kinds of interest (risk management, insurance) predominate? How does increasing divesting and contracting out to commercial enterprises affect the quest for personal and population data? To what extent do commercial pressures encourage the use of data for purposes beyond those for which they were collected?

Equally, understanding how ordinary people experience surveillance in everyday life is a prime task for sociological research. Some studies have already been done, for example of how young persons "act up" in front of video cameras in the street. But many others are needed, of filling warranty or benefit application forms, surfing the Internet, using bar-coded plastic cards, and so on. Such analysis would yield clues as to how far these apparently powerful surveillance systems actually work, and how far their power is curtailed by negotiation, dissimulation, and active resistance on the part of intended data subjects. Under what conditions do social actors trade off personal data against commercial or positional advantages? When might intended data subjects simply refuse to disclose the data? Which classifications are relatively malleable and amenable to modification by data subjects and which are more impervious to bargaining or contestation?

Surveillance studies today is marked by an urgent quest for new explanatory concepts and theories. The most fruitful and exciting ones are emerging from transdisciplinary work, involving, among others, sociology, political economy, history, and geography. Within these, the sociology of technology is particularly important, as it is in the interaction of people with machines that surveillance studies increasingly must deal. But this also draws in colleagues from computer and information sciences, who can explicate, for instance, the vital questions of coding. As similar techniques are applied in different areas – say, the use of searchable databases in policing and marketing surveillance – so theoretical resources from one area may be borrowed in another. As with information scientists, colleagues in law and policy studies will also play a role in surveillance studies, not least because the shift beyond "privacy" also has implications for accountability in legal and organizational contexts.

Surveillance, I have argued, is intensified in a world of remote relations, where many connections do not directly involve co-present embodied persons, and where we no longer see the faces of those with whom we are "in contact" or with whom we engage in exchange. Searchable databases rely on data abstracted from live embodied persons, data that is subsequently used to represent them to some organization. Data thus extracted from people – at cash machines, via street video, in work-monitoring situations, through genetic or drug tests, in cell phone use – are used to create data doubles that are themselves constantly mutating and modifiable. But the data doubles, created as they are from coded categories, are not innocent or innocuous virtual fictions. As they circulate, they serve to open and close doors of opportunity and access. They affect eligibilities for credit or state benefits and they bestow credentials or generate suspicion. They make a real difference. They have ethics, politics.

Sociologies of surveillance will always be produced from some standpoint and it seems to me that such standpoints can hardly be critical if they neglect the relation between abstracted data and embodied social persons. Enlightenment attitudes, embedded in modernity, have fostered facelessness, and electronic mediation has exacerbated this situation today. Rethinking the importance of the face affects how one perceives the issues surrounding the appropriate conditions for self-disclosure (and thus the privacy debate) and also the questions of fairness in the face of automated social sorting. As I argue elsewhere (Lyon 2001a), the missing face offers possibilities as a moral guide at both levels. With respect to social sorting, the face always resists mere categorization at the same time as it calls data users to try to establish trust (see Zureik in this volume) and justice. This does not solve the political question, but it does in my view yield a strong ethical starting point that may serve as a guide for critical analysis.

Notes

1 This chapter was originally given as a paper at the School of Information, University of Michigan, and at the American Sociological Association meetings in Anaheim, CA, August 2001.

Bibliography

Barnett, A. (2000) "Every Move You Make...," *Observer*. Online. Available HTTP: <http://www.guardianunlimited.co.uk/Print/0,3858,4045760,00.html> (accessed 30 July 2000).

Bauman, Z. (2000) *Liquid Modernity*, Cambridge: Polity Press.

—— (2001) *The Individualized Society*, Cambridge: Polity Press.

Beniger, J. R. (1986) *The Control Revolution: Technological and Economic Origins of the Information Society*, Cambridge, MA: Harvard University Press.

Black, D. (2001) "Crime Fighting's New Wave," *The Toronto Star*. Online. Available HTTP: <http://www.torstar.com/thestar/editorial/tech.../20000125 NEWOld_CI-UPFRONT.htm> (accessed 25 January 2001).

Bogard, W. (1996) *The Simulation of Surveillance: Hypercontrol in Telematic Societies*, New York: Cambridge University Press.

Bowker, J. and Star, L. (1999) *Sorting Things Out: Classification and its Consequences*, Cambridge, MA: MIT Press.

Boyne, R. (2000) "Post-panopticism," *Economy and Society*, 29(2): 285–307.

Castells, M. (1996) *The Rise of the Network Society*, Oxford: Blackwell.

Clarke, R. (1988) "Information Technology and Dataveillance," *Communications of the ACM*, 31(5): 498–512.

CNN (2001) "Casinos Use Facial Recognition Technology." Online. Available HTTP: <http://www.cnn.com/2001TECH/ptech/02/26/casino.surveillance.ap/index.html> (accessed 26 February 2001).

Deleuze, G. (1992) "Postscript on the Societies of Control," *October*, 59: 3–7.

Deleuze, G. and Guattari, F. (1987) *A Thousand Plateaus: Capitalism and Schizophrenia*, Minneapolis: University of Minnesota Press.

Ericson, R. and Haggerty, K. (1997) *Policing the Risk Society*, Toronto: University of Toronto Press.

Ericson, R., Barry, D. and Doyle, A. (2000) "The Moral Hazards of Neo-liberalism: Lessons from the Private Insurance Industry," *Economy and Society*, 29(4): 532–58.

Gandy, O. (1993) *The Panoptic Sort: A Political Economy of Personal Information*, Boulder CO: Westview.

—— (1995) "It's Discrimination, Stupid!" in J. Brook and I.A. Boal (eds) *Resisting the Virtual Life*, San Francisco: City Lights.

—— (1996) "Coming to Terms with the Panoptic Sort," in D. Lyon and E. Zureik (eds) *Computers, Surveillance, and Privacy*, Minneapolis: University of Minnesota Press.

Gilliom, J. (2001) *Overseers of the Poor: Surveillance, Resistance, and the Limits of Privacy*, Chicago: University of Chicago Press.

Graham, S. and Marvin, S. (2001) *Splintering Urbanism: Networked Infrastructures, Technological Mobilities, and the Urban Condition*, London and New York: Routledge.

Hafner, K. (2001) "Privacy's Guarded Prognosis," *New York Times*, 1 March. Online. Available HTTP: <http://www.nytimes.com/2001/03/01/technology/01MEDI.html.>

Haggerty, K. and Ericson, R. (2000) "The Surveillant Assemblage," *British Journal of Sociology*, 51(4): 605–22.

Lessig, L. (1999) *Code and Other Laws of Cyberspace*, New York, Basic Books.

Lyon, D. (1994) *The Electronic Eye: The Rise of Surveillance Society*, Cambridge UK: Polity/Malden MA: Blackwell.

—— (2001a) "Facing the Future: Seeking Ethics for Everyday Surveillance," *Ethics and Information Technology*, 3(3): 171–81.

—— (2001b) *Surveillance Society: Monitoring Everyday Life*, Buckingham: Open University Press.

Lyon, D. and Zureik, E. (eds) (1996) *Computers, Surveillance, and Privacy*, Minneapolis: University of Minnesota Press.

Marron, K. (2001) "New Crime Fighter Rides Along with Cops in Cruisers," *The Globe and Mail*, 23 February: T2.

Newburn, T. and Hayman, S. (2002) *Policing, Surveillance, and Social Control: CCTV and the Police Monitoring of Suspects*, Cullompton, UK: Willan.

Norris C. and Armstrong, G. (1999) *The Maximum Surveillance Society*, London: Berg.

Perri 6 (2001) *Divided by Information: The "Digital Divide" and Implications of the New Meritocracy*, (with Ben Jupp), London: Demos.

Regan, P. (1995) *Legislating Privacy: Technology, Social Values and Public Policy*, Chapel Hill: University of North Carolina Press.

Romero, S. (2001) "Locating Devices Gain in Popularity but Raise Privacy Concerns," *New York Times*. Online. Available HTTP: <http://www.nytimes.com/2001/03/04/technology/04LOCA.html> (accessed 4 March 2001).

Rosen, J. (2001) "A Cautionary Tale for a New Age of Surveillance," *New York Times*, 7 October 2001.

Slevin, P. (2001) "Cameras Caught Superbowl Crowd," *Washington Post*. Online. Available HTTP: <http://www.msnbc.com/news/524802.asp> (accessed 2 February 2001).

Stepanek, M. (2000) "Weblining," *Business Week*. Online. Available HTTP: <http://www.businessweek.com: /2000/00_14/b3675027.htm> (accessed 3 April 2000).

TETRAD (2001) "Psyte Market Segments." Online. Available HTTP: <http://www.tetrad.com/pcensus/com/py951st.html.>

Tomas, P. (2000) "Ontario Today Report, July 26." Online. Available HTTP: <http://ottawa.cbc.ca/onttoday/archives/july_26_00.html> (accessed 7 May 2001).

Urry, J. (2000) "Mobile Sociology," *British Journal of Sociology*, 51(1): 185–203.
van der Ploeg, I. (1999) "The Illegal Body: Eurodac and the Politics of Biometric Identification," *Ethics and Information Technology*, 1(4): 295–302.
Virilio, P. (1989) *War and Cinema: The Logistics of Perception*, London: Verso.
—— (1994) *The Vision Machine*, London: The British Film Institute.
Walters, J. (2001) "New Immigrant ID Cards are Proposed to Foil Illegals," *The Toronto Star*. Online. Available HTTP: <http://www.torontostar.ca/NAS . . . /Article_PrintFriendly&c=Article&cid=99119106461> (accessed 30 May 2001).

2 Theorizing surveillance

The case of the workplace

Elia Zureik

Introduction

Until recently, explorations into the nature of surveillance have come to us by way of popular culture, the arts, philosophy, and law. While historically social scientists had little to say about surveillance, criminologists and industrial sociologists researched surveillance in the workplace and society at large. With regard to the workplace, it was Marx and his contemporaries Owen, Ure and Babbage in the nineteenth century (cf. Schaffer 1994), and Frederick Taylor in the early part of the twentieth century, who noticed a series of related trends. They saw in worker monitoring, fragmentation of tasks, the separation between mental and manual tasks, and regimentation of work – through the creation of the factory and eventually the assembly line – the means for increasing profit and reducing the unpredictability of labor, or, as expressed by Marx, for subordinating labor to capital (Marx 1976: 1019–38). This phenomenon, known as the deskilling and disciplining of labor, remains at the heart of the debate surrounding workplace surveillance and computer-based automation.

Current debates in the labor process school were sparked off by the publication of Braverman's *The Degradation of Work in the Twentieth Century* (1974). In spite of its shortcomings – according to some (cf. Burawoy 1978) but not to others (Cohen 1987) – as an objectivist Marxist analysis that paid scant attention to agency and worker resistance, Braverman's book remains a benchmark for understanding the disciplining of labor. It also marks the first time workplace surveillance received serious attention.

It was Edwards (1979) who, in contrast to Braverman, acknowledged in *Contested Terrain* the subjective elements of work and the role of agency in mounting resistance to systems of control. More than two decades ago, Edwards outlined the transition from simple to technical and bureaucratic forms of control in the workplace – leading up to an expanded form of control through the use of computerized monitoring. Playback tapes and numerically controlled machines in industrial programming allowed employers and management to control more efficiently the bodies of workers, pace of work and productivity levels than was the case with direct visual monitoring or the sequencing of automated machinery of the Fordist assembly-line type.

Since the mid-1980s, the most sustained interest and debate surrounding the labor process has been taking place in Britain among a group of sociologists and organization theorists who meet annually under the aegis of the International Labour Process Conference. According to Parker (1999), the debate can be situated around two main camps. The first includes those who see the need to incorporate Foucauldian poststructuralist analyses in order to infuse traditional Marxism with discussions of agency and subjectivity (Knights and Willmott 1990; Willmott 1994; O'Doherty and Willmott 2001). The second camp includes those who retain vital interest in class, power and ideology as central concepts (Thompson and Ackroyd 1995; Thompson and Smith 1998) in the materialist analysis of the labor process. We will turn to a brief examination of this debate in another part of the chapter.

The chapter proceeds by first discussing the various approaches to the study of technology and society, with special reference to the workplace and the accompanying debate over realism and constructivism. This is followed by a synthesis of the literature on surveillance, with special attention devoted to the panopticon as a key metaphor in understanding disciplining and normalization of the self. The third part examines specific aspects of the debate on panoptic surveillance as it relates to the workplace, the various indicators of workplace surveillance, and the nature of subjectivity and empowerment. The chapter concludes by outlining the theoretical and research implications of current issues involving surveillance as they are influenced by computer-based automation in the workplace.

Understanding technology

As will be apparent throughout this chapter, understanding computer-mediated work – indeed any technology-mediated activity – necessitates rejection of monocausal explanations (cf. Burris 1998). In one of the early surveys of the literature covering studies of computerized office work carried out in the 1980s, Kraemer and Danziger (1990) drew a complex, yet inconclusive, picture of the nature of computer "impacts" on organizational centralization/decentralization, worker satisfaction and productivity, job enhancement, stress, and emergence of "intellectual assembly lines." A decade later, Liker, Haddad, and Karlin (1999), in another overview of perspectives on technology and work, remained as inconclusive in their conclusions as previous researchers have:

In the case of technology the social reality is quite complex. Very different technologies are brought into very different social settings for very different reasons, often with completely opposing effects . . . [and] for each study finding that the computer centralizes power, another will find that computer technology decentralizes and democratizes the workplace.

(1999: 592)

In terms of methodology, early research on work and technology tended to be positivist in nature and focused on "impacts" of the technology, as indicated by the title of Kraemer and Danziger's article. More recently, Kling, a key writer on information technology and organizations, expressed similar concerns: "In the 1970s and 1980s, often the questions about computerization were phrased as deterministic impact questions. What would be the impact of computers on organizational behavior if we did X?" (2000: 246). Theoretical innovations in the social study of science and technology have had salutary effects on researching technology in the workplace. For example, Grint and Woolgar (1997: 11–38) outline the dominant approaches to the study of technology spanning a wide spectrum of intellectual traditions, from technological determinism, the socio-technical system, the social-shaping approach, and socio-technical alignments, to actor-network theory and anti-essentialism.

The anti-essentialist approach preferred by Grint and Woolgar draws upon the hermeneutic tradition in which the researcher views technology (its design and use) as "text" that is amenable to discourse analysis. This approach is also recommended by Liker et al. under the label "interpretevist perspective" (1999: 592–3), and adopted by Taylor and Van Every (1993) in their Canadian study of technological innovation and organizational structure. The advantage of this approach is that it avoids the objective/subjective dualism and treats the organization as a "text."

However, the constructivist view of technology-as-text has not been accepted without a challenge. Although the hermeneutic metaphor, according to Hutchby (2001), stresses the role of interpretation and negotiation by the user and designer of the technology and thus has the advantage of treating the "reading" and "writing" of the technology as an open system, it neglects the constraints the technology "affords" as set out in its design and materiality. No matter how flexible and contingent the reading of the "text" is, Hutchby sounds a cautionary note by paraphrasing a typical objection raised by Kling (1992): "a bullet fired from a gun has effects on flesh and bone that are intrinsic to the gun and bullet and cannot be altered by social construction" (Hutchby 2001: 446). In order to remedy the deficiency in the technology-as-text metaphor, Hutchby calls for introducing the concept of "affordances."

Thus, the interpretations and negotiations surrounding the use of the technology should focus on the "interpretations of the affordances of the artifact: the possibilities for action that it offers" (Hutchby 2001: 449).

Kling, who acknowledges the contingent aspects of information technology and its use, takes a different route and introduces the "socio-technical network" model as a substitute for the "tools" model that is typical of the "impact" approach (2000: 249). The social-shaping approach considers the introduction of technology in organizations as a *process* that often involves negotiations among various stakeholders, where the effects of technology are both direct and indirect, and where knowledge is distinguished by its implicit and tacit character.

By now, qualitative research, particularly ethnographic studies, has made headway in the study of computer-based work. The purpose here is to capture the subjectivity of the actor, without losing sight of objective constraints, thus treating research data in a more nuanced fashion by giving voice to agency (Ball and Wilson 2000). It is not a matter of opting for a relativist position over a realist one, or vice versa. Ball (2001) advocates a "materialist-semiotic" approach, by subjecting her ethnographic data to "fine grained" analysis. Thus, although realist analysis of computerized performance monitoring in the workplace (at the procedural and distributive justice level) supported "best practice" results as measured in realist terms, a more "fine grained approach revealed that departmental social relations had a discriminatory topography which favored the younger, male members of the department" (2001: 15). In this particular example, discourse analysis revealed how access to distributive and procedural justice in the workplace was mediated by gender, age, and authority position.

From the micro to the macro

The realist-semiotic position incorporated by Ball remains confined to the shop floor, and does not acknowledge the contribution of the wider politico-economic structure and its relevance to managerial policies and workplace organization. In this respect, and in spite of its methodological sophistication, it shares features with other workplace studies that stop at the office door or factory gate. There is a need to complement this approach by establishing a link between the micro and macro levels of analysis. Vallas (1999), who is conscious of this shortcoming (as we will show later in this chapter), advocates such a link through "neoinstitutional" and "flexible accumulation" analysis – although his analysis is not couched in the language of realism. I provide two examples which attempt to make such a link explicit: Smith's "relations of ruling analysis" (1987, 1999), which is anchored in feminist and Marxist ontology, and Porter's (1993) critical realism approach which has an affinity to both Marxism and structuration theory (Porter 1993: 595). Smith and Porter resort to ethnography to establish the micro–macro link via institutionalism (in the case of Smith) and critical realism (in the case of Porter). Some find the link between critical realism and Marxism, mentioned by Porter, to be problematic at the point of articulation between theory and practice. For Roberts, critical realist statements concerning the similarity between Marxism and critical realism notwithstanding, "by severing the link between theory and practice, critical realism commits fundamental theoretical problems and errors which it initially claimed to have surpassed" (1999: 21).

A main tenet of critical realism is that while there are predetermined or deep structures that constrain the actions of actors, and indeed act in a causal manner, these structures are not always transparent to actors. This is akin to Marx's "hidden abode," in which the intended consequences of capitalism are concealed behind a political and cultural superstructure (cf. Portes 2000: 8). It is the way agency acts on these structures that determines their production and reproduction. This is how Bhaskar (1989), a leading figure in critical realist philosophy, describes critical realism in a language that resonates with structuration theory:

> The existence of social structure is a necessary condition for any human activity. Society provides the means, media, rules and resources for everything we do . . . It is the unmotivated condition for all our motivated productions. We do not create society the error of voluntarism. But the structures which pre-exist us are only reproduced or transformed in our everyday activities; thus society does not exist independently of human agency – the error of reification. The social world is reproduced and transformed in daily life.
>
> (Bhaskar 1989: 3–4; cf. Porter 1993: 593)

In an article that was reprinted in 1987, but originally published in 1974, Smith defines relations of ruling in Marxian terms but anchors this definition in women's experience. Relations of ruling refer to more than political governance. They refer "to that total complex of activities differentiated into many spheres, by which our kind of society is ruled, managed, administered" (Smith 1987: 86). While in capitalism men are alienated from their work, they nevertheless occupy a dominant position vis-à-vis women in the "conceptual mode of consciousness." By being relegated to mediating men's roles in the workplace, women contribute to furthering their own oppression:

> The more successful women are in mediating the world of concrete particulars so that men do not have to become engaged with (and therefore conscious of) that world as a condition to their abstract activities,

the more complete man's absorption in it, the more effective the authority
of that world and the total women's subservience to it.

(Smith 1987: 90)

Subsequently, Smith developed this notion further along the following lines:
first, she resorts to discourse and textual analysis so as to understand the
relations of ruling from "women's standpoint" (1999: 68); second, this
understanding is accomplished by adopting a methodology which focuses
on "people's practical activities" in the tradition of ethnomethodology,
but without subscribing to the latter's insistence on order; third, the focus
on establishing a link between the local and extralocal makes the process of
understanding how consciousness, that is objectified by various organizational, work, scientific, and media discourses, succeeds in constituting its
subjects; fourth, relations of ruling are governed by "historical trajectory"
and capital's abstractions (in Marx's sense) whereby "the individuated
functions of knowing, judging, planning, and deciding are transferred to
organization, ceasing to be capacities immediately of the individual" (Smith
1999: 73); fifth, it is by interrogating the "materiality of the text," i.e., its
objectification, according to Smith, that it will be possible to apprehend
its mediating role between the local and extralocal; finally, she advocates
"institutional ethnography" as a methodology that "seeks to explore and
explicate how the local settings of people's lives are coordinated by social
relations not wholly visible to them" (1999: 76).

To demonstrate the thrust of her approach, Smith examines the conclusions
of a study by Vallas and Beck (1996), who assessed and then rejected the
claims of post-Fordism concerning flexibility in the workplace. Smith seeks
to explain these results by going beyond the workplace and linking workplace
organization at the shop-floor level to changes in capital markets. This is how
she puts it:

> An institutional ethnography would begin at the shop floor, as Vallas
> and Beck do, but be concerned with how the social relations of the
> financial markets enter into changing work organization at the shop-
> floor level. The regulatory functions of the formalized record-keeping
> procedures would be explored, including how their texts are produced,
> where the worked-up texts go, and how they are read at various transition
> points in the organization. Differences of views and experience would
> provide different points of entry into the objectified coordination of
> corporations and financial markets.

(1999: 78–9)

The second example comes from Porter, who turns to critical realism to
examine the relationship between racism and medical professionalism. He

hypothesizes, by means of ethnographic and discourse analysis, that the "structural phenomenon of racism" in the wider society shapes the manner in which racism is manifested at the workplace site. In this case he refers specifically to the relationship between doctors and nurses. He discovers that medical professionalism acts as a restraining factor by filtering out racist utterances in the workplace. Immigrant doctors in this British research setting played an important role in projecting vis-à-vis (white) nurses a rational and professional image, which blunted the public expression of racism by nurses. However, Porter points out that this did not prevent the nurses from engaging in racist remarks in a Goffmanesque backstage fashion.

Surveillance

Definition

The Concise Oxford Dictionary equates surveillance with "supervision, close observation, [and] invigilation" of individuals who are "not trusted to work or go about unwatched" (Fowler and Fowler 1964: 1302). While this definition has a traditional sounding ring to it, by focusing on a direct co-presence form of monitoring, it captures a dimension of surveillance which is increasingly discussed in current debates – that is, the element of trust (Ericson and Haggerty 1997). Surveillance is practiced, particularly in workplaces, public spaces, and total institutions, such as prisons and the military, because those in positions of authority do not trust or are seeking grounds to trust those below them. Nearly two decades ago, a Labor Canada Task Force on Microelectronics and Employment warned that "[C]lose monitoring of work is an employment practice based on mistrust and lack of respect for basic human dignity" (Baarda 1994: 17).

Staples defines surveillance as "the act of keeping a close watch on people" (1997: ix). The "watchful gaze," as he proceeds to label it, is what gives surveillance its quintessential characteristic. Staples's interest in the gaze is confined to "local knowledge-gathering activities" of the everyday variety that take place in workplaces, schools, homes and community. Surveillance involves all sorts of monitoring from the most rudimentary type of visual observation and recording of information, to genetic testing, electronic monitoring and the use of statistical analysis in the construction of categories and prediction of behavior. Staples's interest is not in the "Big Brother" type of state surveillance, but the Foucauldian "micro techniques of discipline that target and treat the body as an object to be watched, assessed and manipulated" (1997: ix).

Lyon, whose main interest is also in the "monitoring of everyday life," defines surveillance as the "collection and processing of personal data, ifiable or not, for the purposes of influencing or managing those ⸻ nave been garnered," and "does not usually involve embodied ⸻s watching each other" (2001: 2). Defined this way, surveillance, whether direct or indirect, is electronically based and relies mainly on information "fragments abstracted from individuals." Under this definition, the stress is placed on the personal and disembodied nature of the gathered information. But more importantly, this definition leaves the possibility open for surveillance to be exercised through databases, thus giving rise to what is called dataveillance – a form of record matching that is practiced by accessing and cross-referencing information stored in multiple data sources (Lyon 2001: 143).

If at one level surveillance-as-power disables the subject, at another level, according to Norris and Armstrong (1999: 5), surveillance is a natural activity in human affairs which endows new members of society with competency. Dandeker considers surveillance as a "feature of all social relationships" (1999: 37), and involves the management of information, supervision of people's activities in specified *spatial* settings, as well as the obeying of instructions in specific circumstances by "subject persons."

Surveillance as normalization

In referring to Foucault's (1979) work on govermentality and disciplinary practice, Clegg highlights the capillary nature of surveillance, namely that it

> is not simply about direct control. It may range from cultural practices of moral endorsement, enablement and suasion, to more formalized technical knowledge. At one particular level of application, these can include the use of new technologies such as computer monitoring of keyboard output and efficiency. At another more general level, one may be dealing with the development of disciplines of knowledge shaped almost wholly by the "disciplinary gaze" of surveillance.
>
> (1998: 38)

The latter practices have their origin in the nineteenth century, which saw the development of statistical knowledge used by the state to count, categorize, and administer populations. Thus, monitoring is subsumed under the general umbrella of surveillance, but surveillance extends beyond the immediate gaze associated with monitoring.

In working within a Foucauldian framework, Castel makes a related point by noting a surveillance shift from the "observable" to the "deduced" in the construction of subjects. The practices of administrative science focus on "risk" rather than "danger." Dangerousness is associated with confining and observing population groups, while risk is based on using statistical techniques in order to deduce or infer profiles of people who are not under the immediate gaze of the observer. In the case of risk, the subject is deconstructed, so to speak, through the use of statistical techniques. Thus, "surveillance is practiced without any contact, or any immediate representation of the subjects under scrutiny" (Castel 1991: 288). As a matter of fact, the subject that is exposed to the "observing gaze" dissolves and is reconstituted in the abstract through categorization and social ordering:

> There is, in fact, no longer a relation of immediacy with a subject *because there is no longer a subject* [emphasis in original]. What the new preventive policies primarily address is no longer individuals but factors, statistical correlations of heterogeneous elements. They deconstruct the concrete subject of intervention, and reconstruct a combination of factors liable to produce risk.
>
> (Castel 1991: 288)

Foucault's reliance on Bentham's panopticon in depicting surveillance in society is a basic element of the surveillance debate, including the workplace, and has led to the adoption of a passive and contested view of individuals in the disciplinary society. Two decades ago, Giddens expressed skepticism about

> Foucault's "archeology", in which human beings do not make their own history but are swept along by it, does not adequately acknowledge that those subject to the power of dominant groups themselves are knowledgeable agents, who resist, blunt or actively alter the conditions of life that others seek to thrust upon them.
>
> (1981: 172)

More recently, Green took a somewhat similar view, when he noted that

> Foucault's analysis is a totalizing story in which resistance and "exteriority" are, by definition, impossible to achieve. Surveillance is deployed for control and achieves its object. It is a story enabled by an unreflective concept of the individual, a lack of any clear identification of what is not power or of who or what possesses it, and a serious inability to locate structural inequality.
>
> (1999: 28)

However, in rejecting the panopticon metaphor, Green borrowed from Foucault another metaphor, that of the "plague management," which "implies the notion of a 'dialectic,' in which contrasting social forces are copresent with the use of surveillance technologies in the market and within the work-place" (1999: 27). If the panopticon is aimed at normalization of the self through the constant gaze, plague management aims to categorize what is essentially a heterogeneous population. In the same manner that the "intendant" operated to surveil urban plagues, where the "ill, the healthy, the vulnerable and the strong is a dangerous, even seditious, social phenomenon" (Green 1999: 32), here too surveillance operates in an imperfect, even inaccurate, manner in information-saturated societies. The heterogeneity of the public creates spaces for resistance. The new "plague victim" in a world of dataveillance is the poor and untrustworthy (excluded) consumer. Green goes further and asserts, contrary to the arguments that consumption is the new form of oppression, that "healthy" consumers can in fact be empowered by the "plague manager's gaze" through "positive awareness of the life-enhancing benefits of material goods" (Green 1999: 35).

In an attempt to further theorize the concept of surveillance, Haggerty and Ericson draw upon the ideas of poststructuralists, notably Deleuze and Guattari, "to suggest that we are witnessing a convergence of what were once discrete systems to the point that we can now speak of an emerging [surveillance] 'assemblage'" (Haggerty and Ericson 2000: 606). What characterizes surveillance assemblages is their "rhizomatic" structure which makes possible "data doubling" and linkages among various databases spanning domains covering the public and private spheres. Thus, the combination of assemblages and rhizomatic structures achieves several things. First, at the center of surveillance are attempts to capture the human body. This technology makes it possible to keep track of the body movement across various spaces and at differing temporal paces. This "decorporealization" of the body, through its reconfiguration into binary digits (bits) of information and its hybridity with machines, the so-called cyborg, renders the human body accessible "beyond our normal range of perception" (Haggerty and Ericson 2000: 611).

In contrast to Foucault's panoptic treatment of the body, then, here the body is not captured in its totality as a unitary entity, but as a collection of discrete pieces of information. The body is reconstituted, so to speak, depending on the nature of the assemblage and the purpose for which the body is targeted – as consumer, worker, patient, citizen, etc. Second, in contrast to the disciplinary nature of the panoptic form of surveillance, electronically based surveillance systems of consumers, for example, "lack the normalized soul training" (Haggerty and Ericson 2000: 615). Third, a key point that is vigorously debated in the discussion over surveillance concerns the empowerment/disempowerment thesis. Advocates of the empowerment thesis argue that this technology is contingent on the context of its use, that its effect should be considered on a case-by-case basis, and that the technology opens spaces for agency to negotiate and adopt counter methods of control (Mason *et al.* 2000), or as Barker and Sewell call it "reverse surveillance" (2001). As suggested by Poster (1990: 16–20), who opts for the "super-panopticon" label, surveillance technology in the shape of databases can be used to mobilize marginal groups in society, such as women and minorities, and empower political movements (cf. Ronfeldt *et al.* 1998). Likewise, Haggerty and Ericson "take exception" to the claim that the powerful and mainstream society is exempt from the electronic gaze:

> And while the targeting of surveillance is indeed differential, we take exception to the idea that mainstream is "untouched" by surveillance. Surveillance has become rhizomatic, it has transformed hierarchies of observation, and allows for the scrutiny of the powerful by both institutions and the general population.
>
> (2000: 617)

Thus, because of the leveling effects of rhizomatic structures, they go on to note that a process of synopticism, and not only panopticism, is at work here (Haggerty and Ericson 2000: 617–18). Lyon weighs the synoptic view of surveillance, where the many watch the few and in which the technology acts as an empowering agent in terms of effecting mobilization and consumer choice, and comes out on the side of the surveillance school where dominant global trends and "information flows" are managed by "remote control" in order to further the interests of international capital (Lyon 2001: 94–5). But as Mathiesen (1997) declares, synopticism of the "viewer society" kind does not challenge or contradict Foucault's panopticism; rather it reinforces it, and makes it even "worse." The mass media, particularly television, provides access by the many to the few, where the few in the shape of media personalities, opinion makers and movie stars legitimate the dominant ideology by shaping the consciousness of the many.

As expressed by Boyne (2000: 299), there are good arguments for supplanting the concept of panopticism with "post-Panopticism." That the concept of panopticism has outlived its utility is summarized in several familiar points: first, now the many watch the few, although, as we have seen immediately above, there is an important caveat to this; second, there is no need for monitoring because of self-surveillance; third, visualization is pre-empted through simulation and prevention techniques; fourth, the fallibility of total institutions is proven time and again, as demonstrated in prison riots and industrial sabotage; finally, there is increasing empirical evidence which challenges the notion that the workforce is becoming docile. Thus, for Boyne, "contemporary Western societies are post-Panoptical" (303). He suggests retaining the panopticon concept as an analytic ideal type, but refining it to take into account the specificity of the site and developments in technology.

Key features of surveillance

What emerges from this overview is that surveillance is (1) an ubiquitous feature of human societies, and is found in both the political (public) and civil (private) sphere of society; (2) associated with governance and management; (3) endemic to large-scale organizations; (4) constitutive of the subject and has a corporeal aspect to it; (5) disabling as well as enabling and is "productive" in Foucault's sense; (6) understood in terms of distanciation, i.e., the control of space and time; (7) becoming increasingly implicated in a system of assemblage which brings together diverse control technologies; and (8) rhizomatic, as evident in the ability of convergent technologies to capture and assemble inordinate amounts of information about people from various sources.

Surveillance extends from the use of obtrusive methods such as electronic recording of information through telephone tapping and interception of electronic messaging, closed circuit television, video monitoring, and genetic testing by means of fingerprinting, DNA analysis, and retinal identification, to the use of less obtrusive measures such as routine gathering of data on population in the name of governance and administration, as for example through census taking and survey research. The variety of surveillance techniques involving obtrusive and non-obtrusive measures, in which monitoring, recording, counting, and categorizing of people, referred to as social ordering, have affected the identity of individuals as workers, hospital patients, citizens, refugees, students, prison inmates, travelers, and neighborhood residents.

The workplace

Introduction

We dealt in the early part of the chapter with the sociological treatment of technology and the workplace, and noted that resolution of the workplace-technology debate escapes the simple yes or no answer. Questions such as: "Does technology determine power relations in the workplace? Does it reinforce existing ones? Or does it diffuse them?" are not particularly helpful. It is not surprising that the most informed answer is couched in the language of contingency theory, i.e. "it depends on the context, type of industry, managerial culture, etc." Expressed in terms of Kranzberg's "First Law" governing the relationship between technology and society, "Technology is neither good nor bad, nor is it neutral" (Castells 1996: 65).

Translated to the workplace, and regardless of how the debate over technology and society is framed, surveillance remains an essential component of the relations of production in capitalist society (Giddens 1987: 175).

In the drive towards increasing productivity and competition, workplace surveillance, whether covert or overt, is emerging as one of the most contentious issues facing employers, workers, unions, governments, and legal experts. In referring to electronic mail as a major form of workplace surveillance, Lessig notes that

> the single greatest invasion of any sensible space of privacy that cyberspace has produced is the extraordinary monitoring of employees in which corporations now engage. On the theory that they "own the computer," employers increasingly snoop in the e-mail of employees, looking for stuff they deem improper.
>
> (1999: 145)

Privacy advocates issue a more ominous warning concerning the implications of genetic screening for the workplace. In the absence of appropriate safeguards, employers have been known to use genetic information to refuse individuals employment, and insurance companies have denied coverage to individuals whose genetic make-up predisposed them to certain types of illness (IPC 2001: 15).

Indicators of surveillance

Discussions of surveillance techniques at the micro-level have received their greatest attention in research about organizations and workplaces of all kinds. This work by organization theorists is innovative, carried out in a multi-disciplinary fashion, is informed by theoretical debates spanning several fields in the social sciences, and a great deal of it is empirically grounded (McKinlay and Starkey 1998). The thrust of recent writings is to argue that top-down vertical surveillance associated with Taylorism is being substituted by new forms of horizontal monitoring in which computerized monitoring is practiced by work teams who evaluate each other's performance on a peer basis (Sewell 1998; 1999). Horizontal monitoring is premised on enhancing worker autonomy and empowerment. However, as Sewell (1998) demonstrates in his thorough analysis, horizontal and vertical control need not be perceived as separate forms of surveillance. By relying on Foucault's notion of "biopower," Sewell is able to show how the two forms of control are articulated in a "chimerical" fashion to insure that the results of individual surveillance are juxtaposed against those derived from team performance, so as to reward high performers and expose or discipline low performers (cf. Vallas 1999).

There is no consensus among organization theorists that peer group monitoring, such as "awareness monitoring," is an indicator of democratization in the workplace or empowerment of workers. It could very well be a reflection of normalization of the self, whereby peer pressure enforces management-inspired group norms on an individual basis (Sewell 1998). To quote the title of Burawoy's book on the same topic, any such worker–management consensus is a case of management "manufacturing consent" (1982).

In an attempt to synthesize opposing views concerning the empowerment and resistance thesis, Mason *et al.* (2000) provide evidence derived from several case studies (call centers, tax collection offices, public health reporting systems, work-flow management in a printing shop, and computer-based training in a maternity ward) which challenges the claims of the labor process school. The cornerstone of their criticism is the acceptance of an *a priori* assumption in most labor process studies that there is an inherent contradiction between labor and capital which management resolves to its advantage by adopting surveillance techniques that result in the exploitation of workers. Moreover, they reject the claim that capital–labor conflict is bound to disempower workers, thus giving rise to various forms of resistance on the part of workers. Whether it is the management school, which paints a rosy picture of the workplace, or the conflict perspective of the labor process school, which is built on the assumption of "basic antagonisms," the authors claim that reality lies elsewhere. With regard to the labor process argument, the authors contend that (1) it is "simplistic" and does not capture the complexities of the workplace; (2) it tends to "conflate" and exaggerate minor acts of resistance by workers; (3) equates "conflict of interest" between workers and management with general "conflict;" (4) ignores the fact that definitions of acts of resistance depend on the managerial level in question; and (5) assumes that any act of non-compliance by workers is defined as resistance, even when management concurs with rule violations by workers.

To correct what they see as the weakness of the labor process approach the authors turn their attention to examining how employers actually deploy surveillance, how employees perceive the boundaries between legitimate and illegitimate surveillance, and how employees perceive and resort to acts of resistance. The authors contend that both workers and unions accept surveillance in the workplace. They see it as an extension of traditional means of monitoring, as long as it is based on transparency, is part of the collective agreement and does not contravene the law. To support their notion of worker endorsement of surveillance under certain conditions, they quote a standard management statement, this time given by a worker who said that, "if you have not got anything to hide then there is no problem with it [surveillance]" (Mason *et al.* 2000: 16). Here the authors contend that workers view the data collected by means of monitoring as "objective" and provides "protection against unfair work distribution or accusation of dereliction" (2000: 16). In several instances, the authors point out that workers had to resort to "collective" work arrangement, even if this meant reestablishing traditional work methods. They admit that the "new technologies characteristically conceive work as individual and standardized," which runs counter to what is being advocated in modern management of human resources with its emphasis on team work. What is striking about these studies is the total severing of the workplace from the surrounding political and economic environment. The received realism, in the form of objective data, is taken at face value. No attempt is made to investigate the reproduction of "relations of ruling," to quote Smith (1999: 68), and how these contribute to concealing various structural constraints operating on workers.

In *The Use of Personal Data in Employer/Employee Relationships* (Office of the Data Protection Commissioner 2000), the official British document makes a distinction between "performance monitoring" which is aimed "at the quantity and quality of an employee's work output" and "behavioral monitoring" which is "directed at checking an employee's conformity with the employer's rules and standards of conduct" (2000: 28). The report reserves the label "surveillance" to describe performance monitoring, or in our context, computerized performance monitoring (CPM). In CPM an employee's performance is assessed by quantitatively measuring the productivity and quality of a worker's output per unit time. Overall, the British report recommends that monitoring should not violate trust nor be excessive and "should not intrude unnecessarily on employees' privacy and autonomy" (2000: 28).

The US Congress's publication *The Electronic Supervisor: New Technology, New Tensions* (OTA 1987) provides a useful summary of the types of jobs and work conditions that lend themselves to electronic monitoring. With regard to the types of office jobs, the report singles out word processors and data entry clerks, telephone operators, customer service workers, telemarketers, insurance claims clerks, mail clerks, and bank proof clerks. Each of these jobs can be timed and the output per worker is measured in terms of time units. The conditions of work most favorable to CPM include routinized work, work involving interchangeable workers, and simple data collection. These conditions facilitate performance of a large volume of simple tasks, low training and skill level of workers, ample supply of labor (hence great tolerance of turnover), and small productivity differences between experienced and inexperienced workers.

Gary Marx (1985) lists several attributes of CPM which set it apart from traditional work supervision: it transcends time and space, is capital rather than labor intensive, substitutes categories for individual workers as targets of supervision, is decentralized and encourages self-policing, has low visibility, is more intensive in terms of gathering inaccessible information about workers, and reveals extensive information beyond the immediate work environment. In a subsequent work, Marx (1999) draws a distinction between monitoring the work and monitoring the worker, and argues that "the information gathering net" has been constantly expanding to encompass aspects of workers' private lives and personal characteristics that are not immediately related to work. Thus, Marx includes under workplace surveillance the measurement of quantity and quality of worker output, measurement of worker physiology such as drug testing and DNA analysis, the gathering of locational data, and the extent of conformity with workplace rules generally, including appearance and dress codes.

Regan (1996) pursues the issue of worker surveillance by focusing on genetic testing and screening in the workplace. The key aspects of such surveillance are that it is individually based (since the genetic make-up of each individual is unique), the focus of surveillance is the worker rather than the work, it is being primarily addressed as an individual privacy issue, and that genetic surveillance resorts to collecting personal information that is not directly related to work, but could be used by employers to assess behavioral dispositions of workers. The latter is particularly salient in cases involving the screening of potential employees.

These components, according to Regan, give genetic testing and screening a "total surveillance" quality (1996: 23). More than other forms of surveillance, genetic surveillance claims to rely on precise scientific evidence, but because these claims are based on statistical probability, with all its inherent risks, genetic surveillance is subjected to further criticism. In addition to the "employment at will" principle, which disarms workers from privacy protection, genetic testing further weakens privacy protection because workers have no control over inherited genetic traits that put them at risk in the eyes of employers. Regan correctly points out that by framing the issue of genetic surveillance in terms of individual privacy rights, two things have happened. First, there is near absence of the public and collective dimension of privacy in current debates. Second, the debate over genetic surveillance has shifted from one involving rights of workers to one centering on the degree of scientific accuracy of genetic claims.

Panopticism and the workplace

The defining feature of workplace surveillance is the issue of empowerment/ disempowerment, with Foucault's metaphor of the panopticon at the center of the debate. In a recent stock-taking exercise surrounding issues of surveillance in the workplace, Barker and Sewell (2001) declared that the debate cannot be settled by appealing to empirical evidence alone, i.e., whether or not workplace surveillance is having the effect that Foucault theorized. There are case studies in the literature where surveillance in the workplace is clearly implemented in order to disempower workers, exploit them, and reduce any appearance of management's concern for employee well-being to a disguise for continued employee discipline. The empowering literature presents workplace surveillance as either endorsed by workers, or at least a segment thereof, or as being carried out with input from workers.

Yet there is a third strand in the literature which rejects the dichotomous view of computer-based monitoring by adopting a more nuanced approach to capturing both the empowering and disempowering experiences of workers. The methodological thrust of this approach is to single out subjectification as a theme in Foucault's writing that moves the researcher beyond the empowerment/disempowerment dualism. Ball and Wilson quote Knights's formulation of subjectification (Foucault's *assujetissement*) in order to understand "those ways in which individuals objectify themselves so as to recognize, and become committed to, a particular sense of their own subjectivity" (Ball and Wilson 2000: 543). Such an approach to understanding "normalization" of workers accomplishes four things: first, it brings agency into the labor studies project, not as a reductionist form of subjectivity but as an active, productive entity; second, it takes context and temporality into account, by creating space for multiple subjectivities to be productive; third, subjectification permits us to examine power through discursive practices; finally, the panopticon is best understood as a trope, rather than having a one-to-one correspondence with reality (cf. Barker and Sewell 2001).

Markussen (1995) draws upon the work of Hirschhorn (1984) and Zuboff (1988). Hirschhorn treats the "post-industrial" organization as a "cybernetic" entity characterized by continuous learning through feedback processes, and Zuboff (1988) treats organizations as "electronic texts" and singles out the importance of "intellective" skills in informated organizations. Changes in computer-based work challenge traditional work boundaries (with special attention to gender relations) through the creation of interdependent organizational structure with ambiguous authority relations. "An informated environment increases anxiety and challenges, where people must manage increasingly sophisticated boundaries. The informating processes erode pragmatic claims that have lent force and credibility to the traditional managerial role" (Markussen 1995: 175; cf. Allen 1994). The crux of the change is that the technology is both enabling and disabling, where "the person is not something just to be disciplined or liberated," and where "the electronic text, with its panopticon possibilities and both local and global reflective monitoring and surveillance, challenges our understanding of what is private and what is public" (Markussen 1995: 176). Thus, the same information and communication technology that promises democratization, decentralization and liberation of the worker (i.e., empowerment), imposes measurement techniques on the worker that by far exceed anything practiced in the name of Taylorism through the application of time-and-motion studies. In Agre's words,

> Measurements are no longer administered from the outside by time-and-motion specialists; rather it is continuous, built into the processes of work by their very design. Management employs these measurements in comparing work performance, identifying "problems", evaluating innovations, and in an unbounded variety of other ways. Empowered work then is just as heavily monitored as rationalized work.
>
> (Quoted in Markussen 1995: 175)

As we pointed out in an earlier part of this chapter, a major drawback to workplace subjectivity studies is their neglect of the surrounding political and economic environment. The boundaries of investigation focus on the shop floor, and while this highlights the politics of management–worker relations, it does not incorporate a critical realist perspective taking into account the political economy of the labor process. After all, as critics of Foucauldian subjectivity studies point out, the labor process is governed in the first instance by class relations in which labor is valorized in the capitalist marketplace. Restructuring of the economy, state policies, and globalization, they point out, have direct consequences for management–worker relations, and indeed the future of work (Thompson *et al.* 2000). In the most consistent defense of the materialist position, Thompson *et al.*, who reject the relativism of discourse analysis in favor of critical realism, argue the following: first, "Foucauldian discourse pacifies and marginalizes labor, neglecting the specific character of labor as a commodity"; second, because of the ongoing changes in the linkages between global capitalism and the production process, it is imperative to examine the workplace and the place of the various actors in it "not as a mirror image" of such changes but to relate these changes to specific contexts of the industry in question and the various levels of authority relations in the workplace; third, because of the commodification of labor as "a willful, artful and living subject," "complete systems of surveillance" (as assumed by some Foucauldians), ignore the day-to-day encounter between workers and management and the potential for resistance, thus leading management to exercise control through "employee consent" (Thompson *et al.* 2000).

The upshot of organizational restructuring, in the eyes of many observers, is a shift towards post-Fordist workplace organization. The assumptions of post-Fordism have ramifications for surveillance. By seeking worker participation, flexibility in work arrangements, job enhancement, decentralization, and team work, post-Fordism signals a movement away from worker control and monitoring towards worker autonomy (Piore and Sabel 1984). Vallas, in reviewing the empirical literature, does not find supporting evidence to the claims of post-Fordism: instead of increased autonomy, there is more worker control; team workers tend to impose "concertive control" on individual team members; the adoption of Total Quality programs is inspired by management's desire to assert more control over product quality, not to secure input from workers; the development of flexible specialization and "lean production" are accompanied by the adoption of "quantification of production standards and standardization of work methods that place important limits on the discretionary powers of rank and file employees" (Vallas 1999: 84). The only supporting evidence for the post-Fordism thesis seems to come from substituting collaborative work and organizational networks in place of hierarchical integration. Even here, Vallas concludes, this tends to "concentrate control over strategy, marketing and finance in the handful of firms lodged at the center of each production network" (1999: 86).

Rather than describe the shift as one from Fordism to post-Fordism, Vallas concurs with other writers who isolate neo-institutionalism and flexible accumulation as more suitable descriptions of the change taking place. Briefly stated, the emerging organizational structure in the workplace is shaped by external legal, political and cultural institutional factors. The institutional approach is complemented by "flexible ways of capital accumulation flexibility" (Vallas 1999: 91), which are reflected in downsizing, delayering, and subcontracting. The upshot of this, according to Vallas, is the creation of a dual labor force and authority structure in the organization: one group of unskilled workers that is peripheral and lacking job and income security, and another professional group that occupies the organizational core.

Writing from within mainstream social science and in criticism of Foucault's panopticon model, Rule (1996) questions the claim that computer-based monitoring is giving rise to a more encompassing form of worker control, compared, for example, to face-to-face supervision. Based on studies he and associates carried out between 1985 and 1989, Rule points out that computer-based monitoring enabled management to conduct performance assessment, but that this assessment was confined to single tasks and could not be labeled disciplinarian in a Foucauldian meaning of the term. He cites instances where monitored workers actually welcomed the technology as a neutral means for judging performance. These findings lead Rule to conclude, by way of recommendation, that computer-based monitoring should be allowed in the workplace as long as the information collected pertains to work-related activities, is not used in an inferential manner, and does not extend to the private lives of workers.

Gender and surveillance

The entrée to any discussion of gender, surveillance, and privacy should start with the literature surrounding gender, space, and authority relations in capitalist society (cf. Smith 1987). According to Markussen, "gender is inextricably interwoven into our images of authority. When interaction and communication across traditional lines of commands are intensified, and when women enter formerly male-dominated work communities, awareness of gender must be involved, if authority relations are to change" (1995: 178). Canadian data, as well as comparative evidence from other countries, point to a general position of subordination of women in the workplace. Overall, women are rarely in authority positions, and when they are, they tend to manage other women workers (Boyd *et al.* 1991; Samper 1997; Adam and Green 1998).

Underlying claims about gender-based surveillance is the unwanted male gaze. In the case of the workplace, surveillance and privacy are associated with authority structures, body representations, and consequent sexual harassment and discrimination (Collinson and Collinson 1997; Trethewey 1999). In the case of gender and space, the discussion centers on the role of surveillance in the use of public and private spaces by men and women, and how men design and colonize the use of public spaces (Coleman and Sim 2000). Time–space surveillance, usually considered a central aspect of labor discipline among the working class, now affects managerial strata as well, particularly middle management (Collinson and Collinson 1997).

In a study of downsizing and delayering in a major British insurance company, the Collinsons discovered that the patterns of time–space surveillance affect women more adversely than men. What is interesting about this study is that surveillance practice was enforced by means of traditional supervisory means. Electronic monitoring was not involved. The authors discovered in the course of their research that downsizing of middle management has created an informal "macho" culture in the organization which adversely affected women. In order to catch up with a mounting back-log at work, junior management found itself compelled to sacrifice leisure and private time with family in order to compete with, or at least conform to, the emerging culture of the organization. For the majority of junior female managers, this meant sacrificing home life for work.

The spatial and temporal separation between private (home) and public (work) life, which sociologists associate with industrialization and division of labor, seems to be blurred here. The world of work encroaches on the home life in a gendered fashion. Employee resistance to time–space surveillance was apparent in various Goffmanesque methods, such as in the "management of appearance." Employees would leave their car keys on their desks in the office, or bring an extra jacket to work, and leave it on the chair behind their desk, thus giving the impression that they are at the office putting in extra hours, when in fact they have gone home. It is not uncommon among junior male managers to fake illness and stay at home, rather than admit that the real cause of their absence was work-related stress. Working hard to be seen working, according to the authors, is a sign that "both employees and managers have subscribed to the 'panopticon discourse' of incessant visibility" (Collinson and Collinson 1997: 400).

From the legal evidence available concerning e-mail in the workplace, as reviewed by Rosen (2000: 80), it is clear that the intersection of gender and e-mail has revolved around cases of sexual harassment, with implications for discrimination. Invariably, the courts ruled in favor of employers who intercepted private e-mail of employees in order to protect themselves against liability suits. Rosen summarized the typical stance adopted by employers concerning workplace surveillance by referring to Robert Post, a law professor at the University of California at Berkeley:

> In a provocative defense of the Supreme Court's liability regime, Robert Post has suggested that the corporate workplace is a "managerial" sphere in which social relations are organized around principles of efficiency. For this reason he [Post] argues, citizens should be willing to accept greater restrictions on their autonomy and their privacy in the workplace than they would tolerate in the public sphere, which is ideally a space of self-governance.
>
> (Rosen 2000: 83)

This exemplifies the "employment at will" principle, and highlights the property basis in the definition of privacy in the workplace.

In an interesting twist with regard to employee dissatisfaction, a front-page story in The *New York Times* (Abelson 2001) revealed that employees have been turning to the Internet message boards to express their anger and frustration at employers and fellow employees. Male workers specifically targeted successful women in managerial positions, with accusations that the rise of female workers to managerial ranks was due to sexual favoritism and not competence. White male employees also targeted minority employees, charging that affirmative action policies advantage visible minorities and discriminate against whites. No doubt the debate will continue as to who is liable for these actions, the employer or the employee.

Conclusions

The debate on surveillance in the workplace cannot be severed from the larger question of political economy. Computer-based technology in the workplace has brought about fundamental changes in the cognitive and organizational aspects of work. It is clear that the old dualisms characteristic of Taylorist methods of social control have been eclipsed by the adoption of new management techniques based on the need to involve workers more substantively in the production process. But this should not be taken at face value to represent a new normative position of management. At one level, constructivist analysis of technology and the labor process reveals that empowerment and disempowerment, skilling and deskilling, control and autonomy can coexist, depending on the context of the technology, its methods of deployment, and the gender and authority structure of the organization. This should caution us from making blanket statements about technology, either that it is good or bad. At another level, discourse analysis provides us with clues on how control through consent is attained on the shop floor, while at the same time rejecting certain Foucauldian assumptions that surveillance in the workplace is total. Power will not automatically invite resistance. This is an empirical question that must be interrogated locally and ethnographically against the backdrop of realist positions reflected in class relations, state policies, and globalization. The challenge facing researchers is how to reconcile a realist approach with a constructivist one in a way that reveals the nature of constraints operating on agency.

Acknowledgement

The author thanks Karen Hindle for her assistance in preparing this chapter.

Bibliography

Abelson, R. (2001) "By the Water Cooler in Cyberspace, the Talk Turns Ugly," *New York Times*, 29 April: A1.

Adam, A. and Green, E. (1998) "Gender, Agency, Location and the New Information Technology," in B. D. Loader (ed.) *Cyberspace Divide: Equality, Agency and Policy in the Information Society*, London: Routledge.

Allen, J. P. (1994) "Mutual Control in the Newly Integrated Work Environment," *The Information Society*, 10: 129–38.

Baarda, C. W. (1994) *Computerized Performance Monitoring: Implications for Employers, Employees, and Human Resource Management*, Kingston, ON: Industrial Relations Center, Queen's University.

Ball, K. (2001) "Organization, Workplace Monitoring and the Classificatory Impulse: The Question of Ethics," paper presented at Surveillance, Risk, and Social Categorization Workshop, Kingston, ON, May 2001.

Ball, K. and Wilson, D. C. (2000) "Power, Control and Computer-based Performance Monitoring: Repertoires, Resistance and Subjectivities," *Organization Studies*, 21(3): 539–65.

Barker, J. R. and Sewell, G. (2001) "'Here's Looking at You': Surveillance as a Trope for Organizational Domination," unpublished paper.

Bhaskar, R. (1989) *Reclaiming Reality: A Critical Introduction to Contemporary Philosophy*, London: Verso.

Boyd, M., Mulvihill, M. A., and Myles, J. (1991) "Gender, Power and Post-industrialism," *Canadian Review of Sociology and Anthropology*, 28(4): 407–37.

Boyne, R. (2000) "Post-Panopticism," *Economy and Society*, 28(2): 285–307.

Braverman, H. (1974) *Labor and Monopoly Capital: The Degradation of Work in the Twentieth Century*, New York: Monthly Review Press.

Burawoy, M. (1978) "Toward a Marxist Theory of the Labor Process: Braverman and Beyond," *Politics and Society*, 8(3–4): 247–312.

—— (1982) *Manufacturing Consent*, Chicago: University of Chicago Press.

Burris, B. H. (1998) "Computerization of the Workplace," *Annual Review of Sociology*, 24: 141–57.

Castel, R. (1991) "From Dangerousness to Risk," in G. Bruchell, C. Gordon and P. Miller (eds) *The Foucault Effect: Studies in Governmentality with Two Lectures by and Interview with Michel Foucault*, Chicago: University of Chicago Press.

Castells, M. (1996) *The Information Age: Economy, Society and Culture. Volume I: The Rise of the Network Society*, Oxford: Blackwell Publishers.

Clegg, S. (1998) "Foucault, Power and Organizations," in A. McKinlay and K. Starkey (eds) *Foucault, Management and Organization Theory*, Thousand Oaks, CA: Sage Publications.

Cohen, S. (1987) "A Labor Process to Nowhere?" *New Left Review*, 165: 34–50.

Coleman, R. and Sim, J. (2000) "'You'll Never Walk Alone': CCTV Surveillance, Order and Neo-Liberal Rule in Liverpool City," *British Journal of Sociology*, 51(4): 623–39.

Collinson, D. L. and Collinson, M. (1997) "'Delayering Managers': Time–Space Surveillance and its Gendered Effects," *Organization*, 4(3): 375–407.

Dandeker, C. (1999) *Surveillance, Power and Modernity*, Cambridge: Polity Press.

Edwards, R. (1979) *Contested Terrain: Transformation of the Workplace in the Twentieth Century*, New York: Basic Books.

Ericson, R. V. and Haggerty, K. D. (1997) *Policing the Risk Society*, Toronto: University of Toronto Press.

Foucault, M. (1979). *Discipline and Punish: The Birth of the Prison*, New York: Random House.

Fowler, H. W. and Fowler, F. G. (1964) *The Concise Oxford Dictionary*, Oxford: Clarendon Press.

Giddens, A. (1981) *A Contemporary Critique of Historical Materialism, Vol. 1, Power and the State*, Berkeley: University of California Press.

—— (1987) *The Nation-State and Violence. Volume Two of a Contemporary Critique of Historical Materialism*, Berkeley: University of California Press.

Green, S. (1999) "A Plague on the Panopticon: Surveillance and Power in the Global Information Economy," *Information, Communication and Society*, 2(1): 26–44.

Grint, K. and Woolgar, S. (1997) *The Machine at Work: Technology, Work and Organization*, Cambridge: Polity Press.

Haggerty, K. D. and Ericson, R. V. (2000) "The Surveillant Assemblage," *British Journal of Sociology*, 51(4): 605–22.

Hirschhorn, L. (1984) *Beyond Mechanization*, Cambridge, MA: MIT Press.

Hutchby, I. (2001) "Technologies, Texts and Affordances," *Sociology*, 35(2): 441–56.

Information and Privacy Commissioner of Ontario (IPC) (2001) *Annual Report 2000*, Toronto: Information and Privacy Commission of Ontario.

Kling, R. (1992) "Audiences, Narratives, and Human Values in Social Studies of Science," *Science, Technology and Human Values*, 17(3): 349–65.

—— (2000) "Social Informatics: A New Perspective on Social Research about Information and Communication Technologies," *Prometheus*, 18(3): 245–64.

Knights, D. and Willmott, H. (eds) (1990) *Labor Process Theory*, Basingstoke: Macmillan.

Kraemer, K. L. and Danziger, J. N. (1990) "The Impacts of Computer Technology on the Worklife of Information Workers," *Social Science Computing Review*, 8(4): 592–613.

Lessig, L. (1999) *Code and Other Laws of Cyberspace*, New York: Basic Books.

Liker, J. K., Haddad, C. J., and Karlin, J. (1999) "Perspectives on Technology and Work Organization," *Annual Review of Sociology*, 25: 575–96.

Lyon, D. (2001) *Surveillance Society: Monitoring Everyday Life*, Philadelphia: Open University Press.

McKinlay, A. and Starkey, K. (1998) *Foucault, Management and Organization Theory: From Panopticon to Technologies of Self*, London: Sage Publications.

Markussen, R. (1995) "Constructing Easiness – Historical Perspectives on Work, Computerization, and Women," in S. L. Star (ed.) *The Cultures of Computing – Sociological Review Monograph*, Oxford: Blackwell.

Marx, G. (1985) "I'll be Watching You: Reflections on the New Surveillance," *Dissent*, Winter: 26–34.

—— (1999) "Measuring Everything that Moves," *Research in the Sociology of Work*, 8: 165–89.

Marx, K. (1976) *Capital: A Critique of Political Economy*, New York: Vintage Books.

Mason, D., Button, G., Lankshear, G., and Coats, S. (2000) "On the Poverty of *A Priorism*: Technology, Surveillance in the Workplace and Employee Responses," Plymouth: University of Plymouth, pre-publication draft.

Mathiesen, T. (1997) "The Viewer Society: Michel Foucault's 'Panopticon' Revisited," *Theoretical Criminology*, 1(2): 215–34.

Norris, C. and Armstrong, G. (1999) *The Maximum Surveillance Society: The Rise of CCTV*, Oxford: Berg.

O'Doherty, D. and Willmott, H. (2001) "Debating Labor Process Theory: The Issue of Subjectivity and the Relevance of Poststructuralism," *Sociology*, 35(2): 457–76.

Office of Technology Assessment (OTA) (1987) *The Electronic Supervisor: New Technology, New Tensions*, Washington, DC: US Congress.

Office of the Data Protection Commissioner (2000) *The Use of Personal Data in Employer/Employee Relationships. Draft Report*. Winslow, Cheshire: Office of the Data Protection Commissioner. Online. Available HTTP: <http://www.dataprotection.gov.uk> (accessed 26 April 2001).

Parker, M. (1999) "Capitalism, Subjectivity and Ethics: Debating Labor Process Analysis," *Organization Studies*, 20(1): 25–45.

Piore, M. J. and Sabel, C. F. (1984) *The Second Industrial Divide: Possibilities for Prosperity*, New York: Basic Books.

Porter, S. (1993) "Critical Realist Ethnography: The Case of Racism and Professionalism in a Medical Setting," *Sociology*, 27(4): 591–609.

Portes, A. (2000) "The Hidden Abode: Sociology as Analysis of the Unexpected. 1999 Presidential Address," *American Sociological Review*, 65: 1–18.

Poster, M. (1990) *The Mode of Information: Poststructuralism and Social Context*, Chicago: University of Chicago Press.

Regan, P. M. (1996) "Genetic Testing and Workplace Surveillance: Implications for Privacy," in D. Lyon and E. Zureik (eds) *Computers, Surveillance and Privacy*, Minneapolis: University of Minnesota Press.

Roberts, M. J. (1999) "Marxism and Critical Realism: The Same, Similar, or Just Plain Different?" *Capital and Class*, 68: 21–49.

Ronfeldt, D. F., Arquilla, J., Fuller, G. E., and Fuller, M. (1998) *The Zapatista Social Netwar in Mexico*, Santa Monica, CA: Rand Corporation. Online. Available HTTP: <http://www.rand.org/publications/MR/Mr994/MR994.pdf/> (accessed 26 April 2001).

Rosen, J. (2000) *The Unwanted Gaze: The Destruction of Privacy in America*, New York: Random House.

Rule, J. (1996) "High-Tech Workplace Surveillance: What's Really New?" in D. Lyon and E. Zureik (eds) *Computers, Surveillance and Privacy*, Minneapolis: University of Minnesota Press.

Samper, M.- L. D. (1997) "An International Division of Labor: Gender and the Information Technology Industry," *International Journal of Politics, Culture and Society*, 10(4): 635–58.

Schaffer, S. (1994) "Babbage's Intelligence: Calculating Engines and the Factory System," *Critical Inquiry*, 21: 203–27.

Sewell, G. (1998) "The Discipline of Teams: The Control of Team-based Industrial Work through Electronic and Peer Surveillance," *Administrative Science Quarterly*, 43: 397–428.

—— "The Possibility of a Sociology of Workplace Surveillance," paper presented at the American Sociological Association Conference, Chicago, IL, August 1999.

Smith, D. (1987) "Women's Perspective as a Radical Critique of Sociology," in S. Harding (ed.) *Feminism and Methodology*, Bloomington: Indiana University Press.

—— (1999) "From Women's Standpoint to a Sociology for People," in J. Abu-Lughod (ed.) *Sociology for the Twenty-First Century: Continuities and Cutting Edges*, Chicago, IL: University of Chicago Press.

Staples, W. G. (1997) *The Culture of Surveillance: Discipline and Social Control in the United States*, New York: St Martin's Press.

Taylor, J. R. and Van Every, E. J. (1993) *Bureaucratic Organization and Management in the Information Age*, Toronto: University of Toronto Press.

Thompson, P., Smith, C., and Ackroyd, S. (2000) "If Ethics Is the Answer, You Are Asking the Wrong Questions. A Reply to Martin Parker," *Organization Studies*, 21(6): 1149–59.

Thompson, P. and Ackroyd, S. (1995) "All Quiet on the Workplace Front? A Critique of Recent Trends in British Industrial Sociology," *Sociology*, 29(4): 1–19.

Thompson, P. and Smith, C. (1998) "Beyond the Capitalist Labor Process: Workplace Change, the State and Globalization," *Critical Sociology*, 24(3): 193–215.

Trethewey, A. (1999) "Disciplined Bodies: Women's Embodied Identities at Work," *Organization Studies*, 20(3): 369–96.

Vallas, S. P. (1999) "Rethinking Post-Fordism: The Meaning of Workplace Flexibility," *Sociological Theory*, 17: 68–101.

Vallas, S. P. and Beck, J. (1996) "The Transformation of Work Revisited: The Limits of Flexibility in American Manufacturing," *Social Problems*, 43(3): 501–22.

Willmott, H. (1994) "Bringing Agency (Back) into Organizational Analysis: Responding to the Crisis of (Post)Modernity," in J. Hassard and M. Parker (eds) *Towards a New Theory of Organizations*, London: Routledge.

Zuboff, S. (1988) *In the Age of the Smart Machine: The Future of Work and Power*, New York: Basic Books.

3 Biometrics and the body as information

Normative issues of the socio-technical coding of the body[1]

Irma van der Ploeg

> Systems of registration, censuses, and the like – along with documents such as passports and identity cards that amount to mobile versions of the "files" [in Max Weber's sense] states use to store knowledge about their subjects – have been crucial in states' efforts to embrace their citizens.
>
> (Torpey 1998: 245)[2]

> In a world of identity politics and risk management, surveillance is turning decisively to the body as a document for identification, and as a source for prediction.
>
> (Lyon 2001: 72)

Introduction

"Information" and the related concepts of informatization and digitization were the buzz words par excellence of the late twentieth century – a fact that did not change with the coming of the twenty-first century. These terms are usually taken to signal a movement away from the physical to the immaterial, a shift in importance, for example, from material production to a service economy and information trade; from congested freeways and polluting transportation systems to the lightness of glass-fiber communication networks and the mobility of frictionless electronic data flow. And on the level of personal identity, the shift was from the gravity of a needy, over-determined bodily existence to the weightless mode of multiple virtual personae.

Writing out these contrasts, however, even if they ring so many familiar bells, makes them recognizable for what they are: the clichés and rhetoric of hype. Of course, material production has not in any way become less important to human existence, nor are the provision of services and the economic centrality of information in any way independent of material production. Similarly, the ubiquitous use of mobile telecommunication and electronic data exchange has not in any way contributed to a reduction of physical transport and travel, or relieved the environment from its polluting effects. We are all very much made aware of this every day and thus able to recognize the ideology of our times for what it is.

Although contemporary developments in information technology (IT) bring along changes and transformations of many kinds, these are not adequately described nor understood in the simple oppositional terms referred to above. Worse than that, these very dichotomous ways of understanding both facilitate and obscure some of the subtler, but nonetheless far-reaching changes that are taking place. In this chapter I want to focus in particular on the pervasive dichotomization of information and materiality. More specifically, I want to address one particular instance of this dichotomy that seems to me to require some rethinking: the dichotomy between embodied identity or physical existence on the one hand, and information about (embodied) persons and their physical characteristics on the other. I want to question in particular the presupposition that there is a self-evident, unproblematic distinction to be made between the body itself and information about, or digital representations of that body, in the context of the rapidly extending practices of registration and processing of digital data on physically identified individuals.

Today, the socio-technical production of social categories and identities through IT-mediated surveillance relies increasingly on a gradually extending intertwinement of individual physical characteristics with information systems (van der Ploeg 1999a). The impetus for this development stems to a considerable extent from governments and government-related authorities facing security problems relating to processes of globalization and increasing mobility of persons. The apt metaphor of states' "embrace" of their citizens in the quote from Torpey's *History of the Passport* used as an epigraph at the beginning of this chapter becomes particularly striking when "the files" of which he speaks show the tendency to include ever more data pertaining to bodily characteristics. But it is in various domains of society and spheres of activity, ranging from work, health care, and law enforcement, to consumption, travel and leisure, that the generation, collection, and processing of "body data" is increasing (Lyon 2001).

I argue that in order to make sense of the normative and socio-political implications of this phenomenon, we may need to let go of the idea that this merely concerns the collection of yet another type of personal information. Instead of consisting of mere information about persons, a proactive understanding of this development may be better served by considering the ways in which this "informatization of the body" may eventually affect embodiment and identity as such. We may need to consider how the translation of (aspects of) our physical existence into digital code and "information," and the new uses of bodies this subsequently allows, amounts to a change on the level of ontology, instead of merely that of representation. As Katherine Hayles writes:

> When changes in incorporating practices take place, they are often linked with new technologies that affect how people use their bodies and experience space and time. Formed by technology at the same time that it creates technology, embodiment mediates between technology and discourse by creating new experiential frameworks that serve as boundary markers for the creation of corresponding discursive systems. In the feedback loop between technological innovations and discursive practices, incorporation is a crucial link.
>
> (Hayles 1992: 163)

Instead of the standard dual picture of the body as an ahistorical, natural entity, the representations of which change over time (due to scientific and technological innovations), we may need to consider how all three terms are caught in a process of co-evolution. With technological and discursive practices converging towards an ontology of "information," it is unlikely that their mediating link, embodiment – even while acknowledging its constraining and limiting power – will remain unaffected. And because embodiment concerns our most basic experience of the body and of being in the world, these developments carry profound normative and moral implications we ought to attempt to uncover.

Starting with biometric identification and verification systems, the next section describes a few examples of the variety of social identities being constructed and reinforced by digital registration and processing of individual physical characteristics. The third section describes several further examples of the informatization or digitization of the body taken from the contexts of medicine and forensics. In the fourth section it is argued that these technology-mediated practices, in which various aspects of bodily existence become integrated in information systems, taken together, signal the emergence of a new body ontology. Fifth, I discuss the significance of this phenomenon in relation to the normative concepts of "privacy" and "bodily integrity," and argue that these two notions are based on a body ontology that does not entirely match the currently evolving one. The final section tries to flesh out this abstract claim by providing some concrete illustrations of this growing discrepancy taken from the legal discourse on bodily searches and DNA-banking.

Biometric identification technologies and social categorization

While primitive forms of biometric registration, mainly for administrative purposes, are known to have existed centuries ago, in modern times, the taking of fingerprints for identification of suspected criminals is by far the most well-known example of biometric identification. Today, the millions of finger-prints collected over the years in the USA, Europe, and elsewhere for forensic identification purposes are being digitalized to form huge, increasingly interconnected databases allowing quick, on-line searches (Cole 1998, 2001). The current capacity to identify a given fingerprint by comparison with hundreds of thousands, even millions, of stored fingerprints is unprecedented in scope and speed. Thus, forensic fingerprinting is rapidly moving beyond its classic function of connecting a suspect to a crime scene by matching a "latent" fingerprint, i.e. a fingerprint found at a crime scene, to a suspect; with the help of the quick searches and comparisons of the fingerprints stored in central databases, the retrieval of a fingerprint may now actually generate a suspect.

Even though in public imagination fingerprinting is still firmly connected to criminality and forensics, this exclusive association is rapidly becoming obsolete. Worries about the "stigmatizing effect" of fingerprinting have been laid to rest after the identities produced by the "stigma" of the fingerprint diversified rapidly. From being a sign of criminality, fingerprinting is rapidly growing in importance as a tool to perfect a far wider range of social categorizations, including, for instance, welfare recipients, refugees, and migrants. Fingerprinting has become one of the central technological aids to immigration and naturalization services, both in the USA and the European Union, in their efforts to control illegal immigration and deal with ever-growing numbers of applications for political asylum. The INS in the United States has a system in operation called IDENT into which the fingerprints of every illegal migrant and asylum seeker are being fed. System users hope to make it compatible with that of the FBI, the largest fingerprint database in the country, as well as that of Customs.

Through a growing number of voluntary systems, fingerprinting is now becoming involved in the construction of the more positive, privileged identities of the law-abiding citizen, the respectable client, cardholder, or club member as well. "Low risk" frequent travelers into the USA, for example, can apply for inclusion into one of the systems designed to facilitate legal border traffic (INSPASS at airports, SENTRI or DCL at geographical borders). They then have to go through a background check that includes the routine taking of fingerprints, used for comparison with the FBI database, and stored in the INS system as well. The programs themselves use hand geometry and facial photographs to identify the legitimate user of the accelerated processing on entering the country (van der Ploeg 2000).

Similar systems are in use in several European airports, while last year a central database containing the fingerprints of every person applying for political asylum in one of the European Union's member states – and those of every other person of "irregular presence" caught on European territory as well – became a reality (van der Ploeg 1999b). The IND (the Dutch INS) at Rotterdam international harbor recently added to this an identification system of iris scanning for asylum seekers. "Regular citizens" will increasingly have biometric features used for identification purposes as well. During the development of a new Dutch passport the inclusion of a fingerprint as an additional security feature has been quite seriously considered, but was dismissed in the end. Other public services and authorities increasingly look towards biometric technologies for identification of citizens as well. Obligatory fingerprinting of every person eligible for public aid programs has been introduced in Illinois, Texas, and Arizona, and many of the other states are following suit. In The Netherlands, a similar experiment with welfare recipients started in 2000. In the same country, political negotiations are taking place about plans to redesign the infrastructure of all currently decentralized "municipal basis administrations" (population databases) to render them accessible for a variety of central governmental agencies like the police, the internal revenue service and so on. Part of this plan is the idea to add a biometric identifier to every personal file in these databases. In health care, the wide trend towards digitization of patient records has yielded various systems that include a patient-held biometrically secured smart card.

Next to these public service and administration applications of biometrics there is a broad trend in the worlds of commerce and work where improved methods of identification, authentication, tracking and logging are sought. The growing electronic mediation in these domains calls forth a feverish search for new ways to secure transactions of all kinds, be they telebanking, ATM cash dispensing, e-commerce, or the logistic management of goods, people, and data in offices, businesses and on the road.

The last example to be mentioned here is the extension of increasingly ubiquitous CCTV systems for crime prevention and surveillance of public spaces with facial recognition systems. The coupling of real-time video images to facial recognition systems and "lookout" databases enables the automatic signaling of the presence of suspect individuals as they move through crowds and streets (Norris and Armstrong 1999; Norris in this volume).

Other forms of digitization of the body

If our daily lives are going to show an increasing mediation of our identities (as workers, suspects, consumers, citizens, migrants, refugees, club members, welfare recipients, etc.) through the interconnection of our bodies with information systems, we can add to this picture a couple of other forms of digitization of bodies. Two large domains traditionally concerned with the legitimate enrollment of individual bodies in the process of generating, storing and processing of (identifying, physical) information are medicine and law enforcement. In both areas, IT has been introduced with revolutionizing and fundamentally transforming effects.

In recent years, the computerization of medical records (EPRs, or electronic patient records) has become an area where the digital registration of information about individuals' physical existence has created an abundance of highly accessible (compared to the locally kept, often handwritten, paper files to be replaced), sensitive, "identifying" information. Health care systems throughout the Western countries are moving towards on-line accessible EPRs into which all data on medical history, medication, test results from a broad variety of diagnostic (often already computer-based) techniques, and therapies belonging to a particular individual's medical biography are accumulated, and can be accessed by relevant care givers. Negotiations over design specifications are focusing on how broad the category of "relevant care givers" to be given access can be defined, and to what extent administrative goals of billing, insurance reimbursements, hospital management, and scientific research can be served by such records, without compromising what used to be known as "patient confidentiality" and privacy too much. Such records, by virtue of the personal and unique nature of the information about an individual body contained in them, are in themselves extended forms of "unique identifiers": obviously, every item added increases the uniqueness of the record.

The connection of a record to a particular individual can be established, besides through "classical" personal identifiers like name, age, insurance number, etc., by biometric identifiers as well. Today several experimental designs of EPRs include biometric data as a means of connecting the record to the right person, thus simultaneously securing disclosure and limiting access to the sensitive, private information contained in them. "Genetic counseling" and pre- and post-natal testing for the presence of an ever-growing set of genetic predispositions – the results of which are to be stored on the EPR – adds to the amount of information about bodies "on file" that is both "identifying" and deeply personal. It provides the material for the generation of more information – about individuals, families and populations, about their histories as well as their possible futures, thus facilitating profiling and categorization into various risk categories.

Secondly, there is the set of technologies deriving from genetics for which grand futures are being predicted. Here the domains of forensic biometric identification and medical information come together: "genetic finger-printing" or "DNA-typing" is rapidly equaling, even surpassing, traditional fingerprinting in providing "absolute certainty" about identity in the legal context (see also Nelkin and Andrews in this volume). Moreover, the enormous potential for improving law enforcement by collecting, keeping, and rendering accessible this type of data for future use has not escaped notice, and many countries are now creating databases with genetic identifying information about every convicted criminal subjected to providing DNA-samples in the course of a criminal investigation.

The threshold for inclusion in these databases is lowered time and again. For example, in The Netherlands the criterion for mandatory giving up of DNA has recently been changed from suspects of crimes with eight-year sentences to those serving four years. News media regularly cover stories about politicians proposing to sample the entire population whenever there is some spectacular crime shocking the public, or about medical institutions that, for years, turn out to have been routinely sampling DNA from every newborn baby coming in for their vaccinations, without even the parents knowing about it. Here, as elsewhere, technology is developing quickly, and beyond mere matching of DNA "fingerprints," it is now becoming feasible to generate from the DNA sample the beginning of an actual profile (gender, ethnicity) of the person from whom the sample originates.

Although not commonly discussed in relation to biometrics – with the exception of DNA "fingerprinting" – these practices do have in common with biometrics that they constitute digital representations of our physical or bodily characteristics as individuals in one sense or another. Moreover, precisely in that capacity they all are functional in the construction and perfor-mance of our identities. The transformation of various aspects of physical existence into digital code, field values, images, graphs, and scores, imply endless possibilities for categorization. Stored, retrievable, and keyword searchable from many different locations, simultaneously or over extended periods of time, these "body data" can become part of information-processing practices in ways that were not possible before, or generate new practices altogether. The extensive potential for new forms of knowledge production, policy making and implementation, targeting, and the development of "prevention strategies" is widely welcomed but will also give rise to new forms of surveillance that may not all be just benign. And, finally, there are many possible cross-connections between the various domains in which these data are produced and used. Some of these connections are already realized, others are still mere technical possibilities; some are only fantasized about by over-zealous law enforcers, others may already be written down as future policy goals; some will be existing only in the fearful imaginations of Big-Brother-watchers, others may become reality faster than most of us think desirable.

The body as information

What all the above-mentioned practices have in common is that in each one, parts or aspects of human bodies are represented in digital code, enabling new ways of performing identities and embodiment. Through these partly connecting and overlapping technological practices, then, a new body ontology is emerging, that redefines bodies in terms of, or even as, information.

The notion of body ontology enables us to describe the way the human body is implicated in a process of co-evolution with technology – information technologies, but also surgical, chemical and genetic and visualization techniques, and combinations of these. Over the past century, various developments, mainly in medical science, have resulted in a set of body ontologies that are not based on the familiar anatomical-physiological ontology of the modern body, but quite explicitly construe the body in terms of flows of information and communication patterns. The endocrinological body, originating in the early twentieth century, for instance, knows the body as a biochemical entity, with an ontology of chemical substances that are characterized in terms of messages, signals, and feedback loops. Later, immunology – with a strong impetus from the AIDS crisis during the 1980s – construed a body that differed significantly from the anatomical body in its construction of body boundaries – the boundary between self and other – as the result of a fight going on beneath the skin. A discourse in many respects quite similar to that of strategic defense and warfare developed, based on a body ontology consisting of networks of communicative patterns between, for example, "T cells," B cells, macrophages, and various mediating molecules such as lymphokines and antibodies (Haraway 1991; Martin 1992). The sciences and practices of genetics, finally, as already hinted at above, have generated a body ontology that takes the building blocks of the body to be "information": the human genome and DNA itself are codes to be broken in order to enable us to "read" the "blueprints of life." The "stuff" of genetics is information – no matter how this stuff can be described in biochemical terms of proteins, its "essence" lies in its coding function.[3]

Thus, according to Haraway,

> An account of the biomedical-biotechnical body must start from the multiple molecular interfacings of genetic, nervous, endocrine, and immune systems. Biology is about recognition and misrecognition, coding errors, the body's reading practices (for example frameshift

mutations), and billion-dollar projects to sequence the human genome to be published and stored in a national genetic "library". [. . .] The biomedical-biotechnical body is a semiotic system, a complex meaning producing field [. . .].

(Haraway 1991: 211)

Perhaps it seems somewhat counterintuitive to speak of new body ontologies, rather than mere changes in ways of representing and knowing the body: mere ways to talk about something that in itself is extra-discursive and remains unaffected. However, the fleshy structure bounded by skin, with an inside made up of organs, muscles, tissues, bones, and various fluids that appears to be the most likely candidate for such an extradiscursive referent, turns out, as the work of various historians of the body has shown, to be a particular historical invention itself (e.g. Jordanova 1989; Lacqueur 1990; Duden 1991; Schiebinger 1993). This body ontology, for which anatomy, and, somewhat later, physiology, provide the building blocks, has been quite precisely dated, and thus recognized as a contingent historical construction. The anatomical body as we know and experience it today emerged in the late eighteenth century. At that time, the practice of anatomy, which had existed for centuries already, coupled with the then emerging epistemology of experimental science, and a variety of new technologies of preservation and representation. A new body ontology came into being, that is commonly referred to as "the modern body" (Foucault 1975, 1979; Gallagher and Lacqueur 1987). This body, laid down in the imagery of the anatomical atlas, became the ultimate reference for what gradually came to be experienced and acted upon as the very nature of our bodies (Hirschauer 1991; Duden 1991). This new body was subsequently performed through and in the fast-proliferating practices, discourses, technologies, and architectures of medicine, law, education, public policy, etc., thus gradually and fundamentally altering the experience of being embodied.

The interesting thing is that even if there is a certain obviousness, or common-sense logic, to equating "the body itself" with the anatomical body constructed along the lines described above, the way this notion runs into difficulties in certain contexts shows that it is not the unproblematic, natural prediscursive referent it is often supposed to be. Rather, it is a particular construction, a specific body ontology, ultimately sustained by pragmatic and operational definitions. The co-evolution of various information technologies and bodies observable from the examples discussed above generates confusions, casts doubts, and generates needs for explication of issues previously considered self-evident.

This comes to the surface in particular when normative implications of contemporary technological developments are considered. The growth in

generation and processing of "body data" regularly generates public controversy, for the recognition of the enormous potential for "misuse" of these
types of information is widely shared. In trying to draw lines, and separate
legitimate use from misuse, concepts and values are invoked and applied in
contexts and discursive spaces they were not invented for. The ensuing
discursive exercises sometimes reveal how the ontologies implied in these
concepts and values do not entirely match with the informatization and
digitization processes currently evolving.

Normative concerns: "privacy" and "bodily integrity"

Predominantly, normative concerns are couched in terms of potential
violations of "privacy" – a fundamental, albeit not in all countries constitutional, legal and moral right. Data protection regimes such as those laid
down in the European Directive on Data Protection (European Parliament
and Council 1995) are morally and legally underpinned by reference to rights
to privacy. The object of protection then is "personal data," that is, data
pertaining to an individual in such a way that they are "identifying."[4]
The kind of privacy involved, then, is *informational privacy*, which is defined
in the ethical and legal literature as having control over one's data.

In speaking about the (sometimes forced) integration of bodies and
information systems, however, the more fundamental concept of bodily
integrity appears relevant as well, and occasionally this possibility is considered. Yet in relation to the generation and storage of digital representations
of individual bodily features, its relevance is considered in a very restricted
way, if it is considered at all. It is generally perceived to be at stake only in
the context of the generation of body data as "input" for the IT systems.

For example, in the context of biometric identification schemes, bodily
integrity is discussed only with regard to the material contact between fingertips, hands, eyes and the various sensing devices used to generate a biometric.
This concern is subsequently quickly dismissed (e.g. Kralingen *et al.* 1997).
In the contexts of law enforcement and forensic identification, however,
with their longstanding traditions of "frisking," fingerprinting, and, today,
DNA typing, and various other forms of bodily searches, it is considered
quite clear that bodily integrity is indeed at stake.

Most countries have quite circumscribed laws and rules pertaining to
"bodily searches" in order to protect the rights of individuals against the
powers of the state and its law enforcement branches. These rules specify
under what conditions (strength of suspicion, severity of the suspected crime)
a person can be required to provide fingerprints, bodily tissue (blood, hair,
saliva) or cooperate in the procedure of procuring such materials. If consent
is required, rules are in place as to what exactly is covered by a given consent;

if forced searches are allowed, specifications are usually given about who may perform the search (medical training, gender).

Similarly, the concept of bodily integrity is a normative notion quite central to normative underpinnings of medical practice and science. The contours of the discussion of bodily integrity in the medical context of generation and storage of information about bodies, however, parallel the set of patient rights as laid down in "informed consent" requirements pertaining to medical interventions. That is to say, bodily integrity is protected as far as the performance of tests, the procurement of "test materials," or the conducting of experiments require physical intervention. The results of these medical proceedings – today often in the form of computer-generated, processed and stored data – are considered "personal information" deserving protection for privacy (patient confidentiality) reasons.

Thus, everything beyond the actual touching and procurement of materials to produce digital representations – be they biometric templates, EPRs, CT-scans, genetic profiles, or digital images of fingerprints – is thought of as sensitive, personal *information*, a concept that rather equalizes and flattens further distinctions. There is ethical or legal difference between these types of information and classic forms of personal data, like, for example, proper name-address-age-gender, religious background, video rental records, or income tax files. The only distinction used is between personal or identifying data and non-personal or anonymous data, a distinction that in itself is not an intrinsic characteristic of the data themselves, but, arguably, a function of its relation to other data (Panel on Confidentiality and Data Access 1993).

Thus a specific "division of tasks" exists that reflects a particular onto-logical dichotomy: bodily integrity applies to "the thing itself," whereas informational privacy is presumed to cover all (digital) "representations" of it. The normative relevance of this difference is clear: in our current moral and legal cosmologies, far less stringent criteria apply to what counts as a legitimate violation of privacy, compared to what is needed to justify a breach of bodily integrity.[5] So, if the underlying ontology is gradually changing through processes of informatization, digitization, and the various new forms of constructing, performing, and manipulating the body these transformations allow, and if because of that the presumed demarcation of where "the body itself" stops and begins being "information" will subtly shift, the moral and legal vocabularies available will no longer suffice.

Bodily searches: body boundaries, information, and integrity

Our current concept of bodily integrity, even though it can be a basically felt and psychologically experienced moral value, functions predominantly in the discourses of law and rights. But even there, it is mostly used as an unquestioned and unquestionable value to be referred to in the last instance, rather than itself being the object of explicit deliberation and definitional exercises. There are a few contexts, however, in which the suggestion of self-evidence regarding the question of what constitutes the body and its boundaries whose integrity must be protected is lost, and debates and definitional exercises ensue. In these instances it becomes clear which body ontology underlies the right to bodily integrity, and significantly, how it runs into trouble.

For our current purposes, legal debates over "bodily searches" (the current rekindling of which is largely due to the development of DNA-profiling and banking) is highly relevant and instructive. Even though national differences abound here, in many countries, specifically West-European ones, upholding a distinction between searches *on* the body ("frisking," searching of clothes, skin, fingertips, face) and searches *in* the body is deemed crucial, suggesting that a there is a self-evident body boundary that determines the normative and legal weight of a particular search (Ippel 1996; Tak 1990).

"Integrity" becomes an issue when insides are involved, and boundaries compromised. Pricking through the skin with a needle to draw blood, for example, though not severe, and often routinely justified (e.g., in traffic alcohol tests), is in principle a violation of the body's integrity. However, this seemingly clear-cut boundary appears far less evident when a more detailed explication is called for. To begin with, natural openings and orifices form an obviously problematic gray zone acquiring much attention and thought. Generally, searches of "the natural body openings" fall within the category of searches on the body, although in Dutch law a further distinction is recently introduced between body openings of the upper and those of the lower body half, because of the "burdensome nature" of searches of the lower body half, both to the searcher and the searched. This provides an example of the way the criterion based on a presumed natural body boundary needs to be supplemented time and again by wholly different types of criteria; here, one that refers to a subjective experience of embodiment.

For our present purposes, however, an additional criterion is even more interesting. X-ray photographs, for instance, are quite hard to categorize in terms of an inside and outside of the body, for they do not involve any actual touching of the body. They score high on the legal scale of relative invasiveness of forced searches, but it is quite unclear whether this is on account of the X-rays being sent through the body, and the health risks this involves, or because of the fact that the resulting picture constitutes a representation of the inside of the body. There is also a general consensus among legal experts that the taking of a DNA sample is to be considered a most serious breach of integrity of the body, even though there are several ways of obtaining a DNA sample that are hardly noticeable to the person involved, and, certainly compared to many traditional kinds of searches, do not in the least appear "burdensome." According to Ten Have and van Welie (1998), the reason for this is that such searches do not have as their goal finding traces or objects related to a crime, but generating information about the identity of the person. It is this difference in purpose that renders the taking of a saliva swab from the inner lining of the mouth a far more serious breach of integrity than, for example, a search of the lower body openings to find smuggled drugs. Clearly, in clarifying the legal and normative status of such searches, a simple reference to a boundary between the inside and the outside of the body has been given up, to allow space for the criteria of purpose and subsequent use of the body data.

The inability to distinguish between "the body itself" and "body information" also explains to considerable extent why the efforts to deal with the issues of DNA sampling and banking of genetic information run into so much trouble and controversy. There are several ways of procuring DNA samples that by all traditional standards would hardly count as a breach of physical integrity. Here it is clear that it is not the actual touching of the body, or crossing of the anatomical-physical boundary necessary for generating the data that accounts for all the fuss. Its meaning as a breach of integrity does not lie there, but obviously in subsequent use of the information thus acquired. Focusing on the act of generating the data, in this case, obscures its significance. Much of the discussions surrounding these databases center on the questions of what exactly should be filed and stored, to whom it should be made accessible, and for what uses. If, for example, the DNA samples themselves are also kept, it will be possible to subject these samples to further analysis in the future, thus adding to the mere "fingerprint" whatever medical-genetic information may be derived from whatever (future) technique will become available. There are immense differences in potential to generate information from DNA samples, or DNA records, and within the latter, between STR profiles or complete genetic profiles, between (what are today believed to be) medically non-coding polymorphisms, and (what are today known as) "health-related loci" (Kaye and Imwinkelried 2000). And, as can be inferred from the remarks between the parentheses, these qualifications may not refer to static characteristics. They are relative to the state of knowledge and technology at a particular moment in time – the enormous effort that today is being invested in the further development of analytic techniques and the "decoding" of the human genome may change such premises in years to come.

The relationship between bodily matter and bodily information, on which the demarcation between the rights to bodily integrity and informational privacy is based, when it comes to genetics and DNA, cannot be adequately understood as a boundary between the thing itself and representations of it. There is no clear point where bodily matter first becomes information. The "essence" of the stuff of DNA, both the reason of its scientific isolation in the first place, and, in watered down version, its forensic significance, is precisely that it is "information."

There are, of course, many forms of searches where the act of generating the information, and the concomitant violation of anatomical-physical body boundaries is indeed what should count. Similarly, many body data generated in the medical context are the result of elaborate, invasive procedures and diagnostic techniques; here, the encounter between bodies and information-generating technologies is more often than not quite painful, risky, or otherwise costly to the person. And if one considers the difference between, for instance, surgically opening the body to gather information about the condition of some organ and gathering the same information by a CT-scan, it is obvious that this difference is extremely significant. Moreover, to express this difference, the notion of bodily integrity is indispensable and must not be deconstructed lightly.

But how should we conceptualize a police search or a medical examination of the body-as-information, a virtual body? The concepts of "privacy" and "data protection" are too much in collusion with the very informatization processes they are supposed to limit. To say that the use of body data merely involves the data or the information, and not the body, or the embodied person denies the constitutive and enduring relation between the data and my identity as embodied person. If the bits and pieces of stored information about my life and behavior as citizen, consumer, worker, my "digital persona" (Clarke 1994), are in a sense constitutive of, and inseparable from, me as a person, then the inclusion of body data to this digital biography is similarly inseparable from my embodied identity. Acknowledging this relation by proclaiming body data "private" or "worthy of protection," just like any other "personal data," goes some of the way, but does not exactly do justice to the fact that embodiment is central to individuality and identity in a way that my social security number or my car rental records are not. It may quite reasonably be expected that these changing practices of dealing with bodies will have some profound transforming effects on the level of embodiment, just as the late eighteenth-century emergence of the modern, anatomical-physical body did during the century that followed it.

If it is already recognized that the severity of breaches of bodily integrity in the context of police searches may lie not just in the physical invasion of body boundaries, but also in the purpose of information gathering about a person's identity, then it is highly relevant that the tremendous impact of today's technological developments on law enforcement capabilities relates precisely to this purpose. The capacity of certain technologies to change the boundary, not just between what is public and private information but, on top of that, between what is inside and outside the human body, appears to leave our normative concepts wanting. The new, intensive forms of monitoring, categorizing, scrutinizing and, ultimately, controlling and manipulating of persons through their bodies and embodied identities that become possible in this new ontology suggest that some form of integrity of the person may be at stake. Maybe not exactly "bodily" integrity in the traditional sense associated with anatomical-physical body boundaries, but a form of integrity yet to be defined. Especially since the gathering of body data, including even DNA samples, becomes ever more easy, inconspicuous, inescapable, and ubiquitous, it seems a bit like "ostrich-policy" to remain too focused on body boundaries belonging to the ontology of anatomical-physical bodies, rather than redevising some concept of integrity adequate to the ontology of informatized bodies.

Notes

1 This project was carried out within the framework of the Incentive Programme Ethics and Policy, which is supported by The Netherlands Organization for Scientific Research. I wish to thank Jeroen van den Hoven, Jos de Mul, David Lyon, and the participants of the international workshop on Surveillance, Risk, and Social Categorization, 3–5 May 2001, Queen's University, Kingston, Canada, for useful comments and suggestions.

2 Thanks to Elia Zureik for pointing me to this extract.

3 It may be important to stress here that these phenomena are not mere metaphors used in popularizations of science, while the "real body" to which such descriptions refer remains unequivocally anatomical or physiological. Whereas it is indeed the case that metaphors are involved here, they can be found in the most "serious" scientific descriptions as well. Such metaphors do not refer to other more literal concepts, but are the very stuff of scientific imagination itself. What may start out as metaphorical – meaning carried over from another context of use – after a while becomes the literal (Rorty 1989; Locke 1992).

4 "'Personal data' shall mean any information relating to an identified or identifiable natural person ('data subject'); an identifiable person is one who can be identified, directly or indirectly, in particular by reference to an identification number or to one or more factors specific to his physical, physiological, mental, economic, cultural, or social identity" (European Parliament and Council 1995: 10).

5 Although bodily integrity in many legal systems is conceptually subordinated to a more general concept of "privacy" or "private life," that is, it is often defined as a special subcategory of a general notion of privacy, it is also generally acknowledged as morally and legally constituting privacy's most basic instance. The contrast between the two ethical/legal regimes I'm drawing out here is therefore not that between bodily integrity and privacy as such, which is a very broad and loosely defined encompassing concept, but that between "bodily integrity" and "informational privacy." I argue that our concept of bodily integrity is too narrow to deal with the broad technology-mediated transformative processes in which our bodies are currently caught, and that it is too readily assumed that mere

"information" or "data" is at stake, however strongly the "personal" or "sensitive" nature of this information is stressed, and however stringent data-protection regulations may be defined. Both with respect to the necessity and the justification of protective measures, there is a morally highly relevant difference between the definition of the object of protection as "identifying data (about the body)" and our personal bodily existence as such.

Bibliography

Clarke, R. (1994) "The Digital Persona and its Application to Data Surveillance," *The Information Society*, 10: 77–92.

Cole, S.A. (1998) "Witnessing Identification: Latent Fingerprinting Evidence and Expert Knowledge," *Social Studies of Science*, 28(5–6): 687–712.

—— (2001) *Suspect Identities: A History of Fingerprinting and Criminal Identification*, Cambridge, MA: Harvard University Press.

Duden, B. (1991) *The Woman Beneath the Skin: A Doctor's Patients in Eighteenth-Century Germany*, Cambridge, MA: Harvard University Press.

European Parliament and Council (1995) *Directive 95/EC On the Protection of Individuals With Regard to the Processing of Personal Data and on the Free Movement of Such Data.* Brussels: European Parliament and Council.

Foucault, M. (1975) *The Birth of the Clinic: An Archeology of Medical Perception*, New York: Vintage/Random House.

—— (1979) *Discipline and Punish: The Birth of the Prison*, New York: Vintage/Random House.

Gallagher, C. and Lacqueur, T. (eds) (1987) *The Making of the Modern Body: Sexuality and Society in the Nineteenth Century.* Berkeley: University of California Press.

Hirschauer, S. (1991) "The Manufacture of Bodies in Surgery," *Social Studies of Science*, 21(2): 279–319.

Jordanova, L. (1989) *Sexual Visions: Images of Gender in Science and Medicine between the 18th and the 20th Centuries*, New York: Harvester Wheatsheaf.

Haraway, D. J. (1991) *Simians, Cyborgs, and Women: The Reinvention of Nature*, London: Free Association Books.

Hayles, K.N. (1992) "The Materiality of Informatics," *Configurations*, 1(2): 147–70.

Ippel, P. C. (1996) *Gegeven: de genen. Morele en jurisische aspecten van het gebruik van genetische gegevens*, Den Haag: Registratiekamer.

Kaye, D. H. and Imwinkelried, E. J. (2000) *Forensic DNA Typing: Selected Legal Issues.* Report to the Working Group on Legal Issues, Washington DC: National Commission on the Future of DNA Evidence.

Kralingen, R. van, Prins, C., and Grijpink, J. (1997) *Het lichaam als sleutel: Juridische beschouwingen over biometrie*, Samsom Bedrijfsinformatie, Alphen aan den Rijn/Diegem, 3–66.

Lacqueur, T. (1990) *Making Sex: Body and Gender from the Greeks to Freud*, Cambridge, MA: Harvard University Press.

Locke, D. (1992) *Science as Writing*, London: Yale University Press.

Lyon, D. (2001) *Surveillance Society: Monitoring Everyday Life*, New York: Routledge.

Martin, E. (1992) "The End of the Body?" *American Ethnologist*, 19(1): 121–40.

Norris, C. and Armstrong, G. (1999) *The Maximum Surveillance Society: The Rise of CCTV*, Oxford: Berg.

Panel on Confidentiality and Data Access (1993) *Private Lives and Public Policies: Confidentiality and Accessibility of Government Statistics*. National Research Council, Social Science Research Council, Washington DC: National Academy Press.

Rorty, R. (1989) "The Contingency of Language," in *Contingency, Irony, and Solidarity*, Cambridge: Cambridge University Press.

Schiebinger, L. (1993) *Nature's Body: Gender in the Making of Modern Science*, Boston: Beacon Press.

Tak, P. J. P. (1990) *DNA en strafproces: Een rechtsvergelijkend onderzoek naar de grenzen van het onderzoek aan en in het lichaam*. Arnhem: Gouda Quint.

Ten Have, H. A. M. J. and van Welie, J. V. M. (eds) (1998) *Ownership of the Human Body: Philosophical Considerations on the Use of the Human Body and its Parts in Healthcare*, Dordrecht: Kluwer Academic Publishers.

Torpey, J. (1998) "Coming and Going: On the State of Monopolization of the Legitimate 'Means of Movement,'" *Sociological Theory*, 16(3): 239–59.

van der Ploeg, I. (1999a) "Written on the Body: Biometrics and Identity," *Computers and Society*, 29(1): 37–44.

—— (1999b) "Eurodac and the Illegal Body: The Politics of Biometric Identity," *Ethics and Information Technology*, 1(4): 295–302.

—— "Borderline Identities: The Enrollment of Bodies in the Technological Reconstruction of Borders," paper presented at the Annual Meeting of the Society for the Social Studies of Science (4S), Vienna, Austria, September 2000.

Part II
Verifying identities
Constituting life-chances

4　Electronic identity cards and social classification

Felix Stalder and David Lyon

Establishing the stable identities of its subjects has been one of the central concerns of the modern nation state (Higgs 2001; Torpey 2000). It is a key means of connecting citizen and state. Social services, law enforcement, and national security are all based on the state's ability to connect embodied people to established records reliably. The goal is to classify each individual in context flexibly yet accurately – for example, as legitimate recipient of child support, repeat offender, or illegal immigrant – in order to determine which administrative procedure to apply.

Each of these domains has powerful institutional interests in expanding the accuracy with which individuals are identified. From the Victorian era, when voting lists and demographic data were sought (Abercrombie *et al.* 1986) to the economic restructuring of the 1980s and 1990s when fiscal management and fraud became prominent concerns, the modern nation state has tried to refine its identification of citizens. Which set of incentives figures most prominently in the public discussion depends on the political climate of the moment, but together they have been the engine of the increase in frequency and accuracy of anchoring individuals within the state's administrative matrix.

In the wake of spectacular "terrorist" attacks in different parts of the world, concerns over national security have often taken center stage. With them, the idea of establishing national ID cards for all citizens – or for a subset, such as immigrants and refugees (see, for example, Zureik 2001) – have resurfaced. This happened, for example, in the UK in the mid-1990s in reaction to bombings of the IRA, in Spain in the late 1990s following a string of assassinations by the Basque separatist group ETA, and in North America in response to the attacks on the World Trade Center and the Pentagon in 2001.

The more recently proposed ID cards stand in marked contrast to those that have traditionally been used in many countries. They are no longer simple paper-based documents but sophisticated high-tech devices using a mix of traditional and advanced identification features (biometrics) and, by virtue of being machine-readable, they can connect more easily with remote databases and authentication mechanisms. Some proposed "smart" cards are not only machine-readable but themselves contain programmable chips that store data.

Whenever ID cards are proposed, privacy concerns are raised, usually under the metaphor of the state becoming an all-seeing "Big Brother." These concerns are often countered with the argument of the existence of a trade-off between civil liberties and national security, and that the loss of civil liberties through ID cards is minor and the gain in national security is major, hence the trade-off, though perhaps regrettable, is, overall, positive. But is this really the case? Is there a trade-off and, if so, to which side is the balance tipped?

In this chapter, we critically examine this recurring interest in ID cards as a means to improve domestic security. First, we review the checkered history of the implementation of and resistance to high-tech ID cards since the early 1990s. Then we examine the collusion of forces that, whenever the public seems willing to accept them, lead to a renewal of interest in these systems despite their questionable usefulness. Thirdly, we analyze structural flaws in ID card systems that limit their usefulness to national security. Finally, given the limited role these cards can play in securing our countries, we look at the unintended consequences in order to understand the true nature of the trade-off that high-tech ID cards present us with. These consequences, whether intended or not, include social sorting of a sophisticated kind.

The development of identity cards

The technological history of identity cards moves from print on paper to PINs and programmable chips on plastic. But the more meaningful story is the socio-technical development of identity cards as symbols of belonging, of citizenship. While the passport makes one eligible to travel across national borders, the ID card indicates that the holder has a legitimate place within those borders. The national ID card is predominantly a product of the twentieth century, although it was known in some forms before then. It is an aspect of the consolidation of modern nation states; a visible sign of a bureaucratic system of administration that keeps tabs on all who are included as members of a bounded territory or jurisdiction.

During the twentieth century ID cards became part of the taken-for-granted apparatus of everyday life in many European countries, a situation that was accentuated by the involvement of those societies in two major world wars. The twentieth century was also a period of major migration to North America, and many who came from Europe were fleeing regimes in which the ID card had been a sinister sign of state control, which helps to explain why there often seems to be greater caution about ID cards in the USA and Canada than in Europe.

In the United Kingdom, for example, identification cards were issued during the Second World War, as means of distinguishing between national citizens and potential enemy aliens. But the system was slowly dismantled after the war – something that never occurred in France – and fairly strong feelings were expressed about not wishing to return to an ID card system. Indeed, not until Britain eventually succumbed to pressure to become a member of the European Community did the issue of ID cards return to the political agenda (Lyon 1991). By then, of course, much government administration was being computerized, such that the surveillance power of any ID card system was bound to be far in excess of those simple print-on-paper cards of wartime memory.

Towards the end of the twentieth century, contemporary forms of globalization began in earnest, and increasing mobility started seriously to challenge the capacity of countries to keep track of their citizens. The desire to be accepted as a citizen, with access to its rights and privileges, was unabated, but the question of who exactly is a citizen of which country began to be moot. The authors of this chapter are cases in point. Stalder is a Swiss-German permanent resident in Canada, while Lyon is a Canadian citizen carrying both a British and a Canadian passport. As John Urry says: "Just at the moment that everyone is seeking to be a citizen of a society, so global networks and flows appear to undermine what it is to be a national citizen" (Urry 2000: 162).

Early in the twenty-first century, the ID card situation was challenged again. Not this time by the collapse of political borders (1989) or economic borders (free trade movements), but by the collapse of the twin towers of the World Trade Center in New York as a result of "terrorist" attacks. The internal response of many countries around the world was to try to tighten security. One key measure proposed by many was to introduce ID card systems that included holograms or biometrics to ensure reliability, or "smart card" programability to increase their range of uses. Some proposals were for national ID cards that would indicate citizen-membership of nation states, while others were cards to be used in especially marginal cases, where belonging is particularly precarious, such as immigrants (Canada) or asylum seekers (UK).

Writing at a time when these debates are ongoing, it is impossible to predict precise outcomes. In two key cases, the UK and the USA, initial proposals for new ID cards have both lapsed and, subsequently, been revived in another form. In situations of high pressure from potential technology providers, public willingness to "pay the price in liberty for security" as shown by opinion polls, and at least some measure of political will to seek blanket "solutions" to the now palpable "politics of terrorism" the chances of some new ID card measures being introduced are, we think, fairly strong. One further factor to note is that some countries (such as Hong Kong) are going ahead with smart ID card schemes and no doubt such experiments will be closely watched by those in other larger jurisdictions. Whatever the outcome, some kinds of struggle over proposed ID cards are likely to ensue. Recent history confirms this likelihood.

Struggles over ID cards: politics, technologies, and events

The recent story of ID cards is one of sporadic struggles centering on universal personal identifiers. Such electronic IDs have been a predictable goal of government administrative and policing systems ever since the whole-sale computerization of bureaucratic departments in the latter part of the twentieth century, in all the technologically advanced societies (Lyon 1994: 104ff). The controversial idea is to use a single number – hence universal personal identifier – that readily identifies an individual over a range of databases. While the efficiency of such a system for ease of administrative functions is obvious, so are the potential threats to civil liberties and human rights.

In 1987 Germany introduced a machine-readable ID card for all citizens, in the face of considerable political opposition. The Greens and Social Democrats opposed it, and even the chair of the police union thought it smacked embarrassingly of "secret police." In the same period, however, a national identity card system was defeated in Australia, and this victory was for some years seen as a significant blow to such schemes. It is possible that opposition – centered on threats to civil liberties and the alleged technical deficiencies of the plan – was more coherently mobilized in Australia than in Germany. But in the end the proposal was defeated less through compelling argument than through the discovery of a legal loophole that halted parlia-mentary debate (Clarke 1992). On the other hand, population groups were mobilized, and at one point 30,000 people demonstrated at the parliament building against the proposed cards.

The early 1990s saw several more ID card schemes emerge, some of which succeeded, others of which failed, but not according to any clear pattern. North Americans tend, it seems, to be more wary of such schemes than Europeans, although the British have held out against machine-readable or other technically enhanced ID cards even though (or perhaps because) to have them would bring them more in line with most other countries in the European Union. Machine-readable ID cards have been suggested in the USA and Canada, usually as extensions of the social security number or the social insurance number, respectively. But successive administrations in both countries have reaffirmed their resistance to national identifiers.

By the turn of the twenty-first century, however, several countries in South East Asia – including Hong Kong, Malaysia, Singapore, and Thailand – are establishing relatively high-tech ID card systems. Singapore has had a card for permanent residents for some years, while in Thailand, Sun Microsystems won a contract for a national registration system in 1997, which is yet to be fully implemented. This includes a smart card that stores basic individual information, and on which drivers' licenses, passports, credit cards, and ATM cards will be added in future. The Hong Kong immigration department recently closed tenders for a smart card which will replace the current fingerprint card with digital imprints of both thumbs, and will have the capacity for other uses, like the Thai card. The $394-million contract was won by a seven-company consortium led by PCCW (Pacific Century CyberWorks) and the roll-out is scheduled for early 2003 (Mailloux 2001). The measure has not been introduced without controversy, and several originally planned features of the card had to be scrapped to make it more acceptable to the public (Landler 2002).

Not to be outdone, Malaysia began to introduce its smart-card identifier during 2001, as a "flagship application" within the much hyped Multimedia SuperCorridor (MSC) project. This is another multi-purpose card with national identity card, driver's license, passport information and e-cash applications, and with health card and public key infrastructure to be added later. Like several other countries in the region, the Malaysian government represents strong authority and its opposition parties have not majored on limiting the ID card. On the other hand, it is not clear how long it will take for the system to be fully implemented. The original targets for more than two million users by the end of 2001 were unrealized, and the only citizens holding the first cards were in the affluent MSC region, Kuala Lumpur, and the Klang Valley (Keong 2001).

But not all East and South East Asian countries have adopted electronic national ID card systems. While Taiwan has an ID card, the smart-card version proposed by the government had to be abandoned in late 1998 amid public protest (Chuang 1999). The Korean smart-card-based ID project suffered a similar fate. In 1997 the Korean electronic national identification card, containing an embedded chip, became a political item. The government legislated its establishment despite strong objections from opposition parties and the public. However, the election of the new president Kim Dae Jung in 1998, who knew the excesses of state repression from years in prison, meant that the scheme was abandoned.

After the "terrorist" attacks of September 2001, ID cards were seized upon in many countries as one plank in a potential protection plan. Following initial excitement, a more skeptical attitude towards general ID cards gained ground for a while. However, as part of stepped-up immigration policies, new cards are being introduced in the UK and Canada for marginal cases, with the USA seriously considering them. Canada opted for an upgraded Immigration Card to replace a notoriously unreliable paper document, and the UK brought in a new smart card – Applicant Registration Card (with photo, fingerprint, and cash card features) – for asylum seekers (Travis 2001). Within a few months other, more far-reaching proposals were again being mooted.

In the USA for many years drivers' licenses have played the part of a *de facto* ID, so not surprisingly it is this system that is most likely to be upgraded. The idea is to create a national identification system linking all state driver databases and use smart cards, or at least cards with a biometric identifier. The American Association of Motor Vehicle Administrators is working with the (new) Office of Homeland Security, the Justice Department, and other federal authorities to plan for the new ID card. Although each state would still issue its own licenses, they would all contain standardized data and security features. Non-driver ID cards would complement the drivers' licenses for those who do not drive (O'Harrow 2001). Meanwhile, the current (early 2002) proposal in the UK is to create new "entitlement cards" which would also be smart cards with biometric identifiers. The entitlement cards are based on the model of the already introduced Applicant Registration Cards (Staff and agencies 2002). The plan is for a card that it is compulsory to own, but that a citizen is not required to carry. In both the American and the British cases, strong opposition is emerging to these new proposals, but whether it can be sustained against the new, post-11 September crisis-generated search for security remains to be seen. As Jon Agar points out, crises and cards tend to go together (Agar 2001).

In other European countries, too, terrorism revived or brought forward plans for ID cards. The existing German cards are to be upgraded with holo- grams and biometric identifiers, and in Spain, the new national ID will be a smart card, introduced by the end of 2003. It is unclear exactly why these countries favor the high-tech cards, but the presence of Al Qaeda members in Berlin and Madrid, and previous involvement with "terrorist" groups (such as the left-wing Red Army Faction [RAF] in Germany and Basque separatists in Spain) could also play a role. In the case of Spain, however, the cards were planned before 11 September 2001, and it seems that they have as much to do with the determination of that country to demonstrate its technological prowess in Europe as it has to do with the threat of terrorism.

ID cards: structural inefficiencies

According to many authorities, however, this renewed interest in ID cards as a means of national security stands in a marked contrast to the actual potential of such a card to contribute significantly to this goal. Although objections always tend to be met with technical rejoinders – that tamper-proof, reliability-enhanced cards are available – this does not answer all the questions that are raised about ID cards. This may be addressed programmatically.

The first step in developing any security measure is to compile a detailed threat profile establishing the exact characteristics of the danger (Schneier 2000). This all-important first step, though, is missing in much of the discussion over ID systems. "Terrorism" – a powerful incentive to increase security – is not sufficiently precise as a basis for a successful defense strategy. However, it is indispensable to precisely map out the threat to see whether the proposed security measure can achieve its own goal, and to assess if this achievement contributes to enhancing overall security. For example, if the goal is to secure a building, installing a new lock on the front door indeed fortifies this door. However, it does little to enhance the overall security if the key is left under the doormat, or if the windows in the back of the building are left unchanged. Nor does it protect against intrusion via the Internet.

(Un)reliable identification

The objective of any ID card system is the reliable identification of each member of the population to which it issued, for example citizens of a country, immigrants, refugees, or welfare recipients. ID cards should make it impossible to obtain and use false identification. It is undisputed that more sophisticated ID cards would be harder to forge than most of the existing ID documents, such as drivers' licenses or paper-based ID cards.

However, tampering even with advanced smart cards is not impossible, and most of the widely deployed smart-card systems have proven to be vulnerable (Anderson and Kuhn 1996; Schneier 1999). Unless a card contains a biometric identifier, such as a digital fingerprint, which is checked in real time against a trusted database, the security of the card is limited against sophisticated and determined attacks. Ross Anderson, a computer scientist at Cambridge University, points out: "You can maybe exert some downward pressure on identity theft by incorporating machine readable fingerprints of some kind or another, but, in this situation, making identity cards harder to forge is solving the wrong problem" (quoted in Knight 2001).

It can be argued that the reason why high-tech ID cards address the wrong problem in the context of terrorism is that they are not only vulnerable against determined high-tech attacks, but, more importantly, also against very conventional low-tech trickery. No matter how sophisticated an ID card is, it is only as reliable as the document on which it is based. Administrative identity is established as a series of references, from one document to the other, all the way down to, ideally, the birth certificate. The reliability of the last document, a new ID card, is defined by the weakest link in this chain of references. If the applicant can present a convincingly counterfeited birth certificate, then a new ID card will show whatever information happens to be on this certificate. The possibility of bribing officials to issue a genuine document containing incorrect information further reduces the overall accuracy of the system. If a new ID card contains biometrics that are checked against a central database, then, at least, the new system can ensure that an individual cannot obtain more than one card. It can still not ensure that the information in this one card is accurate. In other words, compared to existing systems such as state-issued drivers' licenses, new ID cards would improve the accuracy of identification. However, given the vulnerability of the chain of references, they do this much less dramatically than their high-tech dazzle might suggest.

New technologies, new risks

It has been pointed out that inserting high-tech features into cards introduces a set of completely new risks. First, it is unclear whether, given today's technology, it is feasible to build a biometric system that is reliable enough to be implemented on a very large scale. Suppose the system is 99.99 percent accurate. This means that if someone is a terrorist suspect, there is a 99.99 percent chance that the software indicates "terrorist: positive." If someone is not a terrorist, there is a 99.99 percent chance that the software indicates "terrorist: negative." Assuming that one in ten million people who pass through the checkpoint, on average, is a terrorist suspect, the system will generate 1,000 false alarms for every one real terrorist. Every false alarm requires all security personnel to go through all their security routines, quite likely disrupting the flow of people through the checkpoint. Because the population of non-terrorists is so much larger than the number of terrorists, the test is impractical and likely to be disabled in practice (Schneier 2001).

Furthermore, if an ID proposal is linked to a central database containing the master files of the biometric identifiers, the security of this database becomes of paramount concern. What if someone breaks into the database and alters the master file? Given the sensitivity of the stored data, and the fact that this database must have thousands of access points, some perhaps even mobile (in police cars, for example), the additional security risk might be bigger than the previous security gains.

For the sake of argument, one may make the assumption that all of these problems could somehow be solved. Ideally, the system would be 100 percent accurate and invulnerable to tampering or attacks. Even in such a technological utopia, the system would not have caught most of the "terrorists" involved in the attacks of 11 September 2001, for simple reasons. Most of the "terrorists" had valid visas and no criminal record of any sort. All three checks that ID cards can perform – verifying the legitimacy of the document, verifying the link between the person, and conducting a quick background check against a list of suspects – would have turned up negative because the documents were legitimate and most of the individuals were not on suspect lists. Terrorists, particularly the ones willing to kill themselves in the attack, belong to a special class of criminal. They rarely have prior convictions, thus background checks are rarely revealing. There are no repeat suicide bombers.

These structural deficiencies, which exist even if the technology works as intended without flaws, introduce real limitations to the efficiency of ID card systems in the fight against terrorism. These limitations, more than just reducing the usefulness, could turn the ID card itself into a security risk. First, ID card systems, particularly if they involve smart-card features, are extremely expensive, involving several hundred million dollars for smaller countries, and billions for large countries.[1] In a world of limited budgets, committing so many resources to a single questionable project is bound to lead to underfunding in areas in which the money would be spent more efficiently.

There is, however, a second and more significant reason why new IDs could have the inverse of the intended effect. Not everybody will have an ID card. Even if the ID card is issued to every citizen, there is always a population of non-citizens, for example tourists or business travelers, who have legitimate reasons to pass a security checkpoint, say, at an airport, without a card. The security personnel will concentrate on people without an ID card assuming that those with cards will effectively be checked by the system. The human attention will be concentrated on a particular group of people for the sole reason that they do not hold the appropriate documentation. Consequently, less attention will be devoted to people with ID cards. ID cards, then, would ensure the speedy passage of criminals and terrorists who are not on a suspect list. However, to prevent the threat of hi-jacking, it is less important to know who the passengers are than what they carry onto the plane. Consequently, all passengers must be searched, no matter who they are – or who they were when the card was issued.

Who promotes ID cards?

These shortcomings are rather obvious for most people involved in these issues. Nevertheless, ID cards are resurfacing again and again. Why? At least part of the answer lies in the fact that there are powerful actors who would profit from the introduction of ID cards, independent of their actual usefulness in any specific context. This ID card constituency consists of three groups: politicians, high-tech industry and law enforcement.

For politicians, ID cards are an ambiguous issue. On the one hand, there is generally strong popular resistance such cards. However, they can be an attractive measure because they are highly visible. They symbolize, for everyone to see, a new resolve to get tough – on "terrorists," illegal immigrants, welfare offenders, or whoever is the villain of the moment. They are a simple, ready-made solution with which politicians can appear to be addressing the issue. The visibility of the card is an important aspect of their attractiveness to politicians who do not only want to do something, but, perhaps primarily, want also to be seen as doing something. Other measures which might be more effective but less visible are therefore less attractive for politicians seeking to project themselves into the spotlight. In the fight for attention and the public's favor, the actual usefulness to achieve the intended goals is not necessarily of primary concern.

For the high-tech industry, new ID cards, particular those involving smart cards and central databases, represent very significant procurement opportunities. From the industry's point of view, the high cost of any such system is one of its most attractive features. For at least a decade, the smart-card industry has been trying to find a large project upon which to roll out the extensive infrastructure necessary to introduce smart cards to society at large. In the mid-1990s, electronic cash seemed the vehicle to propel smart-card technology beyond niches that it currently occupies, and the attention shifted from the public to the private sector (Stalder forthcoming). However, at the turn of the decade, virtually electronic cash systems have failed, and the industry is again looking at the public sector to initiate the "breakthrough" project.[2]

From the perspective of law enforcement, ID cards are highly attractive. Although they are less potent in the fight against terrorism, or illegal immigration, those issues can be useful in temporarily suspending the public's dislike for ID cards. The single most attractive feature of new American ID cards – from this perspective – is that they would provide a stable and universal identifier (UID) for people that would be much harder to forge than the currently used social security numbers (SSN), and that are not bound by the same legal restrictions that limit what SSN can be used for (Hibbert 1996). An UID could, and most likely would, be used to link databases that have previously been separated. As a result, they would effectively create an *ad hoc* "virtually centralized" database from distributed but integrated databases. UIDs have long been criticized as leading towards comprehensive behavioral profiles of individuals based on controversial data-matching techniques (Shattuck 1996).

It is precisely in an ID card's function as an UID, and its ability to contribute to the compilation of comprehensive profiles of individuals – including movement across security checkpoints and interactions with government, and quite possibly also private institutions – that many think its most dangerous (un)intended consequence lies. And this is a danger not for "terrorists," but for everyone who holds such a card.

Suspicion, innocence, and the surveillant assemblage

Computer-based national identity cards have a longer history as an idea than as reality. But the chance of their becoming realities increases each time pressure from high-tech companies meets panic among politicians and a fearful public. How acceptable they are in a given context depends on a number of socio-technical, political, and cultural factors. But it is likely that once they have been tested "successfully" in one context, this will increase their acceptability elsewhere. Given their structural weakness as tools in the fight against terrorism, it is important to look at the (un)intended consequences in other areas that are likely to be triggered by their introduction.

First, the question of suspicion. If a national ID card is established anywhere, it cannot be a "voluntary" scheme, even though that was suggested in the USA following 11 September 2001 (Ellison 2001). It would have to be universal, to avoid the palpable negative discrimination that would follow for those who do not possess a card. Both supporters and critics of national ID cards make observations about this. Peter Neumann and Lauren Weinstein (2001) point out, "The road to an Orwellian police state of universal tracking, but actually *reduced* security, could well be paved with hundreds of millions of such ID cards." But as communitarian Amitai Etzioni reminds us, certain kinds of discrimination could be removed by having national ID cards. For example, by being obliged to verify that intended employees are legal residents in the USA, employers are currently forced to check on applicants that look foreign. In the USA 61 percent of legal immigrants favor ID cards to prevent their being confused with illegal ones (Etzioni 1999: 132, 2002). However, it must be said that once an ID card scheme is in place, some further negative and prejudicial discrimination is conceivable, if not likely. Why is this?

The evidence that ID cards are likely to increase such forms of discrimination is historical (including contemporary history), circumstantial, and socio-technical. The historical evidence, from situations such as Nazi Germany, South Africa under apartheid, and the contemporary, from the state of Israel or from a country such as Singapore, is that the use of such cards has been – and is – used to single out population groups for special treatment. Jews, blacks, and Palestinians are among the groups who suffer in these situations. In the case of Singapore, pink-colored ID cards are carried by citizens only, blue ones by permanent residents. The official description explains that this system exists to "weed out illegal immigrants and other undesirables" (Singapore Immigration and Registration 2001).

But such evidence is insufficient on its own, because many countries with human rights records superior to those just mentioned use national identity card systems. The likelihood of ID cards being used in prejudicial ways is increased if the circumstances in which they are used may be considered a climate of mistrust and negative discrimination. The Third Reich, and South Africa under white (supremacist) rule are obvious cases. In Europe, the French police have often been accused of harassing North Africans (especially Algerians) using ID cards, and non-Greek Orthodox citizens have suffered similarly at the hands of Greek authorities (Davies 1996).

In North America, too, identity classification systems were used with devastating effect during the Second World War. Although no identity card system was in use, after the attack on Pearl Harbor the US military illegally used confidential census data to round up Japanese-Americans and to "evacuate and relocate" them in desert internment camps. Along with their Canadian counterparts, who were subjected to similar treatment, they lost property, livelihoods, and civil rights (Diffie and Landau 1998: 137–8). More recently, during the Gulf War, when "Arabs" and "Muslims" were constructed as a national security threat in the USA and Canada, widespread harassment took place. In typical cases, CSIS agents unexpectedly visited an Iraqi-born physicist in Vancouver for an interview that violated the Charter of Rights and Freedoms, and a Palestinian auto dealer in Cambridge, Ontario had his bank records checked under suspicion of terrorism (Kashmeri 2000). Even more recently, after the Oklahoma City bombing in 1995 the US Congress passed an anti-terrorism bill that allowed the government to use secret evidence to detain and deport immigrants suspected of "terrorism." The law has been used particularly against Arab and Muslim immigrants.

Following 11 September 2001, a backlash effect occurred in North America and Europe that immediately affected negatively people of "Arab" and "Muslim" background. In Canada, some strong objections to anti-terrorism legislation came from those most closely aware of these issues (such as Liberal Member of Parliament John McKay, whose Scarborough East constituency includes people with "Arab" and "Muslim" backgrounds). In Britain, similar concerns were raised about the proposed national ID card system in October 2001 – even in statements that were otherwise supportive of that scheme (Preston 2001). In the same period, 1,200 people with "Arab" and "Muslim" origins were detained without warrant or trial in the USA as "immigrant suspects," which also led to concerns among American civil libertarians. As it turned out, only a small number had any links whatsoever to terrorism, although some petty cases of credit card fraud or speeding were picked up in the trawl (Firestone and Drew 2001).

This kind of evidence should be sufficient to indicate that negative discrimination is likely to occur in situations where public fear is high (and stoked by media polarization of debate), where high-tech companies are keen to market their solutions (surveillance technology firms saw their share prices multiply after 11 September 2001, at just the time when others, such as airlines, were dropping), and where politicians are in the unprecedented *terra incognita* of large-scale "terrorist" threat. Unless reliable braking systems are developed for the "slippery slope," it is hard to see how the presumption of innocence could be maintained under these circumstances. For, however well-intentioned the installation of advanced ID cards, the resulting classifications of ethnic groups will produce categories of suspicion that will capture innocent persons in their net. It is not only those who have done wrong who have something to fear.

There is another reason why the adoption of national ID card systems would be likely to produce negative discrimination effects. As we have seen, no national ID card proposed in the twenty-first century will be lacking in high-tech enhancements, whether using biometrics, or holograms, or smart cards, or some combination of these. This means that one of the key components of any contemporary surveillance technology – the searchable database – will be central to the system. The increasing focus on searchable databases as the linchpins of such technologies is associated with another important shift in emphasis, towards pre-emptive surveillance. Gary Marx (1988) was among the first to note this, but in the last decade the trend has become unmistakable (see, for example, Ericson and Haggerty 1997, and Norris in this volume).

This kind of anticipatory surveillance may be most clearly seen in what is known as the shift to the "New Penology." While the Old Penology tried to identify criminals to ascribe guilt and blame and to impose punishment and treatment, the New Penology seeks "techniques for identifying, classifying, and managing groups sorted by levels of dangerousness" (Feeley and Simon 1994: 180). Individualized suspicion with reasonable cause gives way to categorical suspicion where, for example, police may stop and search vehicles in a given locality, prisoners or even intending employees may be tested to discover drug use (see Nelkin and Andrews in this volume) or, in the context of the aftermath of "terrorism," persons with "Arab" or "Muslim" appearance or names may be detained for questioning. In the case of police stop-and-search procedures, those in the USA who have suffered what they believe to be harassment now speak of the misdemeanour of "driving while black."

As a prime rationale for introducing ID cards is the heightened state of alert – or panic regime – following "terrorist" attacks, the stated intention is prevention of repeat occurrences. While, as we have shown, new technologies such as smart cards may not be effective in ensuring such "prevention," the goal of prevention is nevertheless likely to ensure that some other processes will be set in motion. It is precisely the use of searchable databases, where records can be cross-tabulated with ease to produce categories of suspicion, that fosters the idea that prevention is possible. The need to anticipate "terrorist" actions by previously unsuspicious individuals requires the creation of profiles out of which suspicion can be extracted. The tracking of movement that high-tech ID cards facilitate is a key component in the compilation of such profiles. The techno-utopian goal is to recognize and apprehend criminals before they have a chance to commit their crimes.[3]

But even without national ID systems in place, enhanced categorical suspicion already features as a major part of a post-"terrorism" regime. It is hard to imagine that the risks of such categorical suspicion – for visible minority groups – would diminish if further means of discrimination were available.

A national ID card system in principle offers a government a single means of entry into the myriad databases that currently incorporate personal records of many different kinds. Analogously (in some ways) to the so-called Clipper Chip, which would have given the US government sole and ultimate access to encrypted on-line messages, national electronic ID cards enhance the power of the nation state. Such systems facilitate searches throughout those flexibly integrated discrete databases that currently – in the USA, Canada, and the UK – have no such single key. Of course, it is correct to argue that in today's increasingly networked information infrastructures no single, integrated, national ID card is needed for such comprehensive searches to be made possible. The unique identifier would just make such searches easier.

In recent years, following the work of Gilles Deleuze (Deleuze 1992; Deleuze and Guatarri 1987), the notion of a "surveillant assemblage" (Haggerty and Ericson 2000) has become popular. This refers to the loosely integrated network of databases that develops, not top-down in panoptic or tree-like fashion, but more like a creeping plant, a rhizome. The difficulty with this model is that it is sometimes presented as if the older, centralized, "Big Brother" surveillance is entirely a thing of the past, supplanted by the "assemblage." But it is clear from the reactions to the "terrorist" attacks of September 2001 that the older model can kick in at any time, and even utilize the remote – for example, consumer or employment – shoots of the rhizome for its own peculiar ends (Lyon 2001). In this case too, without strict limits, the existence of an electronic national ID makes access to multiple records more straightforward. In the end, ID cards can lead to the flexible integration of distributed databases, effectively creating a virtual central register, more detailed than any national government could ever dream of compiling on its own.

Notes

1 Costs of complex high-tech projects are notoriously difficult to predict and depend on the specifics of the project. However, typical high-end smart cards cost around $5. It is typically estimated that the card itself contributes about 10 percent of the overall infrastructure costs, which includes card readers and writers, communication links, databases, etc. These costs do not include the personnel required to run such a system and the training involved to ensure that the system is used properly by those, and only those, who need to have access to it.

2 Among the most vocal promoters of a national ID card in the wake of the 11 September 2001 "terrorist" attacks were industry leaders, including Larry Ellison, CEO of Oracle, who proposed a system based on a large database provided by his company (Ellison 2001). Sun's CEO Scott McNealy proposed a system based on the distributed intelligence of smart devices using Sun's Java to execute authentication algorithms (Coffee 2001). While both offered to provide the technology for free, the ensuing maintenance and upgrading contracts would have turned their "gifts" into very lucrative businesses.

3 The UK has proceeded even further along this logic and announced the establishment of a register of children who exhibit criminal potential so that it can be corrected before it is realized (Scheeres 2001).

Bibliography

Abercrombie, N., Hill, S., and Turner, B. (1986) *Sovereign Individuals of Capitalism*, London: Allen & Unwin.

Agar, J. (2001) "Modern Horrors: British Identity and Identity Cards," in J. Caplan and J. Torpey (eds) *Documenting Individual Identity: State Practices in the Modern World*, Princeton, NJ: Princeton University Press.

Anderson, R. and Kuhn, M. (1996) "Tamper Resistance – A Cautionary Note," *The Second USENIX Workshop on Electronic Commerce Proceedings*, Oakland, CA, November.

Chuang, T. -R. (1999) "To Trade or Not to Trade?: Thoughts on the Failed Smart Card Based National ID Initiative in Taiwan," paper presented at AICE International Conference on Computer Ethics, Melbourne, Australia, July 1999 Online. Available HTTP: <http://www.aice.swin.edu.au/events/AICEC99/papers1/CHU99007.pdf> (accessed 3 March 2002).

Clarke, R. (1992) "The Resistible Rise of the National Personal Data System," *Software Law Journal*, 5: 29–52.

Coffee, P. (2001) "National ID Cards Are Not the Answer," *eWeek*. Online. Available HTTP: <http://www.zdnet.com/filters/printerfriendly/0,6061,281 9922–2,00.html> (accessed 24 October 2001).

Davies, S. (1996) "Identity Cards. Frequently Asked Questions," London: Privacy International. Online. Available HTTP: <http://www.privacyinternational.org/issues/idcard/idcard_faq.html> (accessed August 24 1996).

Deleuze, G. (1992) "The Society of Control," *October*, 59: 3–7.

Deleuze, G. and Guatarri, F. (1987) *A Thousand Plateaus*, Minneapolis: University of Minnesota Press.

Diffie, W. and Landau, S. (1998) *Privacy on the Line: The Politics of Wiretapping and Encryption*, Cambridge, MA: MIT Press.

Ericson, R. V. and Haggerty, K. (1997) *Policing the Risk Society*, Toronto: University of Toronto Press.

Ellison, L. (2001) "Smart Cards: Digital IDs Can Help Prevent Terrorism," *Wall Street Journal*. Online. Available HTTP: <http://www.opinionjournal.com/ extra/ ?id=95001336> (accessed 8 October 2001).

Etzioni, A. (2002) "You'll Love Those National ID Cards," *Christian Science Monitor*. Online. Available HTTP: <http://www.csmonitor.com/2002/0114/ p11s1-coop. html> (accessed 14 January 2002).

Etzioni, A. (1999) *The Limits of Privacy*, New York: Basic Books.

Feeley, M. and Simon, J. (1994) "Actuarial Justice: The Emerging New Criminal Law," in D. Nelkin (ed.) *The Futures of Criminology*, London: Sage.

Firestone D. and Drew C. (2001) "Al Qaeda Link Seen Only in a Handful of 1,200 Detainees," *New York Times*. Online. Available HTTP: <http://www.nytimes. com/2001/11/29/national/29DETA.html> (accessed 29 November 2001).

Haggerty, K. and Ericson, R. V. (2000) "The Surveillant Assemblage," *British Journal of Sociology*, 51(4): 506–22.

Hibbert, C. (1996) "What to Do When They Ask You for Your Social Security Number," in R. Kling (ed.) *Computerization and Controversy: Value Conflicts and Social Choices*, 2nd edn, San Diego: Academic Press.

Higgs, E. (2001) "The Rise of the Information State: The Development of Central State Surveillance of the Citizen in England, 1500–2000," *Journal of Historical Sociology*, 14(2): 175–97.

Kashmeri, Z. (2000) "When CSIS calls: Canadian Arabs, Racism, and the Gulf War," in G. Kinsman, D. K. Buse and M. Steedman (eds) *Whose National Security?: Canadian State Surveillance and the Creation of Enemies*, Toronto: Between the Lines.

Keong, L.M. (2001) "'Smart Card' for Malaysians," *Asiafeatures.com*. Online. Available HTTP: <http://www.asiafeatures.com/current_affairs/0104,1230, 03. html> (accessed 30 April 2001).

Knight, W. (2001) "Malaysia Pioneers Smart Cards with Fingerprint Data," *New Scientist*. Online. Available HTTP: <http://www.newscientist.com/ news/news. jsp?id=ns99991331> (accessed 21 September 2001).

Landler, M. (2002) "Fine-tuning for Privacy, Hong Kong Plans Digital ID," *Guardian*, 18 February 2002.

Lyon, D. (1991) "British ID Cards: The Unpalatable Logic of European Integration?" *The Political Quarterly*, 62(3): 377–85.

——— (1994) *The Electronic Eye: The Rise of Surveillance Society*, Cambridge: Polity Press; Malden, MA: Blackwell.

——— (2001) "Surveillance after September 11 2001," *Sociological Research Online*, 6(3). Online. Available HTTP: <http://www.socresonline/6/3/lyon. html> (accessed 28 February 2002).

Mailloux, J. (2001) "Are We Facing an Identity Card Crisis?" *Computerworld Hong Kong.* Online. Available HTTP: <http://www.idg.com.hk/cw/> (accessed 16 November 2001).

Marx, G. T. (1988) *Undercover: Police Surveillance in America,* Berkeley: University of California Press.

Neumann, P. and Weinstein, L. (2001) "Risks of National Identity Cards," *Communications of the Association of Computing Machinery,* 44(12). Online. Available HTTP: <http://www.csl.sri.com/users/neumann/insiderisks.html> (accessed 5 March 2002).

O'Harrow, R. (2001) "States Devising Plan for High Tech National Identification Cards, *Washington Post,* 3 November: A10.

Preston, P. (2001) "The Case for ID Cards is Now Overwhelming," *Guardian.* Online Available HTTP: <http://politics.guardian.co.uk/columnist/story/ 0,9321,561098, 00.html> (accessed 1 October 2001).

Scheeres, J. (2001) "Keeping a Who's-Naughty List," *Wired News.* Online. Available HTTP: <http://www.wired.com/news/business/0,1367,48637,00. html> (accessed 27 November 2001).

Schneier, B. (1999) "Threats against Smart Cards," *CRYPTO-GRAM, Email Newsletter.* E-mail (15 April 1999).

—— (2000) *Secrets and Lies: Digital Security in a Networked World,* New York: John Wiley & Sons.

—— (2001) "Special Issue," *CRYPTO-GRAM, Email Newsletter.* E-mail (30 September 2001).

Shattuck, J. (1996) "Computer Matching Is a Serious Threat to Individuals' Rights," in R. Kling (ed.) *Computerization and Controversy: Value Conflicts and Social Choices,* 2nd edn, San Diego: Academic Press.

Singapore Immigration and Registration (SIR) (2001) "Identity Cards: A Sense of Belonging," *SIR – SIR Inc.* Online. Available HTTP: <http://www.gov.sg/ mha/sir/sirinc/journey-travel-ic.html> (accessed 5 March 2002).

Stalder, F. (forthcoming) "Failure and Success: Notes on the Development of Electronic Cash," *The Information Society.*

Staff and Agencies (2002) "Government Moves Closer to Implementing ID Cards," *Guardian,* 5 February 2002.

Torpey, J. (2000) *The Invention of the Passport: Surveillance, Citizenship and the State,* Cambridge: Cambridge University Press.

Travis, A. (2001) "Asylum Seekers to be Given ID Cards," *Guardian,* 30 October 2001.

Urry, J. (2000) *Sociology Beyond Societies: Mobilities for the Twenty-first Century,* London and New York: Routledge.

Zureik, E. (2001) "Constructing Palestine through Surveillance Practices," *British Journal of Middle Eastern Studies,* 28(2): 205–27

5 Surveillance creep in the genetic age

Dorothy Nelkin and Lori Andrews

A wad of spit, a spot of blood, a semen stain, or a single hair is all that is necessary to create a DNA "fingerprint." DNA profiles can be extracted not only from blood or sperm at a crime scene, but also from objects touched by a person's hands, and from saliva used to lick stamps. From a tiny sample of body tissue, a forensic laboratory can use an autoradiogram to create an image consisting of a cluster of horizontal bands that form a pattern resembling a bar code.

DNA analysis had been developed in a medical context as a technique to identify the markers that indicate familial disorders. But in 1983, a British geneticist used the technique to identify a rapist. Subsequently, DNA testing spread out of the medical sphere into the sphere of public surveillance. As a non-intrusive and easy procedure, DNA fingerprinting has been used in many non-medical contexts. It appeals to military, law enforcement and other governmental authorities: those seeking evidence to establish the identity of a dead body, a missing person, a biological relative, or the perpetrator of a crime. In 1990, the US Congress authorized and funded a military program mandating the collection of blood and tissue for DNA testing of all military personnel. The FBI and the law enforcement agencies in every state require convicted felons to have a sample of their body tissue banked and tested for purposes of future identification. In some states, non-violent offenders and misdemeanants are included. Some countries require immigrants to provide a DNA sample as a condition of entry. DNA samples are collected and stored for the identification of missing children, or elderly Alzheimer victims, or babies switched at birth, or genetic fathers in child support and paternity disputes. Men have brought their children to genetics clinics and had them secretly tested to determine if they were the "real" fathers or if their wives had an affair.

There are, of course, many reasonable purposes for DNA identification. Why not facilitate crime control by having records of recidivists? Why not develop accurate means of identifying missing persons or the remains of soldiers killed in war? To the military and law enforcement officials who collect body fluids for DNA identification, body material is an efficient means to implement legitimate policy goals and to maintain social order. But the expanding use of DNA identification also reinforces a pervasive trend towards increased public surveillance.

Michel Foucault (1979) conceptualized surveillance as a means of "normalization" and focused attention on the production of knowledge in the service of power. Tests, he wrote, have become a means to "compare, differentiate, hierarchize, homogenize, exclude" (183–4). The early development of computer data systems attracted sociological attention to the possibilities and problems of growing surveillance. James Rule (1974) warned of institutional trends in which powerful bureaucracies would collect and store information on private persons to control their behavior, and he predicted a future of increasingly efficient mass surveillance and control. Responding to the expansion of national information systems in the 1980s, Kenneth Laudon (1986) warned about the implications of a "dossier society" for personal privacy and civil rights. Gary Marx (1988) focused on the use of these powerful data-collection and data-sharing tools in undercover police work, warning of "almost imperceptible surveillance creep" marked by subtle, invisible, involuntary forms of social control (Marx 1988: 2).

The development of DNA tests and banking systems has intensified such concerns about surveillance technologies. For DNA samples are more than just a source of identification. Revealing information about health and predisposition, they can expose a person to workplace or insurance discrimination, creating categories of those "at risk." And they can be used to reinforce race or ethnic stereotypes. How will organizations and political systems use DNA identification? Who will have access to the data? How can those in control of DNA data balance the identification benefits of this technology while protecting the social values of individual freedom and privacy? DNA data banking may be a useful tool for fighting crime and meeting military exigencies, but it is also subject to abuse for political or economic ends.

This chapter describes the expansion of mandatory genetic testing for DNA identification. We focus on the disputes that develop when those required to provide DNA samples raise concerns about loss of benefits, psychological harm, and discrimination based on the information revealed by their DNA. And we use these disputes to analyze the problems of "surveillance creep" as growing numbers of people have their DNA on file (McKewen and Reilly 1994).

The military DNA collection program

In January 1995, Corporal Joseph Vlacovsky and Lance Corporal John Mayfield III, two marines stationed at the Kaneohe base near Honolulu, were ordered to provide blood and cheek epithelial cell samples as part of the military's mandatory genetic-testing program. Their DNA samples would be stored at the Department of Defense DNA Repository in order to facilitate the efficient identification of the remains of soldiers killed in battle. They refused to comply and became "the first DNA conscientious objectors" (Mayfield v. Dalton 1995).

The Department of Defense (DOD) began collecting blood and tissue from every person in the military services in 1992. Included in this program are all active duty and reserve personnel as well as civilian employees and contractors, even though these persons are unlikely to become unknown soldiers. The tissue is collected, analyzed, and then stored in the DOD's DNA Repository in Gaithersburg, Maryland. Each individual is provided with two sealed plastic cards that have a fingerprint, signature, blood stain and oral swab, and a bar code; the cost of this kit, pencil included, is $3.00 (not including the cost of analyzing the DNA). DNA samples are vacuum-sealed and frozen to ensure their survival for forty years. When necessary, bits of bodies can be identified by matching their DNA to the samples kept on file. Over four million tissue samples from military personnel are in the Maryland repository. It is the largest DNA bank in the world.

Military authorities regard the identification of remains as a compelling interest for soldiers and their families. In every war, the military has established departments to identify the dead and developed techniques to assist in identification. Lt. Col. Victor Weedn, the initial program manager of the Armed Forces DNA Identification Laboratory, is a forensic pathologist – a lawyer, MD, and expert on DNA analysis. He has used DNA techniques to identify the skeletal remains of Czar Nicholas II, the victims recovered from TWA Flight 800, and the members of the Branch Davidian cult killed in the fire in Waco, Texas.

Weedn explains the importance of a mandated military testing program: "It's an issue to the soldiers, sailors and airmen. They want to know that – if they pay the ultimate sacrifice – they will be remembered" (Weedn 1996). He talks about the effectiveness of DNA identification and the time it would save in the slow and painful task of identifying human remains. He hopes to make the Tomb of the Unknown Soldier a thing of the past.

The problem of identifying remains was a major issue during the First World War, with its devastating death toll and enormous number of bodies that had been dismembered beyond identification (Bourke 1996). The dead body of the "unknown soldier" became a potent symbol of the horror of war. But Vlacovsky and Mayfield cared less about the identification of their dead bodies than their ability to control the integrity of their living bodies. Explaining his willingness to risk a court martial, Vlacovsky said: "This won't destroy the rest of my life. When this is over, I will still have control over my DNA" (quoted in Essoyan 1995: A1).

The marines argued in court that the taking of their tissue violated their Fourth Amendment right to privacy. They regarded the requirement as unreasonable search and seizure: "I expected to give up some privacy when I joined the military," said Vlacovsky. But he added, "It doesn't say we hereby waive our constitutional rights." "It is our God-given right to maintain possession of our genes" (Mayfield v. Dalton 1995). Having little trust in military authorities, they also suspected that the tissue samples would be misused or used without their knowledge or consent for purposes other than the identification of their remains. Samples could be used to assess soldiers' purported predisposition to homosexuality (Hamer and Copeland 1994), or to a genetic disease and then used against their personal interests. Or their DNA could be used for purposes they oppose, such as the development of biological weapons (Cole 1996). They feared the information collected from their DNA samples could be available to law enforcement authorities in criminal investigations.

The Council for Responsible Genetics and clinician Paul Billings submitted affidavits supporting the objecting marines. They documented cases where access to genetic information revealing predisposition to genetic disease had resulted in discrimination. "Thousands of tests could be done on these samples," Billings said, "The military may have kept the door open as a way to counteract rising benefits costs by excluding coverage for those with pre-existing conditions that can be discovered in DNA samples" (Billings 1995).

Weedn dismissed such concerns: "When you've licked a stamp on your tax return you've sent the government a DNA sample." (Indeed, the FBI had tested the saliva on postage stamps to link a suspect to the World Trade Center bombing and to identify the Unabomber.) Weedn insisted "each specimen is treated as a medical specimen with confidentiality and respect." Questioned about the initial DOD policy of keeping specimens after service members were discharged from the military – a policy later changed – he replied that it would be "extremely costly and time consuming to return or destroy the specimens" (Weedn 1996). Instead, Weedn called for greater trust; he said he would not abuse the information in the DNA files.

Weedn's plea for trust did not convince the marines. "With nuclear testing, they just handed people some dark glasses and said 'here, watch the bomb go off' . . . In the 1950s they gave LSD to army troops . . . In the 1970s they sprayed Agent Orange over their troops" (*Mayfield v. Dalton* 1995). Trust could hardly have been strengthened when Assistant US Attorney Theodore Meeker dismissed the importance of informed consent: "If the military's use of unproved drugs on its personnel does not require informed consent, collection and storage of blood samples and oral swabs for possible use in identifying human remains does not require consent" (quoted in Essoyan 1995: 5).

Though both Vlacovsky and Mayfield had exemplary service records, they were threatened with court-martial proceedings, incarceration, fines, and dishonorable discharge for refusing to obey orders. However, a military judge dropped the charges in light of the fact that there were no existing regulations dealing with the consequences of failing to comply with the program. Thus, both Marines received honorable discharges with veterans' benefits – and they kept their DNA.

By the time of the decision, however, they had become interested in the general issues raised by mandatory testing. So they filed a civil suit in the District Court in Hawaii against the DOD on behalf of all service personnel claiming that the military program ignored existing protocols for confidentiality and consent. The court dismissed their suit, contrasting the "hypothetical" arguments of the marines to the "compelling interest" of the military to account for its troops. The court held that taking a blood sample was not unreasonable seizure and thus did not violate the Fourth Amendment. Taking blood was legally considered a minimal intrusion. And, because there was no immediate plan to use the specimens for research, the Nuremberg Code's requirements for informed consent were not relevant. The DOD did amend the rules for its original banking program. They reiterated that the samples would only be used for the identification of human remains unless they are subpoenaed for a criminal investigation or "other uses compelled by other applicable law."

Other cases quickly followed. In April 1996, Sgt. Warren Sinclair, age thirty-three, a fourteen-year Air Force veteran and medical equipment repairman, refused to submit blood samples for genetic testing. Vlacovsky and Mayfield generally mistrusted military motives, but Sinclair, an African-American, had specific political concerns about the use of his body tissue. He was convinced that DNA samples would be used to support racist claims. "Would we ask Jews to give their genes to Germans? No. . . . Until the issue of racism is resolved, Afro-Americans should maintain possession of their genetic material" (Sinclair 1996). Sinclair recalled the use of genetic testing in the 1970s when blacks in the Navy were tested for sickle-cell carrier status. Though no scientific evidence suggest this would affect a person's health (only reproductive decisions), those found to be carriers were disqualified from certain jobs. Black servicemen interpreted the exclusion as one more way to restrict their opportunities.

The Air Force court ruled against Sinclair, arguing that the interest of the government in assuring the identification of remains outweighed the intrusiveness of taking blood. Sinclair was convicted by court martial on 10 May 1996 and sentenced to fourteen days of hard labor and a two-grade reduction in rank (US v. Sinclair 1996).

In April 1996, Donald P. Power, a 1st class petty officer and navy nuclear technician, refused to give a DNA specimen because it violated his religious principles as a member of a Native American lodge. Power said: "My body is a sacred recipe to me, and I didn't think I should share it. . . . They were not holding a part of me on a shelf . . You find personal power in knowing who you are" (Hinde 1997). For his refusal, Power lost a stripe, security classification, and 40 percent of his income. He applied for a waiver on grounds of religious freedom and it was accepted eighteen months later. But few members of the armed services will be able to make use of the narrow religious exception; moral objections are not enough to avoid military rules.

Those who refused to comply with mandatory genetic testing were challenging longstanding assumptions about the authority of the military over the bodies of its men. The military, after all, sends bodies into battle and soldiers cannot refuse assignments that threaten their bodily integrity. Refusal was in effect a declaration of rights based on a view that DNA holds special meaning for the individual; it was beyond the usual domain of military intrusion. As one of the marines put it: "It's your genetic blueprint, how you were created. . . . Your body is one of the few things that you have control over" (quoted Chadwin 1996: 23). Moreover, the marines mistrusted promises of confidentiality; they believed that their samples would become a resource not just for identification, but also for decisions about promotion, health insurance, and law enforcement.

DNA dragnets

Since the Second World War, law enforcement agencies have been expanding their information systems. But until the 1960s, record-keeping functioned on the basis of local tradition and management of criminal justice information was uneven. By the late 1960s, the increasing sophistication of computers converged with growing fear of crime to encourage experiments with identification and surveillance systems (Marx 1988). In 1968, President Johnson's Commission on Law Enforcement and the Administration of Justice declared that information and systems technology was the most important tool for controlling crime. The Commission also proposed the creation of a national computerized criminal history repository.

But the efforts to implement the system faced public opposition. Attitude surveys suggested that Americans had little confidence in institutional leaders, mistrusted centralized information systems, and feared the implications for liberty and privacy (McClosky and Brill 1986). The idea of a national identity center raised fears that government surveillance would extend well beyond the criminal justice system. Critics emerged to warn of the potential for abuse, the unwarranted tracking of "suspicious" persons, the selective surveillance of particular groups of people, the harassment of political activists, and the leakage of information to private organizations seeking information for employment or credit ratings.

Although proposals to collect and bank human tissue for DNA identification raise similar issues, there has been remarkably little protest against them. Indeed, they have been welcomed as an effective means to lower the cost of criminal investigations. People worry that computer banks store information on their economic status or credit rating, but few believe that the collection of DNA samples will affect their personal interests. And the aura of science underlying DNA technologies contributes to the legitimacy of testing and overrides privacy concerns.

However, those directly affected by mandatory genetic testing have responded by using the courts to challenge mandatory DNA collection. In 1991, six inmates from Virginia's Tazewell Correctional Unit Number 31 challenged the state's DNA testing program (*Jones v. Murray* 1992). Virginia, in 1989, had been the first state to require the collection of blood samples from convicted sex offenders and felons for use in a state DNA database. Law enforcement officials attempted to justify the program by citing a study indicating high recidivism rates.

The inmates claimed that the Virginia program was unconstitutional; in the absence of individualized suspicion, mandatory extraction of DNA samples violated their Fourth Amendment right against search and seizure. Also, they argued, imposing blood test requirements as a condition of release would impose additional punishment for their crimes and interfere with their right to due process by putting extra conditions on possibilities of parole.

Like soldiers, prisoners relinquish certain rights. But the prisoners defined their right to bodily integrity in a distinctive category; their body fluids, their genetic blueprint, should not be violated even in the context of the prison system. The Virginia Court disagreed. It conceded that the state could not meet the standards of probable cause or individual suspicion. But the court balanced the government interests in deterring and detecting crime against the privacy interests of inmates and found the law to be reasonable. Convicted felons, said the court, already lose the right to privacy from routine searches of the cavities of their bodies and their prison cells. Most searches, however, are conducted to determine whether the inmates present a current danger – by, for example, concealing weapons. In contrast, the collection of DNA is to protect against a remote future risk.

Dissenting Circuit Judge Murnaghan concurred with the decision as applied to violent felons, but lambasted the idea of collecting blood from prisoners who had been convicted of non-violent crimes and thus were unlikely to commit violent crimes in the future. He questioned whether the lack of reasonable expectation of privacy in a prison cell should extend to permit searches of the body fluids of every felon, violent and non-violent alike. Perhaps most important, Judge Murnaghan suggested: "The only state interest offered by the Commonwealth for including nonviolent felons is administrative ease." Reviving the 1980s concerns about the social implications of creating computerized criminal history systems, Murnaghan expressed "a deep, disturbing and overriding concern that . . . the Commonwealth may be successful in taking significant strides towards the establishment of a future police state, in which broad and vague concerns for administrative efficiency will serve to support substantial intrusions into the privacy of citizens" (Murnaghan 1992).

Other states also began to develop DNA identification programs, and in 1993, the FBI implemented CODIS, a national program to assist federal, state, and local law enforcement agencies support development of a population statistical database; improve DNA forensic analysis methods; and serve humanitarian purposes such as the identification of missing persons or the human remains from mass disasters. The FBI promoted CODIS on the grounds of "productivity and efficiency." Former Director of the FBI crime laboratory John Hicks had described the computer databank as "nothing more than an information management and screening tool" (Hoeffel 1990: 527). He expected that "It will save time and effort, and courts will have fewer cases to process because investigations can be better focused and coordinated" (FBI 1991). CODIS links the DNA profiles of convicts gathered by scattered state law enforcement DNA labs, encourages uniform standards, and pools DNA data to facilitate identification of criminals across borders. The 1994 Crime Control Act reinforced these efforts through a provision for coordinating nationwide DNA data bank systems. A report, commissioned by the Justice Department to implement the Act, announced an award of $8.75 million in grants to states and city crime agencies to improve their DNA testing capabilities (Butterfield 1996). As a result of that incentive, all fifty states adopted laws requiring specified offenders to provide blood samples for forensic DNA testing.

State statutes vary. Most statutes initially required that saliva and blood samples be obtained from sex offenders on their release from prison, or as a condition of probation or parole. Statistically, sex offenders do have a high rate of recidivism. Strategically, selecting a group with such a negative public image for mandatory DNA testing was unlikely to provoke objections. Once in place, the DNA programs expanded to cover a range of both violent and non-violent crimes. In New York, blood samples are taken from defendants convicted of felony, sex offenses, felony assaults, incest, or prison escape. In four states, blood samples are taken from defendants who have been convicted of any felony, including non-violent offenders, despite their low recidivism rate. At least seven states test misdemeanants, and twenty-nine states have DNA collection statutes that apply to juveniles who commit crimes.

Provisions for access to criminal data banks also vary; the most restrictive statutes allow access only for law enforcement purposes. Maintaining confidentiality is problematic: there are over 19,000 law enforcement agencies in the US and over 51,000 additional criminal justice agencies worldwide, which means over 600,000 employees have direct access to the National Crime Information Center maintained by the FBI.

Law enforcement agencies enjoy access to many other DNA sources. The military is willing to release its data to law enforcement officials (Gill 1997: 185). Many hospitals allow law enforcement access to their diagnostic DNA collections. It is easier for police investigators to gain access to medical records than to bank records, e-mail information, or video-rental receipts – all of which are protected by federal privacy statutes.

Yet law enforcement purposes can be very broadly defined. Indeed, what is a law enforcement purpose? Would it include the identification of a man who failed to provide child support? Ohio explicitly allows its databank to be used pursuant to a court order for proceedings establishing paternity or maternity. Laws in New Jersey and Maryland allow their DNA banks to be used to find genetic parents where the party seeking to search the databank has obtained a court order.

DNA data also could be used to explore whether an individual has a genetic profile that might predispose him to aggressive acts (Andrews 1998). Both political parties have made crime a priority issue, and state legislatures are granting money to build more and higher security prisons in the hope that this will reduce crime. There is increased discussion in the popular and policy media about predicting and preventing crime by identifying those people thought to have "criminal genes" (Nelkin and Lindee 1995). Information that purports to identify those "predisposed" to violent behavior holds considerable policy appeal. Yet many innocent people could be snared in the law enforcement net if their genes suggested they were potentially violent.

The military and prisons are self-contained, or what sociologist Erving Goffman called "total institutions" that operate under special rules with respect to social control and the right to intrude on the privacy of individuals (Goffman 1961). But the attraction of efficiency has also encouraged a wider use of DNA fingerprinting as DNA dragnets are used to search for suspects in serious crimes. These may involve innocent people.

In 1990, the San Diego police department collected blood samples from 800 men during a search for a serial killer. They selected men who matched the description of a "dark-skinned male." In 1993, the two-year-old daughter of an American army sergeant stationed in Germany was kidnapped, raped, and murdered. The murderer was identified after an eight-month dragnet investigation that included DNA screening of 1,900 men who had been near the military housing complex (Atkinson 1995). In 1995, police in Prince George County, Florida, searching for a serial rapist, collected saliva samples from more than 2,300 men, stopping them at random on a road near the scene of the crime. In 1998, 50 hospital employees were asked to provide saliva samples in a dragnet search for the strangler of a popular nursing administrator. The police chief, John S. Farrell, explained his use of the DNA dragnet: "It is a way to focus the investigation efficiently . . . in a more businesslike fashion. . . . It would save time and money [Each DNA test costs only $30] . . . It is an extremely cost-effective tool" (cf. Pan 1998: B01). But the African-Americans on the hospital staff felt they were targets of discriminatory suspicion.

In his dissent in *Jones v. Murray* (1992), Judge Murnaghan contended that efficiency is not a legitimate interest and could be used to justify the testing of any citizen on grounds that it might reduce administrative workloads. He worried that arguments for administrative efficiency could justify DNA testing of all citizens at birth simply because of the likelihood of some future manifestation of violence, even when there is no specific evidence this will occur. Murnaghan also pointed out that, if the state was willing to allow the collection of blood from non-violent offenders, the same logic would allow "the testing of other discrete populations, e.g., racial minorities or residents of underprivileged areas." Under the majority's logic, the state could go into the inner city and demand blood samples.

Benjamin Keehn, a Boston Public Defender, had also pointed to the slippery slope:

Why not round up poor people? Poor people are more likely to have their DNA on file. Of course there are benefits every time you get a cold hit. There are going to be dramatic success stories. But where does it stop? Why not take DNA samples at birth?

(quoted in Goldberg 1998: A12)

Keehn's argument convinced a Massachusetts court to halt DNA testing on prisoners and parolees, but the appellate court reversed this ruling.

Refusal to comply with requests to submit a blood sample in a DNA dragnet is bound to imply guilt. Submission to testing is not necessarily voluntary. In addition, the collection of body tissue for DNA testing presents a distinctive set of problems, for unlike fingerprints, tissue samples expose individuals to the risk that the cells will be used for purposes other than identification. They can reveal information about predisposition to disease or physical traits, a fact that becomes increasingly problematic as public authorities responsible for social control in an expanding range of situations – such as immigration – are attracted to DNA testing as a means to extend surveillance and facilitate investigations.

Surveillance creep

In 1989, the Thatcher government in Great Britain instituted a policy allowing officials to use DNA fingerprint tests on immigrant applicants seeking to prove they have relatives in Britain. Over the next few years, 18,000 tests were carried out on immigrants. Most testing is done in UK consulates in the country of origin. DNA testing is considered a cheap and more effective alternative to hours of questioning. But the British testing program was criticized as racially discriminatory, and as creating "a bureaucratic barrier and financial barrier" to immigration. Officially, applicants have a right to refuse to be tested, but rarely do so. Many do not understand why British officials want their blood, and, as in DNA dragnets, the implications of refusal lead most people to comply (Evans 1995).

The practice of testing immigrants spread to Canada in 1991. The purpose of the Canadian policy was to help immigrants with inadequate documents reunite with their families. But the cost, borne by the families sponsoring immigrants, is high: the government charged $975 for the applicant and $325 for each relative sponsored. A national committee on the status of women called the immigrant testing program a way to discourage Third World immigration. High-priced tests resulted in differential application of immigration policies, thereby

> adding fuel to a growing tide of racism and anti-immigrant sentiment. .
> . . It would be more fair for Canada to come out publicly and say we don't want family sponsorship any more rather than put up all kinds of ridiculous obstacles which cost so much money.
>
> (Rinehart 1995: A16)

The United States has never required DNA testing for immigrants, but in the anti-immigration fervor of the 1990s, pilot projects were set in motion to develop worker ID cards that would be linked to an electronic database. They would include fingerprints, voice prints, and DNA sequences – to assure that only citizens and legal aliens hold jobs (Davis 1995). Under the US Immigration and Nationality Act of 1952, aliens can be excluded from immigration for mental or physical defects, diseases, or disabilities. Information about diseases, disabilities, and predispositions could be gleaned from the applicant's DNA and therefore used as a basis to deny the application. Should genetic testing, then, be required of all immigration applicants?

In an odd extension of genetic testing, an Israeli researcher applied DNA techniques to the identification of the true Cohanim – the Orthodox Jews who trace their lineage 3,300 years back to the first high priest. He found a genetic pattern on the Y-chromosome that is shared by the descendants of the Cohanim (Grady 1997). These descendants are accorded higher status and are the only rabbis to perform certain religious duties. A DNA test could be used to validate a presumption of priesthood.

As DNA replaces other technologies such as HLA blood typing or finger-prints, the collection and banking of body tissue for DNA analysis is becoming mandatory in more and more contexts. It is the preferred technology for identifying recidivists and remains, but its use is expanding. Increasingly, it is not doctors or public health officials who collect tissue samples for identification, but government, law enforcement agencies, the military, and immigration authorities. Private firms are increasingly involved, as collecting tissue becomes a growing business: one company advertises in taxis, subway cars, and on billboards (Call 1–800 DNA TYPE). It collects tissue for DNA identification (at $600) that can establish paternity in child support disputes or family relationships for immigration purposes.

Greater efficiency and reduced costs are encouraging the "surveillance creep" that Marx (1988) had predicted. In 1998, a senior member of the British police force called for a national DNA database of the entire popu-lation, arguing that it would cut the time and cost of investigating crimes (Gammon 1998). Techniques of DNA analysis are improving and costs are declining. The Department of Justice expects that the average cost of a DNA test can be reduced to less than $10. Technological developments have also increased the feasibility of DNA dogtags. A one-centimeter-sized chip can contain all the genetic information needed to identify tens of thousands of genes at a time and to store them on a DNA card.

Why worry?

At first glance, DNA identification programs seem an efficient way of solving crimes, preventing immigration fraud, and identifying soldiers who die serving their country. The increased collection of DNA data and the expansion of centralized DNA banks have evoked little public response. It may seem comforting to law-abiding citizens who view the technology as resolving social problems with little personal relevance. But the cases described above suggest reasons for concern. Just as the targets of DNA fingerprinting have expanded, so too have the uses of DNA information. Yet there are many possibilities for error and abuse – for snaring innocent people in the DNA identification net.

Possibilities of error

In a sociological study of forensic scientists, William Thompson documented ways in which the institutional context in which these scientists work biases "the development and validation of new testing procedures, the interpretation of results, and their presentation in court" (Thompson 1997: 1117). Forensic scientists have professional incentives to adopt the goals of their clients and this may compromise scientific detachment. Keen on justifying the value of their services, they may be reluctant to question the reliability of tests. Furthermore, in ambiguous situations, they may make interpretive errors (Thompson 1997).

In a study of responses to DNA evidence, University of Texas researchers set up a team of mock jurors composed of university students and found they did not appreciate the importance of laboratory error rates. Jurors are often faced with "misleading assurances from forensic science experts that laboratory errors are impossible or nearly impossible." The study indicated to the researchers that DNA evidence "could lead to conviction where acquittals might otherwise result" (Koehler *et al.* 1995).

Errors can also be a problem in the military context. To justify the use of DNA identification in the military, Lt. Col. Weedn argued that 15 to 30 percent of previously collected fingerprint cards could not be used for identification because the cards were smudged. DNA samples, however, are no less prone to error and sloppy handling.

Potentials for abuse

In the cases we have described, plaintiffs feared their samples would be used for purposes other than identification, that military or forensic investigators might also look at health status and other information that could lead to discrimination. To date, forensic DNA bankers have been able to claim they are testing only for identification purposes and that their samples could not be used for revealing health problems. But there are possibilities for abuse in the future: certain markers that were not thought to indicate medical risks may turn out to reveal health information. State forensic departments are buying used gene sequencers from companies, enabling them to sequence genes including those that indicate health risks.

Abuses are likely to increase as interest turns to behavioral genetics, for predictive information about behavior may be useful in both military and criminal contexts. The uses of such data will likely reflect existing stereotypes. The scenarios Judge Murnaghan presented are realistic. If genes associated with aggressive or criminal behavior were identified, it would be easy to envision selective testing of black men in light of current stereotypes associating crime with race. Numerous incidents of selective investigation suggest the way stereotypes might influence data-banking practices. In Pennsylvania, state police instructed bank employees to photograph suspicious-looking blacks, in effect, creating a criminal profile applying to specific race groups. Airport security profiles have also used race as an indicator of potential terrorism or drug-smuggling crimes.

If genetic predispositions were identified for antisocial behavior, social interests could encourage measures to prevent crime by circumscribing the rights of people thought to have criminal genes. This might include keeping them under surveillance, or even preventive detention. Their profiles might be kept on file to be consulted when a crime is committed. In the military context, identification of genetic predisposition to homosexuality could – as the marines suspected – have devastating consequences. Though the military may not directly ask, the genes may tell. Soldiers with that genetic make-up could simply be discharged even when there was no evidence they engaged in homosexual behavior.

Concerns about such misuse of surveillance technologies are not without basis. In the 1960s and 1970s the FBI and local law enforcement officials kept tabs on thousands of citizens who were active in the civil rights and anti-war movements, and in some cases harassed innocent people. Today, the tools of surveillance are improving with the growing capacity of central data banks that include DNA. The Fourth Amendment might protect against secondary use of samples that were collected for purposes of identification, but this is a matter of dispute. Indeed, the concerns about privacy that had been raised by critics in the early days of centralized computer data banks are increasingly urgent when the data are DNA.

Violations of privacy

To the marines, prisoners, and immigrants who challenged mandatory testing, body tissue holds religious, social, and political meanings, and privacy concerns were critical. Warren Sinclair, an African-American, suspected that the military genetic testing program would be used to support racism. For Native American Donald Power, the taking of DNA violated his religious beliefs. Mayfield and Vlacovsky defined their DNA in terms of personal identity. And even prisoners, whose privacy rights are compromised, defined taking DNA as different from searching prison cells or body cavities.

While convicted felons would have lesser rights than other individuals, the potential uses of forensic DNA banks affect more than just criminals. Those tested in a DNA dragnet because they happen to be in an area will then have their DNA samples on file. Victims also have their DNA tested at forensic labs and their samples may be banked. Family members related to the offenders are also affected because health information about the offender (say, a genetic predisposition to cancer) indicates genetic risks to relatives as well.

Collecting tissue samples from an individual who has not been charged or convicted of a crime – as in a DNA dragnet – could violate the person's Fourth Amendment right to be free from unreasonable searches and seizures. However, persuaded by the "scientific" nature of "profiling," courts have allowed the random stopping of individuals thought to fit criminal profiles of hijackers or drug smugglers. One judge, referring to hijacker profiles as "elegant and objective", was convinced that hijackers had characteristics "markedly distinguishing them from the general traveling public" (*US v. Lopez* 1971).

Though the practice of testing and banking DNA is extending to a widening range of people – from soldiers who go to battle to chaplain's assistants, from violent to non-violent felons, from immigrant families to foreign adoptees – there has been little public concern about the practice. The possibilities of error are deflected by faith in science and the promise of genetics. Potential abuses of DNA data are deflected by perceptions that surveillance pertains to "others" – the soldier, the criminal or the illegal immigrant – and a belief that DNA identification is an efficient means to maintain social order and control.

Americans these days have few expectations of privacy, accepting surveillance in many spheres. Shoppers accept television surveillance in department stores, strollers accept camera surveillance in public parks (Nelkin 1995). The dossier society that Laudon and Rule predicted years ago has crept up on us, facilitated by the ability to gather, store, and access information – not just about finances, credit rating, or consumer preferences, but about the body, identity, and health.

In 1972, a legal scholar wrote that the social security numbers assigned to us at birth have become a "leash around our necks, subjecting us to constant monitoring and making credible the fear of the fabled womb-to-tomb dossier" (Muller 1972). Could DNA identifiers eventually replace social security numbers, requiring every person to have DNA on file? Indeed, molecular biologist Leroy Hood has predicted that within twenty years all Americans will carry a credit-card-type plastic stripe that contains computer readouts of their personal genomes. "Your entire genome and medical history will be on a credit card" (quoted in Garrett 1996: 49).

Acknowledgements

We wish to acknowledge the support of the National Science Foundation EVS Program grant #SBR-9710345 and the assistance of Michelle Hibbert. This chapter is adapted from a longer article in *Sociology of Health and Illness*, 21(5) 1999: 689–707, and from our co-authored book, *Body Bazaar*, Crown Books, 2001.

Bibliography

Andrews, L. (1998) "Predicting and Punishing Anti-Social Acts: How the Criminal Justice System Might Use Behavioral Genetics," in M. Rothstein and K. Carson (eds) *Behavioral Genetics and Society: The Clash of Culture and Biology*, Baltimore, MD: Johns Hopkins Press.

Atkinson, R. (1995) "DNA Samples Catch American Killer of Toddler in Germany," *Washington Post*, 1 January: A27.

Billings, P. (1995) Amicus in Mayfield v. Dalton 95–00344.

Bourke, J. (1996) *Dismembering the Male: Men's Bodies, Britain and the Great War*, Chicago: University of Chicago Press.

Butterfield, F. (1996) "US Has Plan to Broaden Availability of DNA Testing," *New York Times*, 14 July.

Chadwin, D. (1996) "The DNA War," *The Village Voice*, 14 May: 23.

Cole, L. (1996) "The Specter of Biological Weapons," *Scientific American*, December: 62.

Davis, A. (1995) "Digital IDs for Workers in the Cards," *National Law Journal*, 10 April: 17.

Essoyan, S. (1995) "2 Marines Challenge Pentagon Order," *Los Angeles Times*, 27 December: A1.

Evans, K. (1995) "Targets of the Genetic Inquisition," *Guardian*, 29 March: 12.

Federal Bureau of Investigation (1991) "Legislative Guidelines for DNA Databases," US Dept. of Justice, November.

Foucault, M. (1979) *Discipline and Punish*, New York: Vintage Books.

Gammon, P. (1998) cited in "UK Police Chief Calls for National DNA Data Base," *Nature*, 393: 106.

Garrett, L. (1996) "The Dots are Almost Connected," *Los Angeles Times Magazine*, 3 March: 49.

Gill, S. (1997) "The Military's DNA Registry: An Analysis of Current Law and a Proposal for Safeguards," *Naval Law Review*, 44: 175–222.

Goffman, E. (1961) *Asylums*, New York: Anchor Books.

Goldberg, C. (1998) "DNA Databanks Giving Police a Powerful Weapon, and Critics," *New York Times*, 19 February: A1, A12.

Grady, D. (1997) "Who Is Aaron's Heir?" *New York Times*, 19 January: 4.

Hamer, D. and Copeland, P. (1994) *The Science of Desire*, New York: Simon & Schuster.

Hinde, J. (1997) "Their Hands on Your Genes," *Times Higher*, 7 March: 19.

Hoeffel, J. (1990) "The Dark Side of DNA Profiling," *Stanford Law Review*, 42: 527.

Koehler, J., Chia, A., and Lindsey, S. (1995) "The Random Match Probability in DNA Evidence: Irrelevant and Prejudicial?" *Jurimetrics*, 35: 201–9.

Laudon, K. (1986) *The Dossier Society*, New York: Columbia University Press.

McClosky, H. and Brill, A. (1986) *Dimensions of Tolerance*, New York: Russell Sage Foundation.

McKewen, J. E. and Reilly, P. (1994) "A Review of State Legislation on DNA Forensic Data Banking," *American Journal of Human Genetics*, 54: 941–58.

Marx, G. T. (1988) *Undercover: Police Surveillance in America*, Berkeley: University of California Press.

Muller, A. (1972) *The Assault on Privacy*, New York: New American Library

Murnaghan, Judge (1992) in *Jones v. Murray*, 962 F.2d. 302, at 313 (dissenting).

Nelkin, D. (1995) "Forms of Intrusion: Comparing Resistance to Information Technology and Biotechnology," in M. Bauer (ed.) *Resistance to New Technology*, Cambridge: Cambridge University Press.

Nelkin, D. and Lindee, M. S. (1995) *The DNA Mystique: The Gene as a Cultural Icon*, New York: W. H. Freeman.

Pan, P. (1998) "Prince George's Chief Has Used Serial Testing Before," *Washington Post*, 31 January: B01.

Rinehart, D. (1995) "DNA Tests Help not Hinder Relatives," *Montreal Gazette*, 10 May: A16.

Rule, J. (1974) *Private Lives and Police Surveillance*, New York: Schocken Books.

Sinclair, W. (1996) "Memorandum to Convening Authorities," 27 June.

Thompson, W. C. (1997) "A Sociological Perspective on the Science of Forensic DNA Testing," *U.C. Davis Law Review*, 30(4): 1113–36.

Weedn, V. (1996) "Stored Biological Specimens for Military Identification," *Oberman Seminars*, 14 June.

Cases

Jones v. Murray, 962 F 2d 302 (4th Circuit, 1992), *cert. denied.* 506 US 977 (1992)

Mayfield v. Dalton, 901 F. supp. (D. Hawaii 7 September 1995). Vacated and remanded, 109.F.3d 1423 (9th Circuit, 27 March 1997).

US v. Lopez, 328 F. Supp. 1077, 1081 (1971).

US v. Sinclair (Central Judicial Circuit, USAF Trial Judiciary, 10 May 1996).

6 "Racial" categories and health risks

Epidemiological surveillance among Canadian First Nations

Jennifer Poudrier

Introduction

Some Canadian First Nations people have been genetically defined as being in higher health risk categories because of a questionable if not spurious racializing of medical research. The Oji-Cree of Sandy Lake, Ontario, are classified as being genetically predisposed to a form of diabetes. Such conclusions could enhance health care programs, but at the same time could be a means of discrimination whereby certain groups are determined to be at risk due to biologically inherent characteristics. These types of findings emerge from a long tradition of "scientific" classification that today is being enhanced by genetic science and computer modeling and has impacts on both the health and life-chances of Aboriginal peoples. This chapter focuses on how race-related genetic classifications are constructed and hints at the less desirable possible consequences for minority groups.

A warning of increased genetic surveillance is captured in the popular 1997 film *GATTACA*, which presents a futuristic scenario of genetic apartheid whereby the genetically altered and enhanced or the "Valids" enjoy extraordinary health, status and employment. The "InValids," "Faith Births" or those conceived naturally and mistakenly, are deemed genetically imperfect and constitute the biological underclass. While human potential and life-chances are written in the unalterable DNA, the social order is kept in check at the GATTACA Aerospace Corporation through the continual genetic surveillance of its employees' blood, urine, skin, and hair. To be sure, this scenario is merely fiction and perhaps only represents our deepest fears regarding the progress of genetic information and technology. However, many current aspirations surrounding the use of genetic information presents a disturbingly similar scenario.

In Australia, an MP has proposed that all Australians (including all newborn children), as well as people entering Australia, must submit a DNA sample which would be added to a crime database (BioMedNet News 2001).

Likewise, Nelkin and Andrews (in this volume) describe a variety of public contexts in the United States where the collection and use of personal genetic information for the purposes of surveillance or identification has expanded. Where a growing range of individuals are being DNA fingerprinted in an ever-increasing array of settings, there are good reasons to be concerned about the potential for mistakes, abuse, social discrimination, and loss of personal freedom.

Debates about the ownership of potentially predictive genetic information have surfaced in countries such as Iceland and the Polynesian island of Tonga where biotechnology companies, deCode and AutoGen Ltd respectively, have received legal access to health records and genetic information of citizens (Hollan 2001). These companies claim that they will combine the genetic information with corresponding health records to help find cures for diseases thought to be specific in those communities. The Icelandic public has generally supported deCode's database and research in hopes of a curative outcome. However, there have also been intense public debates regarding the potential social repercussions including issues of informed consent, confidentiality, and ownership of property (Palson 2001).

Genetic discrimination, a condition under which individuals and/or groups are disadvantaged by virtue of their genetic composition, continues to receive serious legal and political attention, particularly in employment and insurance contexts. Earlier this year, the Burlington Northern Santa Fe Railroad was sued by the US Equal Employment Opportunity Commission on behalf of railroad employees for illegally and secretly testing the blood of employees for a potential genetic susceptibility to carpal tunnel syndrome (Hawkins 2001). Genetic testing in this case was expected to subvert compensatory insurance costs by determining that the onset of carpal tunnel syndrome was the result of genetic abnormality rather than repetitive and stressful working conditions. These aspects of genetic surveillance, privacy, and discrimination are certain to persist as insurance companies and employers continue to press for legal access to genetic information.

An arguably more complex aspect of genetic science is genetic categorization in the context of health care and medical research. The advocates of the US government's Human Genome Project have made magnificent promises about the curative potential of disease-related genetic research. This curative promise is often seen as exceptionally good news for many people suffering with illness who are hoping for a genetic cure. However, there has also a great deal of skepticism regarding the accuracy of the impressive claim (Duster 1996; Lippman 1991; McDermott 1998).

Many biologists, geneticists, medical researchers and social scientists alike argue that there has been an excessive and undeserved hype surrounding this genetic-arrow line of medical reasoning. Referred to variously as geneticization, genetic determinism, geno-mania, or geneticism, this genetic focus identifies DNA as the exclusive component responsible for health and disease potential. Moreover, geneticism in the context of health care and disease not only distracts from the complexity of gene/environment and genc/gene interactions, but also tends to completely ignore the socio-economic, cultural, and environmental conditions implicated in the etiology of disease. In a context where the trajectory of health research and research funding is increasingly diverted toward genetic determinants of disease and away from social and environmental factors (Duster 1996; Lippman 1991; McDermott 1998; Nelkin and Tancredi 1994), the hunt for the elusive gene thrives.

Another element to the quagmire of ambiguity regarding genetic science is the use of "racial" and "ethnic" categories in medical and epidemiological research. In the past two decades, biologists and geneticists have continually confirmed the longstanding anthropological and sociological conviction that "race" and "ethnicity" are not biological categories, but cultural and social ones. In January 2001 the director of the Human Genome Project argued that there is no scientific basis in biology to the genetics of "race" or "ethnicity" and that there is more genetic difference among the members of "ethnic" groups than there are between the groups themselves (Zwillich 2001). However, genetic categories of "race" and "ethnicity" continue to permeate medical research. The critical question is why, or, perhaps more appropriately, how?

Much health-related genetic research is dependent upon population health information, which typically emanates from epidemiology. Additionally, a scientific relationship between genetics and epidemiology seems to be gaining momentum. According to professor of public health Jaakko Kaprio (2000), the future of science and medicine will be the discipline of genetic epidemiology, the study of inherited causes of disease in populations. Its primary goals are "resolving the genetic architecture of disease" and quantifying disease risk associated with genetic variation (Kaprio 2000: 1258). Recent interest in investigating the genetic origin of disease has been motivated by the Human Genome Project where the marriage of epidemiological and genetic science is expected to be a windfall for medical research in the twenty-first century (Khoury *et al.* 2001).

The continuity between the disciplines of epidemiology and genetic science seems analogous to matching the terrain of disease with the archaeology of genetics. However, from a critical point of view, the assumptions in both epidemiological and genetic sciences, particularly in the development and use of categories, are highly problematic. On the one hand, epidemiological science is often criticized for being unreflective in the construction of discrete categories of "race" or "ethnicity" as methodological variables (Fenton and Charlsey 2000; McDermott 1998). These variables or categories often bear little resemblance to the complexity and experience of both cultural affiliation and health. On the other hand, there is a great deal of criticism regarding the construction of racist and discriminatory genetic science, and the implications of discriminatory categories that are further entrenched in biology (Duster 1990,1996; Skinner and Rosen 2001).

What follows is a critique of the biomedical use of "race" and "ethnic" categories that support the presumed link between epidemiological and genetic sciences. I use the scientific hunt for the genes presumed responsible for diabetes among Aboriginal peoples as a case to outline various points of critical inquiry into the practice and potential implications of "race"-related genetic science. I draw upon Aboriginal and sociological critiques of contemporary medicine, epidemiology, and genetic science to address the intersection between health research and genetics in the construction of genetic categories.

Underlying this work is the fundamental notion that scientific research is not value-free, objective, transparent, or disinterested. Neither epidemiological nor genetic sciences are neutral in the questions they ask, the way they go about producing knowledge, and the way their findings are disseminated through public health discourse. The aim here is to chart a set of foundational and critical questions about genetic research and Aboriginal diabetes that would contribute to existing work in the sociology of science literatures geared toward opening the "black box" of genetic science and biological categorization. The more important and overarching goal of this work in general is to speak to the potential implications of genetic science for Aboriginal communities and health.

Sociological and Aboriginal analyses of health and illness

The disciplines of medical sociology and anthropology have provided an expansive assessment of contemporary medicine and health care practice (Bolaria and Bolaria 1994; Bolaria and Dickinson 1994; Clarke 1990; Doyal 1979; Edginton 1989; Fee 1983; Illich 1976; Navarro 1986; Waizkin 1983). The fundamental starting point of this scholarly work is a critique of the biomedical model in research, medicine and medical practice. The biomedical model, it is argued, is typified by an ethos of individualism, rationalization, and reductionism that tends to reduce the human body and illness to the physiological, biological, and cellular level. Biomedical reduction and rationalization views the diseased human body as a broken machine in need of a mechanistic fix. This "fix" is expected to come from the domains of pharmacological correction, technical management, personal self-control and, currently, genetic intervention. General criticism of this biological point of view holds that personal and community health is much more than the lack of genetic or biological illness. In fact, achieving, maintaining or promoting health involves further consideration of social, economic, cultural, and environmental factors and less attention to individual biology. Medical sociology literatures offer a range of analytic foci to address various aspects of the biomedical model and health care practice in general.

A prominent strand of scholarship examines the relationship between knowledge, power, and discourse. Drawing upon the work of Foucault (1973) and the fundamental concepts of power/knowledge, bio-power and governmentality, many social scientists have addressed the way that medical and health care knowledges act as disciplinary power and regulatory control (Lupton 1995; Petersen and Bunton 1997; Turner 1986). Where biomedical knowledges emerge in the context of medical power and vice versa, these discourses of authority form, regulate and rely upon definitions of "sick," "health," "at risk," etc. These authoritative definitions act as forms of power/knowledge through the individual body (emerging as individual self-surveillance) and through the body of the population (emerging as forms of efficient population health). Where bodies are "made up" or inscribed upon by biomedical discourse, "disciplinary power exists through the disciplinary practices which produce particular individuals, institutions and cultural arrangements" (Turner 1997: xii).

Another group of scholars addresses the political economy of ill health, concentrating on the more structural, systemic, and social causes of ill health which health discourses often ignore in favor of a focus on individual lifestyles (Doyal 1979; Navarro 1986; Waitzkin 1983). Others focus upon the general iatrogenic effects of medical and health care practice (Illich 1976) and still others address the health disparities among different groups (Bolaria and Bolaria 1994). Some Canadian scholars address the relationships between minority groups, medicine, and health. Bolaria and Bolaria (1994) argue that class, gender, and racial inequalities have differential effects upon people's health. Elements of racism and sexism in medicine doubly marginalize, problematize, and medicalize the health-related experiences of minorities.

Some scholars see capitalist economic arrangements as crucial. In this view, Aboriginal health may be understood in terms of the dominant mode of production; ideology produces social, economic, political, cultural, as well as spatial marginalization. For example, while acknowledging differential socio-economic, location and class experiences of Aboriginal peoples, Wotherspoon and Satzewich (1993) suggest that ill health is related not only to low socio-economic status, colonizing health policies, and the refutation of traditional holistic models of health, but also, for many living on reserves, to environmental hazards.

Frideres (1994) identifies the structures including policies of colonization and ongoing institutionalized racism, which affect traditional health practices and contribute to ill health. Likewise, Waldrum, Herring and Young (1995) describe the way in which historical colonial processes and policies aimed at absolute assimilation caused the ill health and, often, death of Aboriginal peoples. Some of these practices included forced labor and forced residential schooling, which facilitated the transmission of infectious disease, and the criminalization of healing practices, such as the sweat lodge and the sundance. James Waldrum (1994) argues that cultural and socio-economic factors have contributed to the delivery of health care services and to the current health status of Aboriginal peoples in Canada.

Other scholars are especially interested in the way discursive power advanced colonizing policies. For instance, social historian Mary-Ellen Kelm (1998) describes how Aboriginal bodies were materially affected by Canadian colonial policy (which aimed to immobilize and control). She focuses on the way in which the discursive power of colonial medicine, through the assimilative (and often humanitarian) work of field matrons, missionaries, and doctors, was used to pathologize Aboriginal bodies (Kelm 1998; Waldrum *et al.* 1995). For example, between the turn of the century and the 1950s, when increased contact between Aboriginal communities and European settlers saw the emergence of a tuberculosis (TB) epidemic among Aboriginal populations, Aboriginal peoples were increasingly viewed as inherently primitive. Aboriginal bodies were characterized as racially susceptible to disease and dangerous (Kelm 1998). In order to contain the threat of the Aboriginal body, which was described as a public health hazard by Indian agents and health care workers, many Aboriginal peoples, especially children, were detained in provincial TB sanatoria (Canadian Lung Association 1999). Through processes of colonization, the material control over bodies combined with the discursive construction of the "dangerous" Aboriginal body. This shaped, and continues to influence, contemporary health knowledge about Aboriginal peoples (Kelm 1998).

In the context of contemporary Aboriginal health, several questions emerge. How is the current narrative of Aboriginal health constructed? Are Aboriginal peoples and communities still characterized as inherently (biologically or genetically) sick, dangerous and/or a population health risk? One way to address these questions is to interrogate the fundamental nature of medical and health knowledge about Aboriginal health. The primary producer of health knowledge is the science of population health: epidemiology.

Epidemiology: the science of population health

The word epidemiology is derived from the Latin words for "epidemic" and "knowledge of." While an epidemic suggests the sudden emergence of a dangerous disease or infection, epidemiology is geared toward using scientific methods to define the cause of health-related epidemics in defined populations (Lupton 1995). Fortified with rational hypotheses, statistical and mathematical calculations, risk ratios and control groups, contemporary epidemiology has become the science of general population health.

Where populations are the sum of the individuals within them, quantitative epidemiology seeks to discover statistical patterns of biological disorder to identify the incidence of disease among certain groups over other groups. According to epidemiologists Charles Hennekens and Julie Buring, epidemiology is "the study of the distribution and determinants of disease frequency in human populations which encompass all epidemiological principles and methods" (1987: 3).

Epidemiological work is based upon a certain methodological trajectory or formula. In describing this method, Hennekens and Buring state that "natural progression in epidemiologic reasoning . . . begins with a suspicion" (1987: 3). Through theoretical speculation about a suspicion, combined with scientific methodological rigor, epidemiology provides some information about the frequency and distribution of disease (Hennekens and Buring 1987). This information is used to provide practical knowledge about the determinants of the disease in populations. Determinants of disease are then constructed by comparing certain populations or sub-groups within populations with others, or with the use of control groups. Determinants of disease qualify and, in many cases, quantify the relative risks of developing disease. Through varying statistical risk formulae, risk factors represent a prediction about the potential for onset of disease in a particular population or sub-population (Hennekens and Buring 1987). By way of epidemiological practice, members of certain populations are identified as being "at risk" subjects. While additional diagnostic tests are needed to detect actual illness, schemes of risk classification contribute to and are informed by the detection of potentiality. The increasingly future orientation of surveillance in general is thus seen clearly in this context.

Contemporary epidemiological knowledge emerges in a variety of every-day contexts. As the principal provider of health information to societies and individuals, epidemiology has produced information about healthy sexual behavior and about the relationship between health and physical activity. It offers instruction on how long it is safe to stay in the sun and how many portions of fresh vegetables to consume per day. Certainly, the aim of epidemiological work is benevolent and utilitarian to the extent that it is geared toward improving the health of populations. However, it has received some criticism, particularly for its construction of categories.

Critiques of epidemiology

Epidemiological work has produced some necessary information about the relationship between populations and disease potentiality through the construction of risk categories. Epidemiological knowledge has a very profound influence upon our social world. Fundamentally, it shapes, transforms or "makes up" how we perceive ourselves as healthy and/or productive members of society (Forde 1998). From the Foucauldian concept of bio-power, Lupton (1995) and Petersen and Bunton (1997) argue that health and medical discourses define concepts of health and ill health and that these concepts tend to be disciplinary. Health discourse is disciplinary and moralizing to the extent that it defines categories of healthy and unhealthy behavior. These determinants of healthy and unhealthy behavior tend to correspond intimately with moral concepts of good and bad conduct, as well as virtuous and immoral individuals or communities. In this sense, then, health discourse is not only repressive, but it is also productive (Lupton 1995). It produces subjects or identities that conform to the standards of what may be called healthism. They are thus "made up" by predefined categories. Subjectivities are constituted through the authoritative and moral categories of healthy, unhealthy, diseased, not-diseased, good, bad or simply "at risk." As subjects are interpellated or hailed by these health categories, individuals and groups of individuals come to participate in their own self-surveillance (Lupton 1995; Petersen and Bunton 1997). Formed through authoritative and moralizing (repressive) power, alongside the discursive construction of health identities and self-surveillance (productive) power, health discourse becomes a powerful tool of social control. Again, the fundamental producers of population health knowledge and information are the classifications of epidemiological science. However, health knowledge and the categories it produces are certainly not neutral or objective.

There has been some critical focus upon the way in which scientific work produces knowledge. This form of critique, which characteristically emerges from the sociology of science, emphasizes that scientific knowledge is highly interconnected with social, economic, discursive, gender, racial, and political contexts (Biagioli 1999; Duster 1996; Harding 1998; Kay 1999; Nader 1996; Rabinow 1994; Rosner and Johnson 1995; Skinner and Rosen 2001). The science of population health or epidemiology is no exception. There are several points at which the construction and use of knowledge might be interrogated to address this lack of neutrality and objectivity. These range from analyses of subjectivity and identity through interpellation of risk discourse, to the social, economic, and political determination of "meaning-ful" scientific questions, and to the way in which health knowledge is disseminated.

While there is some qualitative research, epidemiological practice tends to be positivist or quantitative in nature (Fenton and Charsley 2000). Like most modern science, replete with notions of scientific progress, epidemiological work is concerned with methodological rigor and firmly entrenched in a scientific model which privileges rationality and reductionism (Forde 1998; Lupton 1995; McDermott 1998). McDermott (1998: 1193) suggests that reductionist "black box epidemiology" is currently in crisis because of its obsession with taken-for-granted methodological technique, causal models and risk assessment, rather than maintaining a focus upon real-life situations that contribute to the onset of disease. This methodological focus has detracted from ontological and epistemological debate (Forde 1998; Lupton 1995; McDermott 1998) and therefore fails to reflect upon kinds questions it asks, the reasons for asking them, and the ways it goes about finding the answers. Where the goal might be the production of practical health knowledge that reflects the realities of the populations it describes, the means have replaced the ends. The goal has become methodological and scientific perfection (Forde 1998).

Fenton and Charsley (2000) argue that quantitative epidemiology tends to treat its variables as isolated and quantifiable social realities. The construction and abstraction of discrete categories ignores the complexity of social life and healthy social living. This is particularly true of the use of "ethnic" or "racial" categories. Fenton and Charsley (2000) explain that positivistic epidemiology has typically viewed ethnic divisions through the same ontological lens as age classifications and socio-economic status.

However, "ethnic" or "racial" groups are not discrete methodological variables. "Ethnicities" are rather more complex and at the very least should be understood as the contextualized culmination of shifting social, economic, historical, environmental, familial, cultural, and political contexts (Fenton and Charsley 2000). More generally, the interpretation of statistical infor-mation regarding the quantification of race or what race actually means is seriously flawed (Zuberi 2000). Fenton and Charsley (2000) advise quantitative epidemiological practitioners that the uncritical use of "race" and "ethnic" categories is neither an accurate nor an effective way to produce meaningful knowledge about health. Where epidemiological work is meant to contribute to social equalities in health, its conceptual models "may instead reinforce social hierarchies based on gender, race, and class [and] constrain our understanding of health and disease" (Inhorn and Whittle 2001: 553).

In the context of Aboriginal health in Canada, John O'Neil, Jeff Reading, and Audrey Leader (1998) are also critical of epidemiology. They address the way in which epidemiological knowledge operates as a powerful mechanism of regulatory surveillance. Where epidemiological research is a "response to the political problem of regulating potentially dangerous behaviours," epidemiological discourse is a tool of disciplinary power over problematic populations and perilous lifestyles (O'Neil *et al.* 1998: 230).

Contemporary portraits of Aboriginal communities reflect images of misery, disease, and poverty that play a commanding role in the construction of Aboriginal identity (O'Neil *et al.* 1998). Health discourse about Aboriginal peoples reflects sick, disorganized, uncontrolled, and dependent peoples (Frideres 1994; O'Neil *et al.* 1998; Waldrum *et al.* 1995). According to O'Neil *et al.* (1998), this image legitimates paternalistic and regulatory management over Aboriginal health in communities, and further marginalizes overarching efforts geared toward self-determination and development. Arguing that biomedicine is "a cultural system itself, and an appendage of the colonial state structure," James Waldrum and colleagues (2000: 37) warn that current medicine must address cultural knowledge, lest it turn into "another form of assimilative pressure."

However, many Aboriginal communities are increasingly developing research projects to collect health information in their own communities (O'Neil *et al.* 1998). This research aims not only to reflect more accurate and culturally appropriate portrait of health and wellness in communities, but also hopes to resist the disciplinary narrative of existing discourse. In other words, efforts are geared toward the development of an alternative health knowledge that "contributes to the production of knowledge about Aboriginal communities that is liberating rather than repressive" (O'Neil *et al.* 1998: 230).

A fundamental accomplishment of these types of initiatives is the ownership of health research and information. It becomes the property of the tribal organizations as an element of self-government. O'Neil *et al.* (1998) describe a research project in Manitoba, Canada, where, in collaboration with a university-based research team, Aboriginal peoples developed, conducted, and analyzed an Aboriginal population health survey. While the research is reportedly a success in terms of ownership and self-determination, there is some hesitation about its capacity to step outside the disciplinary scientific model (O'Neil *et al.* 1998).

A further consideration for the future of health and medical research is critical attention to development of genetic science and genetic categories. Uncertainty about the resistance to surveilling powers of health discourse and categorization comes into sharper focus in an age of genetic research. Drawing upon the work of O'Neil *et al.* (1998), I extend the critical work from epidemiology to genetic science. In a social, political, discursive, and economic context where genetic science has become a sign of progress and has captured public imagination (Nelkin and Lindee 1995; Van Dijck 1998), genetic science has become a prolific and pervasive explanatory framework for the human condition.

Critical focus on new genetic science

In the past ten years, great scientific strides have been made in genetics. For example, the Human Genome Project has recently charted a map of the human genome and defined the location and structure of every human chromosome. While it has yet to determine what the map means or how genes function and interact, the Human Genome Project promises that ongoing research will eventually produce the knowledge, information, and technology needed to define, predict and prevent genetically related disease.

The increased interest in genetic science has met with substantial concern about its potential ethical, legal, social, and political implications. While there are many issues and several theoretical approaches with which to address them, one element of concern is the negative aspects of genetic determinism. Genetic determinism is defined as the condition under which individuals and or groups become defined as "normal" or "abnormal" by virtue of their genetic, and presumably inalterable, characteristics (Annas and Elias 1992; Nelkin and Tancredi 1994). Abby Lippman (1991) contends that these categorizations emerge from the interplay between techniques of prenatal screening and contemporary genetic discourse. More specifically, she argues that by promoting biology as the major determinant of health, the dominant cultural, scientific, economic, and technical discourses construct the need for genetic prevention, prediction, and cure. These then manifest themselves in social inequality and social control.

The intersection between "race" or "ethnicity" and DNA is extremely problematic in social and scientific contexts. In social contexts, Nelkin and Andrews (in this volume) discuss the potential for racial discrimination in light of mandatory DNA fingerprinting of immigration applicants who are seeking entry into countries such as Great Britain and Canada. Members of ethnic groups are often designated as at risk of particular diseases. For example, Ashkenazi Jews, who have higher rates of Tay-Sachs disease, are thought to be genetically predisposed to it (Lemmens and Austin 2001). African-Americans, who have been characterized as carriers of the sickle-cell trait, have experienced a great deal of discrimination and stigmatization surrounding conceptions of health risk (Duster 1996; Kevles 1985).

In current medical research, there has been an expanding interest in identifying the genetic cause of disease among members of "racial" or "ethnic" groups. These genetic factors are expected to be useful for medical and pharmaceutical development, including the creation of efficient screening tests for genetic predisposition and the production of pharmaceuticals custom-made for members of certain "ethnic" or "racial" groups.[1] The link between "race" or "ethnicity" and genetic susceptibility has become an extremely lucrative area of medical research.

On the one hand, scientific research seems to progress with a notion of "racial" or "ethnic" categories. On the other hand, however, and as indicated earlier, recent scientific analysis of the human genome claims that racial designation has no scientific basis in biology. For example, it was reported that humans survive on about one-third of the number of genes that were previously predicted (Wade 2001) and that there is "often more genetic variation between people classified in the same racial group than between members of 'different' ethnic groups" (Zwillich 2001). So why are "ethnicity" and "race" being used as genetic categories? Francis Collins, director of the Human Genome Project, is reported to acknowledge the continued use of racial categories in genetic research and illusively comments that attempts to reconcile this paradox "will continue to be a heavy burden" (Zwillich 2001). The scientific community seems to be somewhat perplexed, but mostly silent on the continued use of racial categories.

From a sociology of knowledge perspective, Troy Duster (1990) explains the continued use of racial categories in genetic and biological sciences. According to Duster (1990), the biological sciences, which often make assumptions regarding the relationship between "race" and genetic compo-sition, are based upon racist and discriminatory assumptions rather than on scientific evidence. In the current climate where health care decisions are determined by ongoing fiscal crises, disease is often problematized according to already marginalized groups with racial categories. Calling it a conceptual prism, Duster (1990) maintains that heretibility and genetic "fitness" are social constructions emerging out of the already well-established social order that continues to perpetuate the ideology of problematic "races" with problematic diseases.

Drawing on the history of genetic attempts to explain problems like criminality, alcoholism, mental illness and IQ by "race," Duster argues "it is not genetic evidence that drives the engine of scientific inquiry, but the social concerns that drives the engine of the 'scientific' attempt to portray and explain these social concerns genetically" (1996: 123). Where ethnic populations are "at risk" and are considered a financial drain on health care resources, and where medical science is increasingly entrenched (through large investments) in genetics, the hunt for "racial" genetic susceptibility proceeds.

In sum, efforts to find genetic explanations for disease among members of minority groups are decidedly problematic. The focus on genetic research drives health research increasingly closer to the authoritative and narrow realm of biological and biomedical sciences and further away from a more nuanced analysis of historical, social, environmental, cultural, discursive, political, and economic factors. As such, the health knowledge that would emanate from genetic research may not be beneficial to communities since biological categories of "race" are not valid. Even more, categories of racial distinction, constructed through the scientific process (and ironically through the ideal of scientific progress) may become more firmly substantiated as scientific fact. Notions of racial distinction, emanating from medical/genetic science which is presumed to be benevolent and objective, may also produce concerns associated with biological/genetic determinism, racism and especially eugenics (Chadwick 1998; Holzman 1999; Kevles 1985; McLaren 1990; McNally 1998; Paul 1998; Wertz 1998).

Indigenous resistance to genetic research

Indigenous peoples globally have not been silent on the appropriation and use of genetic information in medical contexts or otherwise. There has been a great deal of resistance on the part of Aboriginal groups who are committed to protecting indigenous nations from the colonizing capacities of genetic science in several different contexts. These contexts range from the expropriation of traditional indigenous plants, medicines, and resources in the context of biopiracy, to the archeological extraction and genetic analysis of ancient Aboriginal remains, to the highly publicized Human Genome Diversity Project.

One of the most fundamental dilemmas is that genetic science conflicts with Aboriginal principles of holism and respect for all life forms. While acknowledging the different histories, languages, and cultures of diverse indigenous nations, Harry, Howard, and Shelton (2000) of the Indigenous Peoples' Council on Biocolonialism (IPCB) describe commonly held indigenous worldviews:

> Many indigenous peoples regard their bodies, hair, and blood as sacred elements, and consider scientific research on these materials a violation of their cultural and ethical mandates. Immortalization, cloning, or the introduction of genetic materials taken from a human being into another living being is also counter to many indigenous peoples [*sic*] cultural and ethical principles. Indigenous peoples have frequently expressed criticism of Western science for failing to consider the inter-relatedness of holistic life systems, and for seeking to manipulate life forms using genetic technologies.

Another core issue about which there is a great deal of skepticism is the extent to which genetic research about indigenous peoples will be useful to

Aboriginal communities. A case in point is the highly controversial Human Genome Diversity Project that was seen to meet mostly the desires of scientific communities rather than the needs of indigenous peoples (Awang 2000; Harry 2001; Harry and Dukepoo 1998; Lone Dog 1999; Whitt 1998). In an interview, Debra Harry, Executive Director of the IPCB, has argued that it is naive to assume that genetic science will provide the definitive cure to disease and that a focus on genetics is counter-productive to addressing real determinants of disease:

> The public is led to believe [genetic research] will lead to cures of human diseases, however, cures are not going to be realized anytime in the near future if at all, since most human illnesses are a result of complex interactions between genes and the environment . . . genetic research of this scale hurts, rather than benefits, indigenous peoples because it diverts public funds away from direct health care and prevention programs. [T]he millions of dollars spent on human genome sequencing has diverted attention away from far more current and pressing public health needs. The same amount of attention to insure we have access to basic health care, clean water, safe foods, and a healthy environment is an effort from which we would see real benefits.
>
> (IPCB 2000)

In the same interview, Stuart Newman, Professor of Cell Biology and Anatomy and a board member of the IPCB, addresses concerns surrounding racial categorization and biological/genetic determinism:

> Although there are potentially beneficial uses for the information gathered in the Human Genome Project, there is also the great threat that this information will be used to persuade people that they are not good enough, biologically. This will be justified by promised improvements to human health, but unless carefully monitored and regulated, this emphasis on genetics will have a divisive effect, whereby those categories and groups of people that have traditionally been marginalized will now learn that their genes are inferior and need to be improved.
>
> (IPCB 2000)

The heart of the problem with biological categorization is the fundamental nature of Western science and European history. Harry and Dukepoo (1998) and Shelton and Marks (2001) argue that modern Western science is based upon Eurocentric and discriminatory scientific theory, which is ignorant about indigenous peoples, their knowledges, resources, and histories. The scientific assumption of genetic homogeneity, in fact, runs counter to scientific reasoning considering the complexity of Aboriginal histories. Shelton and

Marks (2001) explain, "tribes have long-standing complex relationships [and] . . . these social historical forces insure that there cannot be any clear-cut genetic variants differentiating all the members of one tribe from those of nearby tribes." So, defining a stable relationship between genetic markers and indigenous people flies in the face of its own scientific logic and is based upon stereotypical assumptions (Harry and Dukepoo 1998). These assumptions seem to be founded upon the commonly held notions of isolation, starkness, and what seemed to be a social, cultural, and political abyss before the arrival of European colonizers.

The presumption of genetic homogeneity flows into medical and health research. As indicated earlier, medical research is persistently geared toward determining the genetics of "ethnicity" or "race" as a component of disease onset among minority groups. One lucrative area of contemporary genetic research is the search for the genetic components responsible for diabetes mellitus. Rates of diabetes and diabetes-related illness have recently been considered epidemic by the World Health Organization and, combined with the overwhelming expansion of the genetic sciences, the genetics of diabetes has become a ripe landscape for contemporary research. Additionally, where rates of diabetes among minority and marginalized populations are characterized as particularly problematic, a critical focus of genetic research has been geared toward isolating "racial" or "ethnic" factors. Research about Aboriginal peoples is no exception. As seen from the following description of research dedicated to determining the culprit gene or genes associated with Aboriginal peoples and diabetes, I will concentrate on the more specific case of genetic research associated with the Oji-Cree peoples of Sandy Lake, Ontario, in Canada.

The new Aboriginal "epidemic: " diabetes

The incidence of diabetes is reportedly on the rise. The increasing prevalence of type 2 diabetes (non-insulin-dependent diabetes or NIDDM) is often described as "epidemic" in proportion. According to Health Canada (1999), diabetes is now one of the most important health problems worldwide and is considered one of the top seven diseases leading to death. While there are three different types of diabetes, type 2 diabetes is the most prevalent and affects nearly 90 percent of all diabetics (Canadian Diabetes Association 2001). NIDDM is not indiscriminate in its victims. Different ethnic groups in developed countries are said to be at higher risk levels for the onset of NIDDM. According to the American Diabetes Association (ADA), people of Latin American, African, Asian, Aboriginal, and Hispanic descent living in North America have high rates of NIDDM and are described as "high risk" groups (ADA 1999).

In Canada, the Canadian Diabetes Association (CDA) contends that First Nations communities have disproportionately greater rates of NIDDM and states that Aboriginal peoples are three to five times more likely than the general population to develop diabetes (Canadian Diabetes Association 2001). More recently, epidemiologists Young and colleagues described the prevalence of NIDDM among Canada's First Nations peoples as "an epidemic in progress" (2000: 561) since in the last decade rates of diabetes among Aboriginal peoples in many communities have increased dramatically. In 1998, acting on the assertion that the prevalence of type 2 diabetes among Aboriginal peoples was an "impending crisis," the Assembly of First Nations (AFN) (2000) prepared a report entitled *Aboriginal Diabetes Strategy*. This report outlined strategies to address diabetes through initiatives based on culturally appropriate prevention, education, treatment, lifestyle supports and surveillance (AFN 2000). In 1995, the National Aboriginal Diabetes Association was formed with the mandate to represent, in a respectful manner, the interests of Aboriginal people and to promote and facilitate diabetes-related initiatives for research, education, prevention, and health promotion at both national and community-based levels.

Scientific efforts to determine the cause of NIDDM have been difficult, and its precise etiology remains unknown. What is known is that NIDDM is associated with environmental and lifestyle factors such as age, stress, poor nutrition, sedentary lifestyles, as well as low socio-economic status, and social marginalization (Joe and Young 1994). There is also a specific area of genetic research that both assumes and tries to tease out the genetic basis of NIDDM among Aboriginal peoples.

This area of research is based on the assumption that distinct genetic characteristics, combined with environmental and historical conditions related to colonization, prove Aboriginal peoples have a particular predisposition to the onset of diabetes. This assumption is often related to a genetic theory named the "thrifty gene" hypothesis, which was proposed in 1962 by population geneticist James Neel. The "thrifty gene" hypothesis is a fairly simplistic but certainly captivating explanation for NIDDM. Originally, it was based upon the notion that hunter/gatherer populations survived feast and famine living conditions because of a "thrifty" genetic predisposition to accumulate and store fat. Neel (1962) further suggested that under conditions of recent rapid Westernization and dietary change, this naturally selected genetic predisposition, which sustained populations historically during times of famine, has led to the onset of obesity and diabetes among contemporary populations.

Twenty years after the 1962 proposition, Neel (1982) published a paper acknowledging the scientific evidence that demonstrated significant flaws in the original theory. Nevertheless, he remained quite adamant about the existence of the "thrifty gene." While the "thrifty gene" hypothesis has loomed in the background, it has attracted very little attention, until recently.

Currently, the hypothesis has resurfaced in the contemporary discourse associated with diabetes among indigenous groups globally. For example, Marchand (1999), reporting for the US-based National Institute of Diabetes & Digestive & Kidney Diseases (NIDDK), reveals that in attempt to explain obesity and type 2 diabetes among the Pima Indians, "scientists use the 'thrifty gene' theory proposed in 1962 by geneticist James Neel."

In the Canadian context, the work of physician and geneticist Robert A. Hegele has been connected to the concept of the "thrifty gene." In March of 1999, Hegele and a group of medical colleagues announced that they had found a genetic link between NIDDM and the Oji-Cree people of Sandy Lake, Ontario (Hegele *et al.* 1999). This research was based upon the extraordinarily high rates of diabetes among members of the Sandy Lake community. They claimed that they had discovered the exact gene variant, namely HNF1A G319S, which was responsible for the onset of NIDDM. The research seemed to demonstrate that individuals who had inherited only one copy of the deleterious gene were twice as likely to develop the disease as those who had no copy, while those who had inherited two copies were more than fifteen times more likely to develop diabetes (Hegele *et al.* 1999). Shortly thereafter, the *British Medical Journal* reported that the "'[t]hrifty gene' [is] identified in Manitoba Indians" (Spurgeon 1999).[7] In a subsequent article, Hegele writes about the Sandy Lake study and states that "[n]one of these findings . . . would be inconsistent with the 'thrifty gene' hypothesis of Dr. James Neel" (1999b: S48).

Although its existence has not been confirmed scientifically, the "thrifty gene" theory often appears as an assumed truth seemingly waiting (almost impatiently) for scientific authorization. While the existence of the "thrifty gene" is certainly not settled, the search for the genetic cause of diabetes among Aboriginal peoples remains. For instance, Hegele states, "finding the genetic determinants of complex human traits such as type 2 diabetes is currently a high priority in medical research" (1999a: 33). However, the ongoing search for these culprit genes opens up several sets of questions.

A first set of questions addresses the emergent scientific link between disease genes and "race." If "race" and "ethnicity" are not biological categories, and if genetic studies rely on the presumption of genetic homogeneity among "ethnic" groups, what is the status of genetic research? In the case of the aforementioned research, there are several theoretical and methodological issues that deserve critical inquiry. These include the conceptualization of comparison groups, the use of "white" genes as standards for normality and the assumption of genetic homogeneity among members of the community.

While an analysis of the research in its entirety is currently underway, I will address only the latter issue here.

There seems to be a presumption of genetic homogeneity among the Oji-Cree of Sandy Lake. Essentially, a relatively homogenous gene pool must exist to proceed with research leading to conclusions about the implications of that particular genetic composition for rates of diabetes. In order to establish the notion of genetic homogeneity, in part, the report describes the community as "isolated and accessible for most of the year only by air" (Hegele 1999b: S43). This isolation is presumed to translate into a very slight degree of genetic diversity. However, the contemporary notion of isolation (determined by air travel) certainly does not account for other possible means of travel before the existence of mechanized vehicles. Did the people of Sandy Lake historically travel by boat, by foot or by any other means? It is also reported "the ancestors of the current residents of this region lived a nomadic, hunting–gathering subsistence" (Hegele 1999b: S43). What did that "nomadic" existence contribute to possible inter-tribal marriage or adoption and, therefore, the homogeneity of the community's gene pool? Are there more complex and local histories of family lineage that might be relevant?

A second set of questions relates to the usefulness of determining the relationship between "Aboriginal" genes and NIDDM. In the face of over-whelming evidence showing that diabetes is a consequence of nutrition, obesity, and physical inactivity, which are highly associated with socio-economic status and levels of marginalization, what are the clinical purposes of genetic research? According to Hegele, the genetic information gleaned would be used to determine levels of propensity or evaluative strategies to assess risk where "genetic markers of type 2 diabetes susceptibility could one day be incorporated into a formula of risk evaluation" (1999a: 33). But how could devising a genetic factor into an already well-established risk formula be of practical use? Hegele continues that perhaps once substantial genetic markers for risk are determined, "appropriate preventive measures could then be targeted towards high-risk subjects, even before the onset of disease and/or complications" (1999a: 33). But what are these "appropriate preventative" measures? What could diabetics or those at high risk of developing it have to gain by learning that they are genetically predisposed to disease, particularly when the general course of preventative action would be the same without knowing that it was in the genes? And alternatively, what are the negative effects of being determined as genetically diseased? Perhaps funding might find a more useful place in the ongoing development of programs which make healthy food affordable and available to diabetics or members of high-risk groups, or, on a more radical note, developing strategies which address factors leading to disparities in socio-economic status, more generally. Does the genetic focus act as a deterrent to proactive curative strategies linked to already well-established risk factors including socio-economic status and level of marginalization?

These two sets of questions remain specific to the research associated with the genetics of diabetes among Aboriginal peoples. Another set of overarching questions surfaces about the development of genetic categories for Aboriginal predisposition to disease. What is this research actually accomplishing? Genetic research seems to proceed with a hazy inclination to isolate a potential gene mutation, which may contribute to a higher risk of developing disease, but only when combined with certain pathologized lifestyle conditions. Accordingly, the purpose of this genetic research appears to presume a scientific trajectory toward a more authoritative and incontestable classification and prediction schema: presumably the genetic code.

However, as Nelkin and Andrews demonstrate in this volume, the methods of genetic testing and identification, in various contexts, leave much to be desired. And as Harry (2001) and Lone Dog (1999) explain, there is an urgency to address the implications and meaning of genetic science for Aboriginal communities and indigenous movements. What does "genetic mutation" or the category of "genetic risk" mean to the people it describes? What is the relationship between new genetic categories of health and illness and medically established categories of health? Will new genetic classifications, a kind that are firmly entrenched within a scientific interplay between biology and potentiality, intensify already existing notions of sickness, dependency, and risk (O'Neil *et al.* 1998: 230)? Will these categorizations lead to an amplified effort toward medical surveillance, classification, and containment?

In this chapter I have drawn out sets of critical questions to begin unpacking the intersection between epidemiological science and "race"-related genetic research in the context of Aboriginal health. By using Aboriginal and sociological critiques of medicine, health discourse, epidemiology, and genetic science, I have attempted to address the potential of this science for Aboriginal communities and health. In a social, cultural, and political context where the "weakest 'genetic' explanations take root" (Duster 1996: 119), the use of "ethnic" and "racial" categories surely warrant further critical inquiry.

Notes

1 Recent studies have shown that "race" is not an indicator of pharmacological performance since observable characteristics such as skin color are not related to genetic ancestry (CBC News Online. 29 October 2001. "Race Won't Predict how Drugs Will Work: Study.")

2 This report also wrongfully identified the "Indians" as being from Manitoba, rather than from Ontario.

130   *Verifying identities*

Bibliography

American Diabetes Association (1999) "American Diabetes Association." Online. Available HTTP: <http://www.diabetes.org/> (accessed 22 February 2002).

Annas, G. and Elias, S. (eds) (1992) *Gene Mapping: Using Law and Ethics as Guides*, New York: Oxford University Press.

Assembly of First Nations (AFN) (2000) *Aboriginal Diabetes Strategy*. Online. Available HTTP: <http://www.afn.ca/health/Diabetes/assembly_of_first_nations_consul.htm> (accessed 1 March 2001).

Awang, S. (2000) "Indigenous Nations and the Human Genome Diversity Project," in G. J. S. Dei, B. Hall, and D. G. Rosenberg (eds) *Indigenous Knowledges in Global Contexts: Multiple Readings of our World*, Toronto: University of Toronto Press.

Biagioli, M. (ed.) (1990) *The Science Studies Reader*, New York: Routledge.

BioMedNet News (2001) "DNA Database Idea Under Fire." Online. Available HTTP: <http://news.bmn.com/news/media?uid=2200&date=010427> (accessed 30 April 2001).

Bolaria, B. S. and Bolaria, R. (1994) *Racial Minorities Medicine and Health*, Halifax, NS: Fernwood Publishing.

Bolaria, B. S. and Dickinson, H. D. (eds) (1994) *Health, Illness, and Health Care in Canada*, 2nd edn, Toronto: Harcourt Brace & Company.

Canadian Diabetes Association (2001) "Diabetes Facts." Online. Available HTTP: <http://www.diabetes.ca/about_diabetes/thefacts.html> (accessed 22 February 2002).

Canadian Lung Association (1999) "The History of Tuberculosis in Canada." Online. Available HTTP: <http://www.lung.ca/tb/tbhistory/> (accessed 22 February 2002).

Chadwick, R. (1998) "Can Genetic Counselling Avoid the Charge of Eugenics?" *Science in Context*, 11(3–4): 471–80.

Clarke, J. (1990) *Health, Illness, and Medicine in Canada*, Toronto: McClelland & Stewart.

Doyal, L. (1979) *The Political Economy of Health*, London: Pluto Press.

Duster, T. (1990) *Backdoor to Eugenics*, London: Routledge.

—— (1996) "The Prism of Heritability and the Sociology of Knowledge," in L. Nader (ed.) *Naked Science: Anthropological Inquiry Into Boundaries, Power, and Knowledge*, New York: Routledge.

Edginton, B. (1989) *Health, Disease and Medicine in Canada: A Sociological Perspective*, Toronto and Vancouver: Butterworths.

Fee, E. (ed.) (1983) *Women and Health: The Politics of Sex in Medicine*, New York: Baywood Publishing Co.

Fenton, S. and Charsley, K. (2000) "Epidemiology and Sociology as Incommensurate Games: Accounts from the Study of Health and Ethnicity," *Health*, 4(4): 403–25.

Forde, O. (1998) "Is Imposing Risk Awareness Cultural Imperialism?" *Social Science & Medicine*, 47(9): 1155–9.

Foucault, M. (1973) *The Birth of the Clinic*, New York: Pantheon.

Frideres, J. (1994) "Racism and Health: The Case of the Native People," in Bolaria, B. S. and Dickinson, H. D. (eds.) *Health, Illness, and Health Care in Canada*, 2nd edn, Toronto: Harcourt Brace & Company.

Harding, S. (1998) *Is Science Multicultural?: Postcolonialisms, Feminisms, and Epistemologies*, Bloomington: Indiana University Press.

Harry, D. (2001) "Biopiracy and Globalization: Indigenous People Face a New Wave of Colonialism," *Indigenous Peoples Coalition Against Biopiracy*. Online. Available HTTP: <http://www.ipcb.org/pub/globalization.pdf> (accessed 22 February 2002).

Harry, D. and Dukepoo, F. (1998) "Indians, Genes and Genetics: What Indians Should Know about the New Biotechnology," *Indigenous Peoples Coalition Against Biopiracy*. Online. Available HTTP: <http://www.ipcb.org/pub/primer.pdf > (accessed 22 February 2002).

Harry, D., Howard, S., and Shelton, B. (2000) "Indigenous Peoples, Genes and Genetics: What Indigenous Peoples Should Know About Biocolonialism," *Indigenous Peoples Council on Biocolonialism*. Online. Available HTTP: <http://www.ipcb.org/pub/ipgg.html> (accessed 22 February 2002).

Hawkins, D. (2001) "The Dark Side of Genetic Testing," *U.S. News & World Report*. Online. Available HTTP: <http://www.usnews.com/usnews/home.htm> (accessed 27 February 2001).

Health Canada (1999) *Diabetes in Canada: National Statistics and Opportunities for Improved Surveillance, Prevention, and Control*. Online. Available HTTP: <http://www.hc-sc.gc.ca/hpb/lcdc/publicat/diabet99/index.html> (accessed 28 February 2002).

Hegele, R. A. (1999a) "The Genetics of Type 2 Diabetes Mellitus," *Canadian Journal of Diabetes Care*, 23: 33–7.

—— (1999b) "Lessons from Genetic Studies in Native Canadian Populations," *Nutrition Review*, 57: S43–50.

Hegele, R., Cao, H., Harris, S., Hanley, A., and Zinman, B. (1999) "The Heptatic Nuclear Factor – 1alpha G319S Variant is Associated with Early-onset Diabetes in Canadian Oji-Cree," *Journal of Clinical Endocrinology and Metabolism*, 84(3): 1077–82.

Hennekens, C. and Buring, J. (eds) (1987) *Epidemiology in Medicine*, Boston: Little, Brown.

Hollan, T. (2001) "Gene Pool Expeditions: Estonians or Subjects of the Crown of Tonga: Whose Gene Pool Hides Gold?" *The Scientist*, 15(4). Online. Available HTTP: <http://www.the-scientist.com/> (accessed 19 February 2001).

Holtzman, N. (1999) "Eugenics and Genetic Testing," *Science in Context*, 11(3–4): 397–417.

Illich, I. (1976) *Medical Nemesis: The Expropriation of Health*, New York: Pantheon.

Indigenous Peoples Council on Biocolonialism (IPCB) (2000) "Indigenous Peoples Council on Biocolonialism Press Release." Online. Available HTTP: <http://www.ipcb.org/news/pressrel.html> (accessed 26 June 2000).

Inhorn, M. and Whittle, L. (2001) "Feminism Meets the 'New' Epidemiologies: Toward an Appraisal of Antifeminist Biases in Epidemiological Research on Women's Health," *Social Science & Medicine*, 53(5): 553–67.

Joe, J. and Young, R. (eds) (1994) *Diabetes as a Disease of Civilization: The Impact of Lifestyle and Cultural Changes on the Health of Indigenous Peoples*, Berlin: Mouton De Gruyter.

Kaprio, J. (2000) "Science, Medicine and the Future: Genetic Epidemiology," *British Medical Journal*, 320(7724): 1257–9.

Kay, L. (1999) "In the Beginning Was the Word: The Genetic Code and the Book of Life," in M. Biagioli (ed.) *The Science Studies Reader*, New York and London: Routledge.

Kevles, D. (1985) *In the Name of Eugenics: Genetics and the Uses of Human Heredity*, New York: Alfred A. Knopf.

Kelm, M. (1998) *Colonizing Bodies: Aboriginal Health and Healing in British Columbia, 1900–50*. Vancouver, BC: University of British Columbia Press.

Khoury, M., Beskow, L., and Gwinn, M. (2001) "Making the Vision of Genomic Medicine a Reality: Public Health Research is Key," *GeneLetter Online*. Online. Available HTTP: <http://www.geneletter.com/05-01-01/features/prn_public health.html> (accessed 1 May 2001).

Lemmens, T. and Austin, L. (2001) "Of Volume, Depth and Speed: The Challenges of Genetic Information," prepared for the Canadian Biotechnology Advisory Committee, February 2001. Online. Available HTTP: <http://cbac.gc.ca/documents/Lemmensfinal_English.pdf> (accessed 28 February 2002).

Lippman, A. (1991) "Prenatal Genetic Testing and Screening: Constructing Needs and Reinforcing Inequalities," *American Journal of Law and Medicine*, 17: 15–50.

Lone Dog, L. (1999) "Whose Genes Are They? The Human Genome Diversity Project," *Journal of Health and Social Policy*, 10(4): 51–66.

Lupton, D. (1995) *The Imperative of Health: Public Health and the Regulated Body*, London: Sage Publications.

McDermott, R. (1998) "Ethics, Epidemiology and the Thrifty Gene: Biological Determinism as a Health Hazard," *Social Science and Medicine*, 47: 1189–95.

McLaren, A. (1990) *Our Own Master Race: Eugenics in Canada, 1885–1945*, Toronto: McClelland & Stewart.

McNally, R. (1998) "Eugenics Here and Now," in P. Glasner and H. Rothman *Genetic Imaginations: Ethical, Legal and Social Issues in Human Genome Research*, Aldershot: Ashgate Publishing.

Marchand, L.H. (1999) "Obesity Associated with High Rates of Diabetes in the Pima Indians," *The Pima Indians: Pathfinders for Health*. Online. Available HTTP: <http://www.niddk.nih.gov/health/diabetes/pima/obesity/obesity.htm> (accessed 22 February 2002).

Nader, L. (ed.) (1996) *Naked Science: Anthropological Inquiry into Boundaries, Power, and Knowledge*, New York: Routledge.

Navarro, V. (1986) *Crisis, Health and Medicine: A Social Critique*, New York and London: Tavistock Publications.

Neel, J. V. (1962) "Diabetes Mellitus: A 'Thrifty' Genotype Rendered Detrimental by Progress?" *American Journal of Human Genetics*, 14: 353–62.

—— (1982) "The Thrifty Genotype Revisited," in J. Kobberling (ed.) *The Genetics of Diabetes Mellitus*, London: Academic Press.

Nelkin, D. and Lindee, M. S. (1995) *The DNA Mystique: The Gene as a Cultural Icon*, New York: Freeman.

Nelkin, D. and Tancredi, L. (1994) *Dangerous Diagnostics: The Social Power of Biological Information*, Chicago: University of Chicago Press.

O'Neil, J., Reading, J., and Leader, A. (1998) "Changing the Relations of Surveillance: The Development of a Discourse of Resistance in Aboriginal Epidemiology," *Human Organization*, 57(2): 230–7.

Palson, G. (2001) "The Genetic Saga of Icelanders," *GeneLetter Online*. Online. Available HTTP: <http://www.geneletter.com/08-15-01/features/iceland.html> (accessed 15 August 2001).

Paul, D. (1998) *The Politics of Heredity: Essays on Eugenics, Biomedicine, and the Nature–Nurture Debate*, New York: State University of New York Press.

Petersen, A. and Bunton, R. (eds) (1997) *Foucault, Health and Medicine*, New York and London: Routledge.

Rabinow, P. (1994) *Essays on the Anthropology of Reason*, New Jersey: Princeton University Press.

Rosner, M. and Johnson, T. R. (1995) "Telling Stories: Metaphors of the Human Genome Project," *Hypatia*, 10(4): 104–29.

Shelton, B. and Marks, J. (2001) "Genetic Markers – Not a Valid Test of Native Identity," *Indigenous Peoples Council on Biocolonialism*. Online. Available HTTP: <http://www.gene-watch.org/magazine/vol14/14-5nativeidentity.html> (accessed 1 May 2001).

Skinner, D. and Rosen, P. (2001) "Opening the White Box: The Politics of Racialised Science and Technology," *Science as Culture*, 10(3): 285–300.

Spurgeon, D. (1999) "'Thrifty Gene' Identified in Manitoba Indians," *British Medical Journal*, 318: 828.

Turner, B. S. (1986) *The Body and Society: Explorations in Social Theory*, Oxford: Basil Blackwell.

—— (1997) "From Governmentality to Risk: Some Reflections on Foucault's Contribution to Medical Sociology," in A. Petersen and R. Bunton (eds) *Foucault, Health and Medicine*, New York and London: Routledge.

Van Dijck, J. (1998) *Imagenation: Popular Images of Genetics*, New York: New York University Press.

Wade, N. (2001) "Genome Analysis Shows Humans Survive on Low Number of Genes," *New York Times*, 11 February 2001: 1/1. Online. Available HTTP: <http://www.nytimes.com/> (accessed 15 February 2001).

Waldrum, J. (1994) "Cultural and Socio-Economic Factors in the Delivery of Health Care Services to Aboriginal Peoples," in B. Bolaria and R. Bolaria (eds.) *Racial Minorities, Medicine and Health*, Halifax, NS: Fernwood Publishing.

Waldrum, J., Herring, A., and Young, T.K. (1995) *Aboriginal Health in Canada: Historical, Cultural and Epidemiological Perspectives*, Toronto: University of Toronto Press.

Waldrum, J., Whiting, J., Kornder, N., and Habbick, B. (2000) "Cultural Understandings and the Use of Traditional Medicine among Urban Aboriginal People with Diabetes in Saskatoon, Canada," *Canadian Journal of Diabetes Care*, 24(2): 31–8.

Waitzkin, H. (1983) *The Second Sickness*, New York: Free Press.

Wertz, D. (1998) "Eugenics Is Alive and Well: A Survey of Genetic Professionals Around the World," *Science in Context*, 11: 493–510.

Whitt, L. A. (1998) "Resisting Value-Bifurcation: Indigenist Critiques of the Human Genome Diversity Project," in B. B. On and A. Ferguson (eds) *Daring to Be Good: Essays in Feminist Ethico-Politics*, New York: Routledge.

Wotherspoon, T. and Satzewich, V. (1993) *First Nations: Race, Class and Gender Relations*, Toronto: Nelson.

Young, T. K., Reading, J., Elias, B., and O'Neil, J. (2000) "Type 2 Diabetes Mellitus in Canada's First Nations: Status of an Epidemic in Progress," *Canadian Medical Association Journal*, 163(5): 561–6.

Zuberi, T. (2000) "Deracializing Social Statistics: Problems in the Quantification of Race," *The Annals of the American Academy of Political and Social Science*, 568: 172–85.

Zwillich, T. (2001) "Human Genome Project Director Peers into the Future," *GeneLetter Online*. Online. Available HTTP: <http://www.geneletter.com/ news/ article.epl?id=265> (accessed 22 January 2001).

Part III
Regulating mobilities
Places and spaces

7 Privacy and the phenetic urge

Geodemographics and the changing spatiality of local practice

David Phillips and Michael Curry

Introduction

First the United States and then Canada and Europe have witnessed the development of what are termed "geodemographic systems" over the past thirty years. Direct marketers use these computerized systems to pinpoint mailings, and business planners use the systems to inform their planning for the best sites for new businesses and other facilities. Born through the merging of public data with private computing resources, the premise of geodemographics is that one can profitably divide the landscape into discrete spaces occupied by homogeneous groups of households and individuals. This has become a guiding practice of the marketing industry.

The developers of the systems have abjured the use of related academic work in geography, sociology, and political science, as they have sought to develop credible systems. Rather, they have appealed to the widely accepted principle that "You are where you live." In the end, it has been asserted, what is needed is simply a system that will describe individuals, households, and neighborhoods in terms of the categories to which we know they certainly belong.

Although they have continued to claim the truth of the central premise that you are where you live, users of geodemographic systems have gradually reinvented the systems, in concert with changes in the availability of different kinds of data, in computing power, and in the practitioners' understandings of society. Less noticeable has been that these changes have implications for the changing face of the lived interaction with the landscape and for the sorts of social opportunities that people in the landscape have. Even seemingly trivial changes in the systems are occasionally underlain by dramatic changes in how individuals and neighborhoods are conceptualized. Such changes may – in subtle and not-so-subtle ways – define who people are and what they can do, just as they may preclude people's involvement in the construction of those definitions.

This chapter considers these issues in four parts. The first section chronicles historical changes in the practices of the geodemographics industry. The second section describes current trends in these practices, and offers some predictions of their future shape. Both of these sections relate the practices of the industry to the availability of technology, to the availability of state-supported data collection practices, and to intra-industry corporate alignments. In the third section, we relate geodemographic practice to sociological theories of place. We suggest how and why geodemographic practice is informed by those theories, and how, in turn, those theories can help us to understand the implications of the practice, especially in terms of social categorization. The fourth section relates these practices to ideas of privacy. Our goal here is to show how geodemographic systems elicit privacy-related responses that may have broader social implications. We conclude by questioning whether privacy is an adequate principle for guiding policy and other forms of activism in response to these systems.

History of geodemographic systems

First developed in the United States, geodemographic systems are technological outgrowths of two government systems. The first is the ZIP (Zone Improvement Plan) code. Mandated as an element of President Kennedy's attempt to rationalize government, the ZIP code allowed the quantification and easy organization of both residence and business addresses for the first time. Under the ZIP code system, households were aggregated into units served by a single post office, serving at most perhaps 15,000 people, each indicated by a five-digit number. The US Postal Service simultaneously established a numbering system for postal carrier routes. Each postal carrier was assigned a two-digit number, so that ZIP codes could in turn be divided into units of approximately 800 people. As an incentive to use the systems, the Postal Service (or, actually, its predecessor, the Post Office Department) gave a discount to mass mailers who sorted their mail by carrier route. That geographical unit, defined by the daily path of the individual letter carrier, came to be the preferred unit of division.

The direct marketing industry immediately saw the advantage of directing its efforts at this geographical scale, and by 1967 articles in journals like the *Harvard Business Review* (Anonymous 1967) and *Direct Marketing* (Baier 1967) extolled the virtues of ZIP code-based marketing. In a sense, however, the systems were operating blindly. Although it was possible on the basis of carrier routes and ZIP codes to create lists of targeted households or individuals, it was not easy to translate those lists into a form that could be easily viewed and grasped.

But by the 1960s the roots of such a system were in place. The US Bureau of the Census had begun to establish first the GBF-DIME files and then the (currently used) TIGER files. These files were designated initially for urban areas, and then for the entire country, and became the basis of a computerized mapping system. The government used it for the first time in the 1970 decennial census.

More to the point here, these computerized files, consisting in part of latitude and longitude values for the four corners of every block in every city in the US, allowed – through a process of matching with the Postal Service's ZIP code files – the determination of the geographical coordinates of every mailing address in every city in the US. (Rural addresses created special problems, which have only recently begun to be resolved through new rural addressing systems, driven by the perceived need to rationalize and support emergency response, or 911, systems.) This in turn allowed the creation not merely of lists, but also of maps of ZIP codes, postal carrier routes, and so on.

By the mid-1970s two companies, CACI and Claritas (they disagree about who was first), took advantage of these developments and created what they termed "geodemographic systems." The two systems were fairly similar. Both began with census data at the level of the block group. (In the 1990 census there were 229,192 block groups, of about 1,100 people each.) Having divided the country into these 230,000 or so geographical areas, both systems used numerical taxonomy to sort and classify block groups, dividing them into a small number of like groups.

Numerical taxonomy is a sophisticated way of clustering similar individuals by imagining them to be in an N-dimensional space, where "n" is the number of socioeconomic variables. Using the roughly 600 socioeconomic variables available at the block-group level, creators of the geodemographic systems determined the distance of each of 230,000 block groups to all the others in 600-dimensional space. The ones that were "closest" were characterized as being most alike, just as the ones farthest from one another were deemed least similar.

Using the aging data from the 1970 census, and then the newer data from the 1980 tabulation, CACI and Claritas claimed that their newly created geodemographic systems proved that the roughly 230,000 block-group areas within the US consist, really, of about forty types. These can be discerned at the block-group level, or can be discerned at higher levels by aggregating block-group data to the carrier-route or ZIP-code (or other, for example, census tract, municipality, or county) level.[1]

These earliest systems, developed in an era before the advent of desktop computing, relied on computationally intensive numerical taxonomy, and ran on mainframe computers. Software was inevitably written specifically for the project at hand, and customized results were consequently expensive.

This limited the use of the systems to list filtering for mass marketers, where the postage savings for pre-sorted mail made up for the cost. Individuals and corporations also used these systems to conduct site location analyses when they wished to establish new stores or, later, to establish profitable service regions in the growing cellular-telephone market.

By the early 1990s the systems had proliferated, and their developers, now larger in number, took advantage of greater computing power, but also of a wider range of available data. In part, this involved a greater use of public records, but the systems increasingly relied upon data supplied by consumers, such as the surveys included on product registration cards. Claritas, for example, claimed in 1995 that its "analysis is drawn from as many as 500 *million* individual consumer purchase records" (Claritas 1995), while Metromail relied upon its "BehaviorBank® file containing detailed information on over 25 million survey respondents" (Metromail 1995).

At the same time, the systems began to direct their attention to smaller and smaller measurement units, down to the individual and household level. Arguing that the block-group and carrier route were so large that they inevitably were socially heterogeneous, system producers suggested that this heterogeneity was costing the users of their systems money.

The solution was to drill down, to focus on smaller geographical units. Where before 300 or 400 households seemed an appropriate unit of measure, systems users now claimed that a unit of 20 or 30 households was a better scale. Such a unit would be more homogeneous and thus more likely to produce better results. Indeed, one company asserted that any region larger than a building lot would lead to inaccurate results:

> DNA assigns households with similar characteristics to one of 104 Cells that recognizes those characteristics using individual data about that specific household, combined with relevant geo-demographic data. So you can separate the David Larsons of the world from the newlyweds next door and the retired army sergeant across the street.
>
> (Metromail 1995)

This period also saw a proliferation of producers of the systems. CACI and Claritas were joined by R. R. Donnelley (a mass mailer), which produced Metromail, by R. L. Polk, which presented a product called "Niches," and significantly, by credit reporting veterans Trans-Union and Equifax. Trans-Union marketed its "Solo" product as, like Metromail's DNA, "using individual-level spending and payment data – plus an individual's age and income – to create clusters of people whose behavior reflects a particular lifestyle and buying pattern" (Trans-Union 1994). And Equifax's "MicroVision" was the result of combining aggregated consumer demand data with census data into a system built at the ZIP+4 level of geography. This creates an exact profile of your best customers and allows you to target as few as five to 15 households, instead of the 300 households or traditional targeting systems.

(Equifax: National Decision Systems 1991)

Trends

The geodemographic industry was founded upon resources generated by public programs. These programs – ZIP codes, census data, and 911 address standardization – produced standardized regions as well as locational data (that is, latitude and longitude information) for particular entities. These standard regions were not developed for the specific requirements of the geodemographic industry. Nevertheless, the industry used these legacy regions as the foundation of their marketing analysis. System improvement was marked by the ability to define, categorize, and target smaller and smaller fixed regions.

Through most of the 1990s, even as the geodemographic industry appealed to regions that were smaller and smaller, it was practically committed to a system based on these stable, well-defined regions, and a relatively small and stable set of classificatory types with which to categorize those regions. Through the mid-1990s there was an increasing number of producers of geodemographic systems, but the producers nonetheless tended to create systems that were similar to one another. Focused on site location and on direct marketing, they provided results, in the form of maps or lists, to queries posed by their customers. They promoted their products by attending to the quality of the final product itself. And they shared the view that the world can be divided into regions that are, in effect, containers of like-minded and like-lifestyled households and individuals.

But current trends in geodemographics are moving from this view of the world as consisting of fixed places – at any scale – within which people live similar lifestyles. Rather, the systems increasingly embody – and promote – a different way of thinking about the behavior of individuals and households.

Here we in fact see two trends. The first is a new attention to what are viewed as temporally fluid regions. Alongside its traditional household-based Prizm clustering system Claritas has developed "Workplace Prizm," a geodemographic system that for the first time recognizes that the demographics of American cities during the day are dramatically different from their demographics during the evening and night. In effect – although the application of the systems is still remarkably primitive – Claritas has recognized that they can only understand certain elements of people's behavior if they first acknowledge that people are mobile, and that they routinely move from home to work and back (as well as, of course, to school, and so on).

The second trend is the development of location-based services (LBS). These services are primarily designed to coordinate or assist the activities of mobile individuals as they pass through stable regions. LBS uses GPS (Global Positioning System) or other means to obtain locational information from their clients and chart the course of their activities using existing maps. These services range from call-center services, mobile-resource dispatch, and fleet and asset monitoring, to mobile marketing. This market is poised to increase rapidly both in size and scope. Predictions are that within the next several years (i.e., 2004–6) it will be a $20 to $40 billion dollar market, with perhaps 18 million subscribers in the US alone. Moreover, analysts predicted that only 50 percent will use the automobile-mounted devices, like OnStar, that account for virtually all of the market today; the remainder will use hand-held or body-mounted devices, such as cell phones or wireless, web-enabled Personal Digital Assistants (PDAs) (Gibbons 2001).

These two developments – the recognition of temporal changes in the character of regions and the interest in tracking mobile individuals – are obviously closely connected. Each involves the development of systems capable of tracking the movement of individuals. And each points to the possibility of collecting information about those movements, or of sending information to people based on their locations.

Two factors have been especially influential in the latest development of geodemographic systems. The first is the role of government-subsidized information. Especially critical here have been global positioning systems, the development of which was originally financed and implemented by the US Department of Defense. Also, US Federal legislation now mandates that mobile telecommunications devices transmit, under certain circumstances, their location. Both of these systems, but especially the latter, have the potential not only to provide enormous amounts of raw data to the marketing industry, but also to enhance their ability to deliver messages to particular types of people in particular types of places at particular times.

The second factor has been economic, in the form of a dramatic shakeout in the industry. By the year 2000 a number of companies (Polk, for example) had gotten out of the business. Claritas had acquired a number of products, notably Equifax's National Decision Systems (NDS) and Microvision, from former competitors. Claritas itself had become a unit of VNU Marketing Inc., which also owns A. C. Nielsen. As a consequence, the current market is dominated by two original geodemographic-system providers – Claritas and CACI – and by consumer-credit giant Experian. In Great Britain Experian is the prime purveyor of the systems, and in Canada Compusearch, now owned by US-based MapInfo, is the industry leader. At the same time, each company has developed connections with other supporting companies. Claritas, for example, relies upon the US Postal Service for address lists. It also calls upon Geographic Data Technologies, whose founder, Don Cooke, is often seen as the father of geodemographics, for enhanced geographic boundary files. It has an agreement with Oracle for database support. And it has a strong connection with MapInfo, one of the leading producers of a wide range of mapping systems, including classic geographic information systems, web-based consumer systems, and systems for support of Enhanced 911 and other public-service applications. And so, while the government has been an active player in the development of geodemographic systems through its promotion of global positioning and emergency response systems, the industry itself increasingly consists of corporations that have access to and work with a wide range of data, from emergency response and intelligent transportation systems, to census data and consumer credit and purchase data. These data increasingly exist in databases in which they are or may easily be geocoded.[2]

Marketers as practical geographers

The previous sections have placed geodemographic trends in a technological and economic perspective. In the following section we introduce certain ideological claims. That is, we wish to trace the ways in which the sociological and geographical understandings of the developers of these systems and the systems themselves have been mutually influential.

Before the early nineteenth century, spatial segregation in American society was quite complex. In some cases it was vertical, with the poor living on upper floors of buildings, and the wealthy on lower floors (Warner 1968). In other cases, there was substantial differentiation at the local scale, with wealthier people living in front lots and the poor in back lots on the same street (Groves and Muller 1975; Pessen 1976).

Indeed, the now-familiar forms of horizontal segregation, emblematic of the idea that you are where you live, developed only through the nineteenth century, as a result of a growing middle class wishing to express its new status. At the same time, they wished to attain a degree of distinction from the less well-off people whom they had economically left behind (Johnson 1978). Each small region or neighborhood came to be seen as a place wherein a like-minded group could attain a degree of separation from others – outsiders – while remaining assured in the belief that their neighbors were, in fact, like them.

The ideal, if not the practice, of locational marketing can be found in this historical moment. Regional space was considered a container people occupied without really affecting. This ideal was based not only on sociological theory (or mythic perceptions of America) but also on the technological constraints of geodemographic systems. These systems were built upon legacy definitions of particular regions – the ZIP code, the census tract. Although any entity could access specific locational data, longitude and latitude data for instance, these entities were already organized and constructed as a set of relatively stable geographic regions. Each of these neighborhoods could be conceptualized as a container, within which there were households and residents who occupied that neighborhood, much like sardines in a can. That is, their inhabiting a neighborhood was simply a matter of being there; it was fundamentally passive. Computational energy was spent, not in redefining regions, but in defining a set of classificatory categories, and assigning the extant regions to those categories.

But with the 1960s, even as the flight to the suburbs continued, and even as this sociological ideal was being implemented in working geodemographic systems, the nation was increasingly rent by schism. The notion of the suburbs, or of any segment of American life, as united by a set of core values or ideals, was increasingly challenged. The very premise of locational marketing – the social cohesion of neighborhoods – was increasingly questionable. Marketers responded with the technological means at their command, and within a conservative ideological framework. They made their locational analysis more and more precise in the desperate belief that at some level – if not 40,000 people then 1,000 people, and if not there, well, then 40 people – they could discover and resuscitate the ideal refuge of a like-minded group of neighbors.

The increasing availability of ever more precise locational data as well as ever more abundant personal information, and marketers' sense of devolving social cohesion, have gradually led to a constantly narrowing definition of the "where" of "you are where you live." Now, only your skin marks the boundaries of your physical extension.

Thus, "lifestyle" marketing has, in a sense, reached both the logical extreme and the antithesis of locational marketing. In carrying "you are where you live" to its technological and analytic extreme, it has turned on itself. The spatial container is no longer recognized as the primary definer of its individual contents. In response, marketers and demographers have begun to understand regions themselves as constituted by the patterns of activity of individuals.

Technological advances, in the forms of GPS and other location data gathering and delivery systems, facilitate and encourage these new understandings. Meanwhile, scholars of a wide range of philosophical and political predispositions have also come to argue for a way of thinking about geographical space that recognizes that said space – the neighborhood, the block, and so on – is in fact a social construction, and one inevitably in the process of reconstruction (Augé 1995; Curry forthcoming; Harvey 1989; Tuan 1977). Indeed, this view has been expressed in a range of scales, from the local, where it has been explicit at least since the work of Jane Jacobs, to the global, where Castells has argued for an understanding of a new economy of flows (Castells 1997).

Motivated, it would seem, by a dramatically different set of concerns, the new geodemographics is nonetheless an expression of that same view. For here the focus has moved to the individual, one who is sometimes at home, sometimes at work, and sometimes in between. The individual is an active geographical agent, making decisions on the fly, as opportunities arise. And here those decisions seem inevitably to occasion responses on the part of the users of the systems, just because the systems for the first time allow immediate validation of their worth. If a store uses a geodemographic system to offer electronic coupons to people walking by, or if a digital sign promoting a sale is set to appeal to an especially large group of people with certain tastes, again known to be walking or driving by, the utility of the system is immediately evident. Thus, just as from a philosophical point of view the new systems are fulfillments of the desire for a richer way of understanding people's geographical behavior, they are also themselves active agents in manipulating that behavior to create "ideal" geographies.

"Privacy" and geodemographic systems

If the mutual construction of ideal individuals, behaviors, and places in the service of market efficiency is an issue of some public concern – and, like other contributors to this volume, we believe that it is – then it is legitimately the focus of media attention. The quality of this attention is important in that it will "frame" the systems in the public consciousness. These "issue frames" act partially to circumscribe public understanding and "promote a particular problem definition, causal interpretation, moral evaluation, and/or treatment recommendation" (Entman 1993: 52). Frames both reflect and constrain the social response to these systems. To be effectively mobilizing, issue frames should place practices within a cognitive schema of social life that is as familiar, compelling, complex, and robust as possible (Gamson 1988; Snow *et al.* 1986). Yet it appears that the discursive framing of geodemographic systems has promoted a narrow and simplistic understanding of their social importance.

Privacy has served as a primary coordinating concept that frames concerns about geodemographic systems. Privacy is, admittedly, an overloaded word. We may in fact identify at least three recent forms of privacy concern. The first concern is primarily about intrusion into personal places or "space."

From this perspective, privacy is a matter of individual rights and autonomy, and privacy can be "invaded." More recently, in response to corporate practices of automated data collection, collation, and analysis, privacy activists have come to believe that the most important privacy concern may be not the invasion of one's personal space, but rather bureaucratic market management through social discrimination (Gandy 1993). "Redlining" and demographic profiling have come to be seen as privacy concerns. Finally, some sociologists and political scientists have argued that the critical privacy issue is what informs the decision to appropriately distinguish between public issues and private issues (Boling 1996).[3] All of these meanings of "privacy" may be implicated in our understanding of geodemographic systems.

The historical and geographical root of these systems, that is, the construction of and flight to homogeneous suburban neighborhoods, reflects the first type of privacy concern – a concern with the isolated and protected home, a desire for sidewalks free from the jostlings of the other. It was this concern with the protection of the homogeneity of the neighborhood that in fact led to the practice of redlining. This practice was widely criticized – and often rendered illegal – as recently as the 1960s. Yet at the time, redlining was understood not as a privacy issue at all, but rather was viewed as an issue of discrimination.

The early development of geodemographic systems in the 1970s was barely noted. Indeed, it was not really until Michael Weiss's (1988) admiring series of books, beginning with *The Clustering of America* in 1988, that the average person would have had the slightest reason to know of their existence. In a way, this is remarkable, since the systems seem on their face to be little more than high-tech means for redlining, which, as we have mentioned, was an issue of some public salience. However, the invisibility of the systems, and hence the public silence about them, can perhaps be explained by the institutional context of their operation. As we have mentioned, they were special-purpose programs, written to order for particular clients, and they ran on largely invisible mainframes.

During the 1980s, techniques of personal data collection and analysis insinuated themselves more strongly into everyday life. Scholars began to link the historical problems of redlining with the reawakened concern for personal privacy, and so introduced social discrimination to the realm of privacy issues. However, scholarly concern rarely focused on geodemographics in particular; instead it concentrated on more general concerns of individual profiling and categorization.

Since the 1970s, and especially since the explosive popularity of the Internet in the mid-1990s, the popular media has linked new data-collection techniques with privacy concerns. However, rather than building on the scholarship linking bureaucratic social management, personal data collection, privacy, and discrimination, media discourse employed and continues to employ what can only be termed regressive privacy frames. That is, the discourse has focused on the personal affronts associated with personal data collection – identity theft, high-tech "peeping Tom"-ism, and annoying telemarketing calls. At the same time, it has ignored structural effects – the management of taste, increased inequity in market knowledge, and the creation of a society fractured into increasingly precise and exclusive market segments. The discourse has identified the victims as unrelated individuals, rather than as members of a social order.

There are some signs that this trend is shifting. Occasionally, popular press articles address the use of personal information in the manipulation of consumer tastes, especially in the targeting of children as consumers. But in geodemographics we see an interesting and almost paradoxical counter-trend. As the creators of geodemographic systems have begun to shift their data-collection and delivery mechanisms to a cell phone or PDA carried on a person's body, they have come more into the public consciousness, and have in this way begun to make privacy issues appear salient. But because the collection and delivery mechanism is so intimately connected to the body, the focus of those privacy issues has reverted again to the personal affront. The collation and analysis of personal data, and the discriminatory classi-fication of individuals, has taken a back seat to issues of trespass and nuisance. This is in marked contrast to the issues of redlining and community harm the public raised when geodemographics first attained recognition.

It would be an overstatement to suggest that the discourse is devoid of concerns about the processes of discrimination and categorization. A geo-demographic system linked to a realtor's home page which directed inquirers to neighborhoods "similar" to the ones in which they were currently living raised considerable public ire and accusations of racial discrimination, and was quickly removed from the host site (Helperin and Doocey 2000). A geodemographic system used to locate ATM machines based on neighbor-hood crime statistics was clearly identified as a technology for redlining, though the discrimination was considered reasonable since it was formally unrelated to racial markers (Lubove 1999).

Nevertheless, we see the dominant regressive trend in the privacy discourse shaped by the producers' product literature, which pays considerable attention to the need to avoid "violating a person's privacy" by sending unwanted advertising to her cellular telephone or other wireless device. These concerns are echoed in the business press (Fawcett 2000; Hawkins 2000; Mack 2000; Nobel and Callaghan 2000), which also emphasizes the privacy violations that occur through incessant tracking of an individual's movements (Montfort 2000). The business press also refers to the three-inch square PDA screen as valuable "real estate," not to be trespassed upon by uninvited ads (Black 2000; Weisler and O'Brien 2001). It is shaped by policies that suggest the solution lies in the control of "personally identifiable information." Such solutions suggest that the problem lies in the identification of individuals, not the categorization and characterization of groups or regions. Indeed, when social categorization is mentioned, it is lauded as the ideal goal, that which will make the problems of privacy disappear. In a perfectly managed consumer environment, desires are predicted (or manufactured) and sated before they have fully entered the consumer's consciousness (Williamson 2000).

So, recognizing the constitutive roles that individuals play in shaping the character of regions, geodemographic systems increasingly focus on the individual as the source of data and the object of persuasion, while the instrumental goal of that persuasion is rationalized, idealized, and manageable social landscapes. Meanwhile, discourse about these systems, by employing a narrow understanding of "privacy," focuses attention only on the individual, obscuring the power of geodemographics to model, characterize, and categorize individuals and social relations, and to reify those models.

Finally, we turn our attention to the third sense of "the privacy problem." What, in fact, is a legitimate public issue? Specifically, we believe that in a vibrant democracy the social, economic, and cultural implications of the wireless 911 system should be the subject of robust debate. Like the ZIP code, the census, and land-based 911 systems before them, they are a publicly funded mandate to generate and rationalize vast amounts of data concerning social activity. Yet there is no evidence that editors of popular news outlets even consider them newsworthy. They cover these systems, but as far as we have found, only in terms of political intrigue or conflicts between competing telecommunication companies.

There are alternative solutions to the wireless 911 mandate, and these solutions have enormous implications for the ability to collect locational information. Briefly, one type of solution has locational capabilities embedded in the handset. The owner of the handset can, theoretically at least, control whether to release that locational data. The other type of solution places all locational capabilities with the network operator, which tracks handsets willy-nilly. The latter potentially throws off a gusher of valuable data. The business press acknowledges the private value of locational information, made available in part by the publicly mandated E911 system (Savage and Stirpe 2000; Stirpe 2001), but the popular press has failed to follow their lead.

There is another sense in which the public domain becomes privatized through new developments in geodemographic systems. That is the degree to which the character of lived regions becomes the product of the goals and strategies of ever fewer, more interlinked, well-capitalized, and private corporate interests. Corporate and state bodies have always been significant actors in the social construction of place. Historically, though, the mechanisms of those actions have at least been visible and – to a certain degree – opposable. Highway projects loom large on the fiscal and public horizon before they are actually built. The effects of redlines are enduring, relatively stable, and noticeable. However, new systems have the potential to allow the instantaneous reconfiguring of spatial elements toward any emergent strategic end. The spatial contours of places will become more fluid, and the means by which the existence, the meaning, and the social importance of places are negotiated will become more fast-paced, and less visible to their inhabitants.

Conclusion

We have outlined several contradictory, and even paradoxical, trends in geodemographic practice. The sociological belief that "you are where you live" has fostered a drive to understand "where you live." Using whatever computational techniques and data that were currently available, marketers have been able to define place more precisely – from ZIP code, to census tract, and finally to houschold – until the notion of a social and spatial context for individual action virtually disappeared. Locational marketing, in a way, contained the seed of its own demise.

Recently, there has been a resurgence of interest in the spatial contexts of individual action, especially as those contexts change as individuals move through them. This interest has been awakened in part because new technologies permit the tracking of mobile individuals. In this case, geographical theories have been appealed to because measurement techniques at last make them operationally viable. So, just as a focus on region devolved into a focus on the individual inhabitant, the focus on the individual has been replaced by an interest in the space of the individual.

The region, then, has renewed interest for demographers and marketers. However, there is an important distinction between the old and new understandings of region. Where once regions and neighborhoods and places were seen as stable containers for certain populations and activities, they are now understood as fluid, both temporally and spatially, and even as products of their inhabitants' actions. Since regions are created by the behavior of individual inhabitants, the goal becomes to influence those behaviors through direct, persuasive appeals. Regions are managed by managing individuals.

This constant play between the construction of the individuals and of their social contexts is mirrored in the privacy discourse associated with these practices. The social discrimination connected with old geodemographic practices – redlining, for example – was adopted into privacy discourse as geodemography became more and more concerned with defining the individual, rather than the region. The "issue frame" of social discrimination permitted privacy activists to suggest that the problem was deeper, more important, and more complex than invasion of "private" territory. Whatever rhetorical and theoretical ground this frame has provided, it is in danger of being whittled away, as marketers and news providers focus on the intrusive, rather than classificatory and discriminatory, aspects of the locational tracking and targeting of individuals. It is ironic that this frame may be losing its power just as marketers return their attention to the construction of regions, from which the frame derived its power in the first place.

The evolution of marketing and demographic practice has been fundamentally influenced by national policy. ZIP codes, census data and 911 addressing have all contributed to the data collection and message delivery process. More importantly, though, they have provided the "legacy" regions upon which the geodemographic industry was built and continues to prosper. As the industry moves away from those regions, however, it is turning again to a font of data provided as a byproduct of wireless 911 systems. Again, geodemographics prospers through federal mandate.

These findings have implications for policy makers and activists. First, 911 policy should recognize the privacy implications of the technological systems that are implemented. Moreover, the definition of privacy concerns should include not merely tracking or intrusion, but the value, and the effects, of data as they are collected and collated, even without reference to a particular individual. Activists might take advantage of the heightened interest in privacy, even as that interest is expressed through the limited frame of intrusion, to broaden definition of privacy to include social well-being and the autonomy and power to create community.

Acknowledgement

This research was partially funded through the National Science Foundation Award #SES-0083348 and through the Academic Senate of the University of California, Los Angeles. David Phillips would particularly like to thank Karen Gustafson for her invaluable assistance.

Notes

1   In what has come to be an emblematic difference between the two corporations, CACI categorized these in dull numerical and socioeconomic terms, such as "IV.3. Upper middle class," while Claritas used categories like "furs and station wagons" and "Archie Bunker's neighborhood."
2   MapInfo's MapMarker, for example, allows the user to "Geocode your entire Oracle database – matching address information with map coordinates,

transforming it into spatial data. MapInfo's MapMarker® gives you complete geocoding information for the entire U.S., and other solutions are available internationally" (MapInfo 2001).

3 For an extensive discussion of the many social meanings of "privacy," see Zureik in this volume.

Bibliography

Anonymous (1967) "Zip Code – New Look in Mail Marketing," *Direct Marketing*, 30(4): 30–2.

Augé, M. (1995) *Non-Places: Introduction to an Anthropology of Supermodernity*, London: Verso.

Baier, M. (1967) "Zip Code – New Tool for Marketers," *Harvard Business Review* 45(1): 136–40.

Black, J. (2000) "Old Ads, New Metric," *Internet World*, 16(5): 28.

Boling, P. (1996) *Privacy and the Politics of Intimate Life*, Ithaca: Cornell University Press.

Castells, M. (1997) *End of Millennium. Vol. 3: Information Age: Economy, Society, and Culture*, Oxford: Blackwell.

Claritas (1995) "Prizm: The Precision Tool for Neighborhood Lifestyle Segmentation," Ithaca: Claritas.

Curry, M. R. (forthcoming) "Discursive Displacement and the Seminal Ambiguity of Space and Place," in L. Lievrouw and S. Livingstone (eds) *Handbook on New Media*, Beverly Hills, CA: Sage Publications.

Entman, R.M. (1993) "Framing: Toward Clarification of a Fractured Paradigm," *Journal of Communication*, 43: 51–8.

Equifax: National Decision Systems (1991) "Microvision: The Microgeographic Consumer Targeting System," Atlanta: Equifax.

Fawcett, A. W. (2000) "Media Eye Mobile Marketing," *Advertising Age*, 6 March: S24.

Gamson, W. A. (1988) "A Constructionist Approach to Mass Media and Public Opinion," *Symbolic Interaction*, 11: 161–74.

Gandy, O. (1993) *The Panoptic Sort: A Political Economy of Personal Information*, Boulder: Westview.

Gibbons, G. (2001) "Location-Based Services," *GPS World*, 12(4): 30.

Groves, P. A. and Muller, E. K. (1975) "The Evolution of Black Residential Areas in Late Nineteenth Century Cities," *Journal of Historical Geography*, 1: 169–92.

Harvey, D. (1989) *The Condition of Postmodernity: An Enquiry into the Origins of Cultural Change*, New York: Basil Blackwell.

Hawkins, D. (2000) "Will Cellphones Be Stoolies?" *US News and World Report*, 129(21): 74.

Helperin, K. and Doocey, P. (2000) "Wells Fargo Online Service Accused of Redlining," *Bank Systems + Technology*, 37(9): 19.

Johnson, P.E. (1978) *A Shopkeeper's Millennium: Society and Revivals in Rochester, New York, 1815–1837*, 1st edn, New York: Hill and Wang.

Lubove, S. (1999) "Redlining Software," *Forbes*, 5 April: 53(1).

Mack, A.M. (2000) "Unplugged," *Brandweek*, 41(36): 50.

MapInfo (2001) "Spatialware." Online. Available HTTP: <http://www.mapinfo.com/community/free/library/spatialware_brochure.pdf>(accessed 30 April 2001).

Metromail (1995) "DNA: Defining the Individual," Oakbrook, IL: Metromail.

Montfort, N. (2000) "You Are Here – Location-based Services and GPS Gadgets are Homing In," *Ziff Davis Smart Business for the New Economy*, 1 October: 42.

Nobel, C. and Callaghan, D. (2000) "Wireless Services Hit Snags," eWeek, 18 December: 15.

Pessen, E. (1976) "The Social Configuration of the Antebellum City: An Historical and Theoretical Inquiry," *Journal of Urban History*, 2: 267–306.

Savage, M. and Stirpe, A. (2000) "Under Surveillance: Location-based Wireless Technology Raises Privacy Concerns for Solution Providers," *Computer Reseller News*, 4 December: 32.

Snow, D. A., Burke Rochford, E., Worden, S. K., and Benford, R. D. (1986) "Frame Alignment Processes, Micromobilization, and Movement Participation," *American Sociological Review*, 51: 464–81.

Stirpe, A. (2001) "Location, Location, Location: Solution Providers Make Use of Tracking Technologies," *Computer Reseller News*, 12 February: 51.

Trans-Union (1994) "Solo: Bringing New Focus to Market Segmentation," Chicago: Trans-Union.

Tuan, Y. (1977) *Space and Place: The Perspective of Experience*, Minneapolis: University of Minnesota Press.

Warner, S. B. (1968) *The Private City: Philadelphia in Three Periods of its Growth*, Philadelphia: University of Pennsylvania Press.

Weisler, M. and O'Brien, J. (2001) "Establish Trust – or Bust," *Brandweek*, 42: 13.

Weiss, M. J. (1988) *The Clustering of America*, New York: Harper and Row.

Williamson, D. A. (2000) "Forget about Wired, the Future Is Wireless," *Advertising Age*, 6 March: S18.

8   People and place

Patterns of individual identification within intelligent transportation systems

Colin Bennett, Charles Raab,
and Priscilla Regan

Introduction

One of the most interesting and perhaps ambitious applications of geographic information technologies is the development of Intelligent Transportation Systems (ITS). Implementation of ITS requires the application of technologies to both roadways and vehicles to perform surveillance, communications, data processing, traffic control and navigational tasks.[1] The range of ITS is extensive, and includes services such as the wireless provision of traffic information to drivers, law enforcement, the management of commercial vehicle fleets, environmental regulation, the provision of route and location information to the traveler, and – the topic of this chapter – electronic toll collection.

In this chapter,[2] we compare the implementation of three current systems of road toll collection: the 407 Highway system in Toronto, Ontario; the Smart Tag system in Virginia; and, more briefly, the Dartford River Crossing in England. Potentially, the systems allow an almost unparalleled level of tracking of vehicle users. A host of questions are relevant: To what extent is this actually occurring? What sorts of data are collected, and to what extent do vehicle users know about these collection and processing activities and have control over them? Are data matching and integration occurring, and what are the implications for individual privacy? Are these systems tracking vehicles as they cross geographically situated toll collection centers? What are the intended and unintended consequences for power relations between public and private agencies, on the one hand, and individuals, on the other?

These questions frame a partial agenda for investigating ITS, and geographic information systems (GIS) generally. Such investigation is important because the implementation of surveillance systems to track human movement is rapidly becoming a common practice. Its trajectory has outpaced the ability of theory, research and regulatory policy adequately to comprehend or control it, although ITS has attracted attention in academic as well as regulatory policy circles (Agre and Harbs 1994; Wright 1995). Empirical studies of how ITS works, and of its contexts, are not yet so prolific as to confirm or reject the forebodings of those who directly, and in our view incautiously, read off human consequences from the technological possibilities of ITS and GIS. Yet human processes related to mobility – movement through space – have become a focus of attention in a wide variety of organizations and jurisdictions for which mobility is either a problem or an opportunity.

Data-handling systems for locating, identifying and recording persons' behavior and preferences, including the authentication of individuals' claims, provide the infrastructure for many processes. These include electronic commerce and the electronic delivery of public services, but with more particular reference to ITS, they include the control of physical movement across borders and the control of access to premises and other spaces. Within or alongside these processes are further examples: the provision of services or goods to those on the move, the extraction of payment for the movement itself, the monitoring of the volume and speed of movement, and the tracking of criminal suspects in transit.[3] "Surveillance" is the term that most usefully embraces these activities.[4]

Although we cannot here explore the complex issues involved in human identity and identification, they are at the heart of our inquiries into ITS and other applications of GIS. They also reinforce a view of the broadly political nature of ITS and GIS insofar as these systems affect the distribution of values within and across societies, and affect the fate of persons and groups. More concretely, the "politics" of ITS and GIS – which we barely touch on here – involves decision-making concerning the application of technologies to the purposes of government and the economy, and the implementation of rules for their use. But the significance of these systems goes beyond the political into more intimate realms of identity, and into the relationship between persons and the larger structures of states, economies, and – in the present case – systems for allowing, constraining and keeping track of human physical mobility.

Among other observers, sociologists and anthropologists have long viewed human identity as multiple and fluid. Individuals routinely act differently in different contexts, adopting different roles in different social settings. The ability to negotiate social contexts is essential to sociability and individuality (Goffman 1959). At the same time, cultural and social geographers have shown that in many cases the contexts within which identities are established are places and, to a large degree, human identity is tied to the places within which people work, shop, play, and carry on many other activities central to their lives (Duncan and Agnew 1990; Tuan 1982).

Moreover, students of bureaucratic and industrial processes have shown that knowledge of social and geographical identities has come to be seen as essential to the management of these institutions (Beniger 1986).

As a consequence, government and industry have become increasingly interested in the development of technological systems that will be able to organize, and make accessible in a geographically coded form, information about individual activities. If these information systems constitute an institution's way of knowing individuals, their relationships, and their contexts, these organizations themselves inevitably develop within institutional milieus that favor particular ways of knowing and particular purposes for knowing. Individuals and locations are understood, classified, and acted upon according to the needs and abilities of the designers and operators of the information systems.

The concept of personal identity is a problematic and theoretical focus in several of the social sciences as well as in philosophy. Checking identity is also an issue for states, governments and public policy. Is it worrisome and regrettable that the way in which "identity" features in discourse and practice differs so widely between these two domains, the academic and the practical? Moreover, the values, views, and goals which information systems facilitate may be very different from those of the subject population itself. Where theorists problematize identity, and often take the individual's perspective from the bottom up, practitioners seek to stabilize it through an administrative perspective in which identities are attributed, recorded and categorized in ways that are often independent of place, time and context. Once assigned to a category, it is difficult to transfer to another, or to invoke the situational subtleties that belie categorization (Bowker and Star 1999). With regard to movement, identity is never straightforward. Persons who seek to travel across national borders are normally required to reveal their identity and thus establish their right to travel from one country to the other. What are they required to reveal about themselves? Or, to put it another way, what can be said about the categories within which the person's identity is established? Are these definitions incontestable, and can they ever be definitive?

Information systems instantiate the values, epistemologies, and ontologies of their creators and impose them on their subjects (Agre 1994). Indeed, if these systems are often invisible to their subjects, they very often operate in terms of schemes of categorization that would be quite foreign to those subjects. Social identities "do not derive from the self-reflexive acts of individual egos, but from traces of behavior pertinent to the apparatuses of consumer and state surveillance" (Frohmann 1994: 9). Individuals may not even be aware of their inclusion in particular groups. Similarly, in geographic information technologies, places are seen as locations to which individuals are only contingently attached . . . [T]he traditional practices of place formation and sources of attachment to place disappear . . . to be a part of a place is simply to maintain the right set of socioeconomic characteristics.

(Curry 1997: 682)

Thus the processes of ascribed identification, and the geographic information technologies that sustain them, implicitly challenge the possibility of consent, an important requisite of liberal societies and political systems. Yet users of GIS must come to terms with the requirements of data protection, including consent, if individuals can be identified in locational data. This is especially true where such data are matched in order to profile groups and individuals according to categories that are commercially or governmentally relevant. This reconciliation may be particularly problematic as data-protection laws, rulings and interpretations of the principles of fair information practice change in the direction of more stringent requirements or of broader coverage. Among the most salient conflicts that relate to GIS and other systems of data is that between the acknowledged usefulness of these databases and technologies in commerce, planning, policy-making and daily life, and the right or claim of individuals and groups to the protection of their privacy. These conflicts may turn upon questions of identity: users of categorization schemes "know" a person by these devices, yet the person "knows" who she is, and perhaps disputes the users' "knowledge." How can conflicts be resolved between "we tell you who you are" and "I tell you who I am"?

These scenarios and questions usually imply a context of stable social phenomena and more or less settled identities by which persons are known, but other contexts are of increasing importance. David Lyon argues that "[m]obility creates a world of nomads and unsettled social arrangements . . . it is not surprising that in transit areas, such as airports, surveillance practices are intense" (Lyon 2001: 19). He draws particular attention to one consequence of movement: because we are in very frequent contact with strangers, both parties require "tokens of trust," such as identity documents and other stable proofs of who we are (Lyon 2001: 81–2). Of particular relevance to this chapter is that information about mobile persons is also collected and transmitted in situations where the need for fast, efficient implementation of certain functional requirements, such as road-toll payment, has stimulated the development of systems to replace cash with other transactional methods.

These are less dramatic circumstances than the scenarios of nomads, migrants, and unsettled social arrangements. For them, the rationale for surveillance and tracking is related to the maintenance of public order and perhaps also to sovereignty questions of policing national borders. Yet with toll payments, it is important for road operators to verify the vehicle's payment by collecting and matching its classification and registration (license) number plate, in order to detect violations and fraud. These technological mechanisms thus record and allow the use of data capable of identifying individuals and tracking their movements. ITS technologies, however, can be applied not only to payment functions, but also to communications, traffic management, and navigation. Global positioning systems (GPS) provide the driver with the vehicle's location, but may also allow a surveillant to track the vehicle's movement. Sophisticated technological devices provide route guidance to drivers, as well as information about traffic and weather conditions, accidents and hazards, and the vehicle's proximity to services and goods.

All these technologies, in principle, could allow anonymity by concealing the identity of the traveler. In practice, however, information can be processed in ways that violate the traveler's reasonable expectation of privacy. As an attorney with the USA's Federal Highway Administration observes: "While driving is a public behavior, the ability to compile information about an individual's driving behavior, travel patterns, toll payments and other travel activity creates the potential for a database which has not previously existed in an easily accessible format" (Dingle 1995: 18–19). ITS systems therefore pose sharp challenges to regulatory regimes that are concerned to protect privacy, but they also provide possibilities for designing privacy protection into the technologies themselves (Agre 1995: 129–33; Alpert 1995: 115–16; Halpern 1995: 70–2).

With these theoretical issues in mind, we now turn to the comparative analysis of three contemporary road toll collection systems in Toronto, Ontario, Virginia and Southeast England.

The 407 Express Toll Route in Toronto

The 407 Express Toll Route (ETR) runs east–west just north of the city of Toronto, Ontario. It was begun in 1993 and since 2001, the extensions now stretch 108 km through one of Canada's most densely populated urban environments and busiest transportation corridors. It has the most frequent interchanges (every 2.3 km) of any similar highway in existence.[5] Around 97 percent of current users are from within the province of Ontario.

The original purpose was solely to relieve traffic congestion. The Ontario government developed the highway from the outset as an electronic toll route, however, to reduce the burden on taxpayers and to expedite construction. The government created a separate Crown Agency, the Ontario Transportation Capital Corporation (OTCC), to complete the highway by working in partnership with a variety of private sector corporations (407 ETR

2001). In 1999 all responsibility for the management of the highway and the collection of tolls was passed over to a private corporation, 407 International Inc., which is now the sole shareholder, operator, and manager of the highway (407 ETR 2001). The government still owns the land, leased to 407 ETR, and is involved in case of any wider land usage issues. The Ontario Ministry of Transportation also maintains an auditing role under the controlling legislation (the 1998 "407 Highway Traffic Act"), and the concession lease agreement.

The technology is innovative, and to date unprecedented. The ETR's toll collection technology has five main components: the vehicle transponders (leased by the vehicle owner and portable between vehicles of the same class); the vehicle recognition and identification system; the roadside toll collection system; the toll transaction processor; and the revenue management system. The 407 ETR is currently the only multiple entry and exit automatic toll road in existence. Instead of tollbooths or plazas, 28 separate interchanges on the highway, each defined by an overhead tolling gantry, automatically record the beginning and end of the trip. The equipment logs the entrance and exit of the vehicle from the highway by reading the transponder attached to the inside of the front windshield. On exit, a green light on the transponder and four short beeps indicate the toll transaction has been successfully completed. Highway 407 users are billed once a month.

Transponders are mandatory for any heavy vehicle (over 5 tons) traveling the 407 under the Ontario Highway Traffic Act. There are both practical and economic reasons for this. The rear license plate of any training vehicle is not necessarily registered to the driver or owner of the truck itself, so the license plate would not necessarily match with the registered owner. Moreover, rear license plates are often obscured from video cameras on heavy vehicles. The OTCC also wanted to ensure a level playing field for all commercial vehicles, and did not want to put domestic industry at a competitive disadvantage with out-of-province or international vehicles. Owners of lighter vehicles who are frequent users of the highway are strongly encouraged, but not required, to register and lease a transponder from the 407 ETR Corporation. On registration, the vehicle owner is asked for basic contact details as well as the plate number, make, model and year of the vehicles registered to that owner. The applicant is then asked to select a payment option: pre-payment, post-payment, pre-authorized bank withdrawal, or charging to a credit card.

Owners of lighter vehicles may choose not to lease a transponder, in which case trips are logged by using a license plate recognition system. The system is located on each overhead gantry and sends up to five video images of the rear plate to a central processing computer, housed in the 407 Corporation, whenever such a vehicle enters and exits the highway. A $2 non-transponder charge per trip is added for this process. The central computer checks to determine if an account exists for that license plate. If not, an electronic search is made of the Ontario Ministry of Transportation's License and Control Branch database for the name and address of that license plate holder.[6] The number of account holders has increased since its inception, and the processing of non-transponder usage has declined.

The question of personal privacy was a priority from the time Project Request for Proposals for the 407 ETR was issued in September 1993. Since 1994, the Office of the Information and Privacy Commissioner (OIPC) has been actively involved in discussions with the Ontario Transportation Capital Commission (OTCC) about how individuals could travel along the 407 ETR and still maintain their privacy. If residents of Toronto were to use this new system, it was necessary to gain their trust by building in strong safeguards against the inappropriate collection, use and disclosure of personal information. The OTCC worked closely, therefore, with the OIPC to ensure that the toll and billing system did not compromise personal privacy.

They claim that the result is the first Intelligent Transportation System in the world to allow users to travel the road anonymously. This is accomplished through three features. First, the plate recognition system (for vehicles without transponders) only records the rear license plate of the vehicle; the OTCC agreed that it was not necessary to collect any more information for toll collection purposes. Thus, like "photo radar" programs developed in other parts of Canada to catch speeding drivers, the cameras have a fixed geometry and do not take images of the interior or the front of the vehicle.

Second, the governing legislation only permits the ETR corporation to use any personal information it collects for toll collection, traffic management and for its own marketing purposes. The 1998 407 Highway Act stipulates that personal information may only be collected

1   To assist the owner in the collection and enforcement of tolls, fees and other charges owing with respect to Highway 407.
2   To assist the owner in traffic planning and revenue management with respect to Highway 407.
3   To assist the owner in communicating with users of Highway 407 for the purpose of promoting the use of Highway 407.
4   To assist an entity with whom the owner or the Ministry of Transportation has an agreement relating to the collection and enforcement of tolls (407 Highway Act 1998: c.28 s.54[5]).

In addition, tight contractual clauses between the Ministry of Transportation and 407 International Inc. ensure that the confidentiality of personal information is protected and that it is not used for any purpose not referred to in the legislation.

Finally, potential travelers have the option of obtaining a transponder and travelling the 407 without providing any personal information. The user can effectively open a pre-paid cash account at which point he or she receives a transponder and a booklet of payment slips pre-printed with the anonymous account number. The user is reminded to replenish the account when the transponder flashes yellow, rather than green, as the car travels under one of the 407 gantries. The user simply visits any chartered bank to deposit funds into the account number that appears on the payment slip. Those funds are then electronically transferred into the user's 407 account. Of course, if users wish to remain anonymous, they cannot allow their balances to fall below zero. If they do so, the rear license plate identification and the recognition system will be activated (Information and Privacy Commissioner/ Ontario 1998). To date, very few individuals have taken advantage of this anonymous option. Nor is this option encouraged, as it significantly increases the processing costs for the corporation.[7]

These relatively tight controls mean that, with few exceptions, the information gathered on the 407 ETR is only used for toll collection purposes. Aggregate data on patterns of overall traffic flows are reported to the government, as are accidents. Law enforcement agencies, however, cannot obtain personal information from the 407 corporation on, for instance, stolen vehicles, unless under warrant. No information is transferred to the police on more minor traffic infractions such as speeding. At first glance, the 407 seems to have been designed, developed and implemented with extensive safeguards against the inappropriate use of information about vehicle movement. The system does constitute a tracking technology, but it is one that has been clearly designed to prevent widespread secondary uses of personal data.

The 407 ETR system, while touted as "state-of-the-art" is, however, expensive to operate and use and not suitable for wider traffic management purposes. The Ontario government has installed a new system (COMPASS) on other Toronto freeways to respond to traffic congestion problems caused by accident, breakdown or peak rush hour use. This system collects no personally identifiable information but can warn motorists of incidents and delays. The system is fully integrated with emergency response procedures.

It is apparent, however, that these contemporary intelligent transportation systems may eventually be overtaken by cellular and GIS technologies. Currently, 28 percent of vehicles traveling on Canadian roads contain cellular devices. Private sector providers may soon have the ability and incentive to collect that tracking information which might then be purchased by government for traffic management purposes. The amount and specificity of the traveler information that might be available is then enhanced. Drivers may get real-time information on congestion, emergency services and routing (i.e., the best way to get from A to B on this particular evening when there is a ball game and bus strike). The collection and processing of this kind of information may also obviate the need for automatic toll collection systems such as the 407 ETR, and indeed will reduce the need for jurisdictions like Ontario to build traffic loops, on-ramps and install video cameras.[8] The smart vehicle of the future will record location information, and cellular operators will collect it for governmental use. The efficiencies of on-board cellular and GIS tracking technologies for a range of public and private purposes will likely present far greater challenges to individual privacy than the relatively discrete and manageable highway system on Toronto's route 407.

The Smart Tag System in Virginia[9]

Smart Tag is an electronic toll collection (ETC) system used at five locations in the State of Virginia: the Dulles Toll Road in northern Virginia; the Dulles Greenway in northern Virginia; the George P. Coleman Bridge on the eastern shore of the middle peninsula; the Powhite Parkway Extension in the Richmond area; and the Expressway System in Richmond. The Smart Tag system has been phased in at these locations beginning with the Dulles Toll Road in April 1996; the Dulles Greenway in May 1996; the Coleman Bridge in August 1996; the Powhite Parkway Extension in July 1999; and the Richmond Expressway System in July and August 1999.

As of the summer of 2000, there were more than 257,000 Smart Tags in use: 175,000 in northern Virginia, 32,000 on the Coleman Bridge, and 50,000 in Richmond (Smart Tag Statistics 2001). In each location, usage of the Smart Tag system exceeds original expectations. On the Dulles Toll Road, over 60 percent of cars use Smart Tag during rush hour with about 40 percent usage overall. On the Dulles Greenway, about 80 percent of the cars use Smart Tag during rush hour with over 50 percent usage overall. The Coleman Bridge reports the highest usage with 90 percent of cars using Smart Tag during rush hour and about 80 percent usage overall. The newer Smart Tag systems in the Richmond area were heavily subscribed from their inception and have about a 50 percent rush hour usage.

The Dulles Toll Road system was initiated in March 1994 when a contract was awarded to Castle Rock for installation of an ETC system called FASTOLL. The genesis for the system was the Virginia Department of Transportation's (VDOT) March 1993 strategic plan (Smith 1993) for Virginia called PROGRESS, VDOT's Intelligent Vehicle-Highway Systems (IVHS) Program for an Efficient and Safe System. Beginning in 1991, the federal government also encouraged the implementation of ETC systems such as Smart Tag through the Intermodal Surface Transportation Efficiency Act of 1991 (ISTEA) program. ISTEA provided federal funding and incentives for automatic toll facilities in order to reduce congestion at toll plazas. As in Toronto, VDOT recognized the potential of IVHS to increase the efficiency and lower the expense of surface transportation. But it was equally impressed with the potential of IVHS to enhance economic growth through development of an IVHS industry, which might benefit high technology firms in Virginia. The plan spoke enthusiastically of new potential for innovative public–private partnerships. Although the FASTOLL system was originally to be completed during 1995, it did not become fully operational until April 1996. In January 1998, VDOT changed the name to Smart Tag as part of its overall Smart Travel system.

The Smart Tag system, like most ETC systems, uses several key components (*Electronic Toll Collection* 1998). Automatic Vehicle Identification (AVI) uses a radio frequency device located in a transponder, which is designed to link the account on the transponder to the toll equipment. As in the Toronto system, the Smart Tag transponder is read electronically, and the toll is deducted from a pre-paid Smart Tag account. The Smart Tag transponder can be used at any Smart Tag collection plaza in the state. A Video Enforcement System (VES) can capture the license plates of vehicles that do not have a valid transponder or sufficient funds. On the Coleman Bridge, motorists who get a "blue light" when driving through the Smart Tag Only lanes have their license plates recorded and retained, and toll violations can be issued to those motorists. Video enforcement for toll collection for the Dulles Toll Road is not yet in operation but is an enhancement project that was proposed in the 1999–2000 Six Year Plan.

Any ETC usually requires a communications and database system. A lane controller receives input from the AVI, VES and AVC (Automatic Vehicle Classification) equipment and records the customer's toll. All Smart Tag systems in Virginia use a compatible ETC system (Mark IV reader). There may also be a toll plaza computer, which consolidates data and checks the validity of toll tags. A Customer Service Center receives toll transactions and posts these transactions against the customer account, as well as storing data on valid accounts. VDOT owns and operates a Customer Service Center with two satellite locations; this one center manages all Smart Tag accounts throughout Virginia.

The current marketing literature and the 1993 strategic plan promote six fairly typical advantages of Smart Tag. First mentioned are efficiencies in terms of traffic flow. VDOT currently reports that on the Dulles Toll Road, lanes with attendants collecting tolls process 525 vehicles per hour; exact change lanes process 650 vehicles per hour; and Smart Tag Only lanes process 1,400 vehicles per hour. A second benefit is that there is less need for capital construction to widen or reconfigure toll plazas to accommodate increased traffic volume. Indeed, some ETC systems eliminate toll plazas altogether or streamline them to require little capital construction. A third advantage is that ETC systems are seen as being environmentally friendly because cars release fewer pollutants as they idle for less time at toll plazas. A fourth benefit involves freeing personnel from the monotonous and hazardous job of collecting tolls. Fifth, ETC systems provide a more accurate and comprehensive accounting system. Finally, ETC systems can encourage travel at off-peak times by reducing tolls. New federal legislation, the Transportation Equity Act for the 21st Century (TEA-21), promotes more sophisticated uses of ETC systems, promoting, for example, variable pricing in order to reduce peak hour traffic volumes.

In addition to marketing these advantages, the state has endorsed the use of several incentives to encourage drivers to adopt Smart Tag. Smart Tag users receive a 10 percent discount at toll collection sites on the Richmond Metropolitan Authority Expressway System. In August 1999, the Dulles Greenway announced a toll increase of 25 cents, to $1.75, for those who are not using Smart Tag. The rationale for the increase was to help ease traffic backups at toll plazas (Blum and Hedgpeth 1999). When the Dulles Toll Road opened HOV-2 lanes, it designed them so they fed directly into the Smart Tag Only lanes at the toll plaza.

Privacy concerns are not visibly addressed or acknowledged in the Smart Tag literature. The twenty-item customer agreement for Smart Tag does not mention information collection, disclosure or use practices. In the Smart Tag brochures, two items have privacy implications but are not presented as privacy issues. The brochure mentions that if people want to pay cash instead of using their Smart Tag, they should remove the Smart Tag from the vehicle or wrap it in aluminum foil. Smart Tag developers recognize that drivers may want to be anonymous on some trips, but they do so by implication only, and not by addressing the privacy concern directly. Second, the brochure states that receipts are not provided when someone uses a Smart Tag, but a customer can obtain a detailed statement from the service center "starting at $2.00 a month." By implication, the brochure acknowledges that records containing date, time and location for Smart Tag uses are compiled and retained, but implies that Smart Tag owns this information and customers must pay for access. The question of who other than the customer might have access either by court order or request is left undefined.

The Smart Tag Application Form states: "All information is personal and confidential," but there is no indication of how a customer can verify that statement. The personal information supplied on the application form is technically information supplied to the state for an administrative purpose. Because of concerns about requests for access to that information, personal information related to toll facilities, particularly ETC information, is exempt from the state's Freedom of Information Act. Custodial control for the information is assigned to VDOT and could be released in response to a subpoena. According to Smart Tag personnel, information is not released for marketing or other purposes. This is not spelled out on the application form or customer agreement in part because of the difficulty of crafting language that takes into account all contingencies; the statement quoted above, that "all information is personal and confidential" is regarded as the overarching policy.[10]

This statement is very similar to that made by the Massachusetts Turnpike Authority's Fast Lane which says the Turnpike "shall hold all customer account information confidential." When asked about the possibility that law enforcement authorities would subpoena this information, a Turnpike Authority responded that they would resist releasing information but that they thought such demands unlikely (Kerber 2001). The E-ZPass toll system in New York, however, has complied with such demands. In one case, E-ZPass locating records allowed authorities to find the body of a kidnapping victim by using E-ZPass records to track where and when his car had traveled (Sipress 2000). New case law in Massachusetts, New Jersey, and New York requires law enforcement officials to demonstrate that they are investigating a serious crime to obtain toll records. Bills have also been introduced in state legislatures to protect the privacy of toll records and to specify the conditions under which they could be released for law enforcement purposes (Most 1998).

The Smart Tag brochure indicates that Smart Tag transponders can be used by other vehicles with the same number of axles. From a privacy standpoint, this means that the transponder may not be recording the movements of the individual account holder. The account holder could authorize its use for a child or friend. In such a case, the account holder may want to know when and where the transponder was used. This feature of the transponder also makes it a target for stealing. If it is stolen, the account holder, Smart Tag officials and the police may all have an interest in accessing the records.

Another privacy implication of the Smart Tag system is that it is designed to encourage customers to use a credit card. If travelers do not use a credit card and automatic replenishment on the Smart Tag account, they must pay a $15 refundable security deposit. The automatic replenishment system is the easiest and least expensive method, but it does entail an authorization to allow Smart Tag to charge a credit card account. It also means that some information about road travel may become incorporated into one's credit history and could be used for profiling purposes. Smart Tag offers alternatives to automatic credit card replenishment. Customers can add money to the account by mailing a check, visiting customer service, or calling in a credit card authorization.

The institutional and management arrangements for Smart Tag are particularly interesting in three respects: within the Smart Tag system itself; between Smart Tag and the I-95 Corridor system in which use of E-ZPass is dominant; and between Smart Tag and the larger Smart Travel system in Virginia.

Although all the Smart Tag road systems are located in Virginia, the organization and management of each road system involve different configurations of government and private involvement. For example, the Dulles Greenway is privately owned. The Dulles Toll Road is owned and operated by VDOT. The Richmond Metropolitan Authority (RMA) owns and operates the Expressway System, including the Powhite Parkway, Downtown Expressway, and Boulevard Bridge. Each of these road management authorities contracted with a private sector partner to build the Smart Tag system. MFS Transportation Systems, a subsidiary of MFS Network Technologies, built the RMA Smart Tag system. The project covers fifty-five lanes of the system and includes toll plaza infrastructure modifications, upgrades to computer and communication systems, replacement of audit systems, integration with current customer service centers, and a five-year maintenance contract (ITS America 1998).[11] Castle Rock Consultants advised on the design and implementation of the FASTOLL/Smart Tag system on the Dulles Toll Road.

Despite the fact that the road systems are managed differently and that the Smart Tag systems have been built by different contractors, the technical configuration of each of the Smart Tag systems is compatible. Most importantly, the actual operation and management of Smart Tag is organizationally separate from road management. The real operation of Smart Tag occurs in the Smart Tag Customer Service Center, which is owned by VDOT. VDOT then contracts for its services. This Center serves as the financial and administrative clearinghouse. All five Smart Tag systems in Virginia feed their ETC transaction and customer accounts through this one central office.

The pivotal position played by the financial management center explains, in part, the relationship that the Virginia Smart Tag has with other ETC systems on the East Coast. The Regional Consortium, comprised of five transportation agencies representing Delaware, New Jersey and New York, manages the E-ZPass system. These Consortium Member agencies are part of a larger E-ZPass Interagency Group (IAG), an association of sixteen northern toll agencies spanning seven states (E-ZPass Network 1999). The IAG allows travelers with E-ZPass transponders to use them on member toll roads in New York, New Jersey, Delaware, Pennsylvania, Maryland, Massachusetts, and shortly West Virginia (ITS America 1999). One of the components of the Northern Virginia District's Smart Travel vision is that

"VDOT will implement a toll tag that will be usable throughout Virginia and the member states of the I-95 Corridor Coalition. Similarly, electronic toll tags used by the I-95 Corridor Coalition states will be usable throughout Virginia" (Tang 1999a: 13).

At this time, the Smart Tag system is technically compatible with the E-ZPass system. Smart Tag readers can read information from E-ZPass transponders and vice versa. But the Smart Tag and E-ZPass financial clearinghouse systems are not compatible, and transactions cannot be made between the two systems. Although the readers can get information from the transponders, they cannot interact with the transponder.[12] This is not a technological problem, but an institutional one. The VDOT, as well as Smart Tag and E-ZPass users who travel in both systems, want compatibility between the systems. An additional factor that may hasten compatibility is that TEA-21 includes a requirement that agencies demonstrate "consistency" with the National ITS Architecture to be eligible for federal ITS funds.

The third institutional and management arrangement is between Smart Tag and Smart Travel. As noted above, the name Smart Tag replaced FASTOLL in 1998 to symbolize the unity of all ITS applications under one umbrella concept (Tang 1999b: 1–4). The plan is to develop interrelated systems so that, for example, surface street management, freeway management, incident management, traveler information, customer service, and payment systems can work together. The vision entails a statewide network of Smart Travel centers that will provide the intelligence for the system.

The Dartford River Crossing in England

As a brief comparative illustration of an existing electronic toll-payment system in Europe, we look at the Dartford River Crossing of the Thames in southeast England, near London. The new privately financed Queen Elizabeth II Bridge opened in 1991 as part of the densely traveled M25 motorway around London, which already included the Dartford Tunnel. Tolls are meant to recover construction costs, and the physical infrastructure for collecting them from the estimated forty million vehicles using the crossing each year includes a new £2.5 million system, DART-Tag, described as "Europe's most advanced toll system" (HHS Online 1999; Flowchart 2001). The tag, a microwave transponder, is free. Drivers pay in advance by setting up a direct debit facility in the bank. Some lanes are reserved for the use of DART-Tag users.

When a vehicle approaches, the tag is interrogated by an antenna to obtain a customer number and retrieve a customer record. If the driver's account is in credit, the barrier automatically opens. Traffic lights at the barrier tell the driver roughly how many credits are left, and a red light means the account is empty in which case the barrier will not open. Passing through the open barrier updates the driver's account record. Drivers receive a monthly statement itemizing the entries. As in the Smart Tag and 407 ETR cases, there is a price incentive to obtain the tag, in this case a 7.5 percent discount. An estimated 20 percent of vehicles using the crossing are subscribers. Travelers have the option of throwing coins into a basket or going through a staffed booth if they require change. A central computer keeps a count of every vehicle using these services, presumably to compile simple tallies for financial and management purposes.

Whereas Smart Tag's Customer Agreement is vague about information practices, the Dartford River Crossing company's terms of conditions and use contains a privacy policy statement. It describes the information required when an account is set up, why it is necessary, how it will be used (including use in an aggregated form for flow-monitoring purposes), and how the user can opt out of third-party use. It explains that the web site used for transactions contains security software (certification system provided by BT Trustwise in connection with Verisign) including encryption for all communications with customers and banks, firewalls, and secure premises. Information is kept confidential, with internal company procedures to guard against unauthorized disclosure. If the privacy policy changes, customers will be informed on the web page and consent will be sought for any substantive changes of use of information. Subscribers automatically consent to the passage of their information outside the European Economic Area during use (Dartford River Crossing Limited 1999).

Concluding observations

It is apparent that each of these three systems is both a reflection and a precursor of future ITS. At a policy level, these cases offer some insights into the evolving nature of the privacy issue and how it might best be addressed in the context of current and future ITS applications. Four conclusions are relevant about the protection of privacy.

The first lesson concerns the business case for these systems. Often the logic of these systems is framed in terms of speeding the flow of traffic. Efficiency, therefore, is the goal, and the architecture is crafted in terms of relating intelligence directly to traffic management. Moreover, the economics of these systems, based on complex public–private partnerships, favors more extensive and intensive uses and sharing of personal data. The logic then favors surveillance. In order for privacy to be taken into account, it has to be addressed in the development of that architecture, but those involved in the process are transportation specialists and contractors. There are few natural entry points for the privacy interest even in the presence of an overriding legal privacy framework.

The second lesson relates to the importance of technical standards and how the standard-setting process can institute protocols that embody privacy protective or invasive measures. European developments are instructive.[13] As a result of the need to promote the free flow of goods and services throughout the EU, there has been considerable standards activity in Europe concerning transport telematics applications, including ETC (sometimes known as electronic fee collection – EFC). The European Commission has played a large part in coordinating and supporting research and development, and in addressing major issues, of which the interoperability of these systems has been perhaps the largest. The Fourth Framework Programme is an example of this effort. Interoperability exists within, but not across, countries with EFC systems. The international and European standards organizations (ISO and CEN) have also been closely involved in these developments. While current standards do not ensure interoperability of payments, work was proceeding in that direction, for instance within CEN TC278, and through an agreed Applications Interface Definition for an EFC based on Dedicated Short-Range Communication (DSRC). Technical standards decisions about the various elements of toll collection systems can have profound policy consequences for the collection of personal information.

It is too soon to say whether systems in European countries or any future common system will make extensive use of advanced GIS, including geo-positioning through satellite communication. Countries that have invested in particular toll collection infrastructures and technologies may be more reluctant to move towards a new system. These fixtures include toll plazas, payment lanes, roadside or overhead equipment, etc., as well as personnel. The calculation of tolls by means of distance traveled, involving "virtual" toll collection points rather than a system of lanes, overhead gantries, and the like, would involve the collection of such data through these GI technologies. That, in turn, depends on the standardization work that might be undertaken by a working group in CEN TC278.

By contrast, there has been less need for standards-setting activity in Canada and the United States. Indeed the incremental, state-by-state use of E-ZPass on the I-95 corridor would indicate that interoperability in US systems is not an initial goal but became a later addition to the policy agenda when significant incompatibilities arose. Toll systems in North America tend to develop locally to meet local traffic management needs by state and provincial departments of transportation and local/regional transportation authorities.

Thirdly, we would stress the importance of an overriding legal framework for the collection and use of tracking information. Such frameworks exist in

Canada, the United Kingdom and in the rest of Europe. In Canada, specific data protection provisions were introduced into the enabling highway legislation for the 407 ETR. In the UK, the collection of personal information for toll collection purposes is regulated under the aegis of the Data Protection Act 1998 and the Information Commissioner, though to date there have been few if any policy pronouncements or regulatory actions by the Commissioner on this issue. In the Netherlands, the *Registratiekamer* (the Dutch Data Protection Authority) has been involved in considering the privacy implications of road-tolling proposals for managing intra-urban traffic congestion. A related point, then, is the active involvement of a privacy watchdog office at the outset of system development. The significance of privacy in the context of the development of the 407 ETR is explained to a large extent by the early involvement of the Office of the Ontario Information and Privacy Commissioner, and to the very public way in which that office raised privacy concerns.

In the US, there is no overriding legal framework, perhaps accounting for the less stringent controls over possible secondary uses of electronic toll information, and for the less prominent mention of privacy in the materials provided by the Smart Tag system. Most states have laws addressing the privacy and confidentiality of state records but these, of course, are not tied explicitly to information related to ETC. ITS America, an advisory committee of the US Department of Transportation, has, after a lengthy period of consultation with stakeholders, finalized a set of Fair Information Principles for personal information related to ITS. But these are voluntary guidelines and have no binding force (Voccola 2001: 4).[14]

The fourth lesson is that complex technologies do not necessarily require complex privacy-enhancing solutions. No doubt, a range of encryption solutions can be advanced to protect the integrity of the tracking information generated within toll collection systems. It is instructive, however, that the solution adopted on Toronto's 407 involved no major changes to the existing infrastructure of collection. It merely allowed a payment and accounting process that did not require the submission of personal identifiers. The fact that very few individuals have so far taken advantage of this system suggests, however, that the administrative burden is not something that most users of the highway would tolerate in order to protect the privacy of their movements. Similarly, in the Smart Tag system, the cash payment option is inconvenient compared to the credit card payment process.

In the Dartford River Crossing and the Smart Tag System in Virginia, where there are controlled points of entry and exit, privacy can still be maintained through the anonymity of cash payment at a traditional toll plaza. Thus far, therefore, any privacy pressures have been translated into privacy solutions by the retention of traditional payment devices, although the more convenient way to use both systems is to supply valid credit card information and thus surrender a measure of privacy. There are legal and political pressures to retain this sort of facility, but with the application of advanced ITS technologies, perhaps especially on multi-lane roads where the channeling and slowing of traffic for toll payment is to be avoided, traditional processes may be highly vulnerable.

We now return to the more general questions and issues raised at the outset of this chapter. The implications of ITS for these matters of identity, surveillance, and the categorical sorting of persons and groups are not yet particularly evident in the toll-road applications we have studied so far. From the analysis of these systems, it is apparent that the range of personal data collection is still quite limited to essential payment-related information. Systems vary in terms of their transparency and general concern for privacy-related questions. But the overall picture is one in which the payment collection technologies are usually confined to the simple purpose of making sure that the right people are charged the right amount for the journeys they have completed. The most obvious sorting in toll collection systems is among those using electronic tolls, those using exact change and/or tokens, and those needing change. The electronic toll systems represent the most expeditious way of negotiating the toll plaza but in most instances involve some divulgence of personal information and use of a credit card to open and update an account.

The matching and sharing of personal data obviously vary according to the number of organizations within the contractual arrangements surrounding these systems, and also according to the number of jurisdictions from which travelers might originate. Thus far, the opportunities for policy intervention to protect values such as privacy are present, though variable, because of the relatively discrete and bounded character of the data processes involved. The latter's significance for politics and policy has been relatively modest to date; ITS has not been an important site for the kinds of overt or covert conflict between institutions and individuals, the watchers and the watched, that are projected in many scenarios concerning technology and human movement.

However, it is also apparent that each of these systems is under pressure for the secondary uses of the data collected. So far, those pressures have tended to originate from public sector agencies and been motivated by various traffic management and law enforcement interests. Aggregate data collected through these systems might be useful in managing traffic flows, physical and environmental maintenance, and in reducing congestion. Individual-level data might also be valuable in tracing stolen vehicles, enforcing customs rules, catching speeding and dangerous drivers, and apprehending criminals. But wider commercial pressures for the use of these data to profile, for example, the kinds of people who drive particular vehicles along specific routes at specific times, have not yet been significant or have been resisted by policy intervention.

This preliminary research, however, has also revealed that these systems are rapidly being overtaken by more advanced technologies that will enable a more intensive and extensive surveillance of vehicle movement, and thus may broach the larger social, political and privacy questions. For example, the European Commission listed thirty-five telematics applications projects for transport in 1997–98 (European Commission 1999). These covered a variety of land, water and air transport applications, of which only a small number concerned tolling and related road applications of ITS.[15] Some applications are of particular interest. VERA (Video Enforcement for Road Authorities, using video records as evidence to prosecute road traffic offenders throughout Europe) has a law-enforcement purpose, including harmonized approaches to enforcing traffic laws by employing video and digital imaging technologies. The objective of SANSICOM (High-Technology GNSS Satellite Navigation System with Integrated Communication Link for Road Applications) is to integrate a communication link for various road applications into a satellite navigation system with a communication capability. This will be used to monitor road situations, including in-vehicle systems for safety. Applications will relate to fleet management for road haulers, container and car tracking, stolen vehicle recovery, search and rescue operations, and road traffic control.

In the US, the 1991 ISTEA encouraged the development of what was first termed Intelligent Vehicle-Highway Systems (IVHS) and then was extended to Intelligent Transportation Systems (ITS). In 1995, the Department of Transportation spoke of bundling these systems into six groups: travel and transportation management; travel demand management; public transportation operations; electronic payment; commercial vehicle operations; emergency management; and advanced vehicle control and safety systems. New projects continue to be developed in these areas and many reflect new technological advancements in GPS and wireless systems. Development of these systems is accelerated by federal funding and policy, most recently by TEA-21, as well as by states and private communications and transportation vendors (US Department of Transportation 1995).

The incentive to suppliers as well as to road users, of the added functionality that advanced GIS tracking technologies may make possible – targeted information about weather, goods, services, etc. – will obviously raise additional privacy issues. These may well bring into play a more intensive development of sorting and classification systems in order to tailor messages and services to the known, or presumed, characteristics and preferences of drivers. With existing systems, toll payments may be based on the measurement of the physical dimensions of the vehicle as it traverses the payment point, with the dimensions related to classification systems of vehicle types with associated levels of charges. But they may also be based upon license plate number capture, or through information transmitted from the vehicle's on-board unit. So far, the main interest of the ITS community in classification has been in terms of vehicle types.

However, quite a lot can be known, or at least inferred, about vehicle owners and drivers. Data reveals who drives what vehicle, where and when, and allows analysis of the previous travel behavior of individual road users; those data can also be linked to other sources of information for profiling purposes. Commercial pressures to use tracking information have so far been limited, but we can foresee them intensifying as the convergence of on-board telematics and GIS technologies increasingly become adopted for toll collection and traffic management functions. That convergence will also continue the erosion of the distinction between the public and the private realms, and between the individual and the vehicle, as commerce extends the assumption that "we are what we drive."

Notes

1 These technologies and user services and their implications for various privacy interests, based upon the US Department of Transportation's Program Plan, are discussed in Alpert (1995) and Glancy (1995).

2 This chapter is part of a larger project, funded by the National Science Foundation in the USA (*Grant No. SES-0083271*), which attempts to gain an analytical understanding of the implementation of personal identification in geographically coded information systems, and an appreciation of the effect that identification practices have on individual privacy, sociability, trust, and risk. This will involve, in part, locating and clarifying contradictions and ambiguities in common notions of identification and privacy, conceptually systematizing practices of iden-tification, and theorizing the effects of these practices on social equity amongst individuals and on the individual's relation to political and economic com-munities. The research project analyses particular types of geographic information systems, and performs a series of comparative case studies – in the USA, Canada, and Europe – of the processes by which identification practice is incorporated within those systems. A companion paper in this volume by our project colleagues, David Phillips and Michael Curry, reports initial findings concerning another field of application, geodemographic systems.

3 Discussion of a wider range of technological applications for location and tracking, including systems that are not necessarily related to movement, can be found in Clarke (2000).

4 For seminal explorations of surveillance, see Lyon (1994, 2001).

5 The authors are grateful to Peter Walker for his research assistance on this section of the chapter.

6 Interviews with staff at the Ontario Ministry of Transportation, 2 March 2001.

7 Interviews with staff at the 407 Corporation, 2 May 2001.

8 Interviews with staff at the Ontario Ministry of Transportation, 2 March 2001.
9 We acknowledge the research assistance of Brendan Crowley for this section of the paper.
10 Interviews with staff at the Virginia Department of Transportation, 12 April 2001.
11 MFS Transportation Systems has implemented a number of other ETC projects including the Denver E-470, the California 91 Express Lanes, and the Regional Consortium for Toll Collection (NJ, NY and DE) as well as projects in South America, Canada, Europe and the Pacific Rim.
12 Interviews with staff at the Virginia Department of Transportation, 12 April 2001.
13 In mid-1999, there were at least 17,000 km of tolled motorway in Europe, operating in nine European Union (EU) and other countries, and including Electronic Fee Collection (EFC) in France, Italy, Spain, and Norway. Some two million EFC subscribers were involved; this accounted for about 10 percent of toll transactions in places where EFC was available. The French system is TIS, the Italian is TELEPASS, the Norwegian is the 5.8 GHz system, and the Portuguese is Via Verde. New EFC systems were being planned for introduction in several other countries: the Netherlands, the Nordic countries, Germany, Switzerland, and the UK. Different national requirements meant that these were designed in a non-interoperable manner, and influential opinion did not consider it feasible or desirable to harmonize the existing systems. Yet it was thought possible to work towards a migration of the different EFC systems, in stages, to a common system through the enlargement of the diverse national ones. See EC – DG XIII, Telematics Application Programme, Transport Sector, CARDME -3 (Project TR 4102), *Deliverable 5.1. Review of Current Possibilities for Migration of EFC Systems (Doc. D5.1, Version V2.01, Draft)*, 1 June 1999
14 See also www.itsa.org. Regulations are noticeably absent in the United States, perhaps accounting for the less stringent controls over secondary uses on the Dulles toll road, and for the less prominent mention of privacy in the materials concerning the Smart Tag system.
15 Among these projects are ADVICE (Advanced Vehicle Classification and Enforcement Systems, involving electronic fee collection on toll motorways), CARDME -3 (Concerted Action for Research on Demand Management in Europe, on convergence of motorway tolling systems throughout Europe), and INITIATIVE (Industry Initiative To Introduce Automatic Tolling In Vehicles in Europe, concerning a search for the optimal electronic fee collection system on toll motorways). There are important overlaps and collaboration among several of these, including a network of technical personnel from public and private organizations. A further grouping is the Nordic countries' MÅNS (Objective-oriented Nordic Co-operation on Interoperable Payment for Transport Services).

Bibliography

407 ETR (2001) "407 ETR History." Online. Available HTTP: <http://www.407etr.com/html/history.html> (accessed 7 December 2001).
407 Highway Act 1998, c. 28, s. 54 (5). Province of Ontario, Canada.
Agre, P. E. (1994) "Surveillance and Capture: Two Models of Privacy," *The Information Society*, 10(2): 101–27.
—— (1995) "Reasoning About the Future," *Santa Clara Computer and High Technology Law Journal*, 11(1): 129–33.

Agre, P. E. and Harbs, C. A. (1994) "Social Choice About Privacy: Intelligent Vehicle-Highway Systems in the United States," *Information Technology & People*, 7(4): 63–90.

Alpert, S. A. (1995) "Privacy and Intelligent Highways: Finding the Right of Way," *Santa Clara Computer and High Technology Law Journal*, 11(1): 97–118.

Beniger, J. R. (1986) *The Control Revolution: Technological and Economic Origins of the Information Society*, Cambridge, MA: Harvard University Press.

Blum, J. and Hedgpeth, D. (1999) "Dulles Greenway Raises Weekday Toll: Drivers Will Pay 25 Cents More Without Smart Tag," *Washington Post*, 3 August: B03.

Bowker, G. C. and Star, S. L. (1999) *Sorting Things Out: Classification and its Consequences*, Cambridge, MA: MIT Press.

Clarke, R. (2000) "Person-Location and Person-Tracking: Technologies, Risks and Policy Implications." Online. Available HTTP: <http://www.anu.edu.au/people/Roger.Clarke/DV/PLT.html> (accessed 21 March 2001).

Curry, M. R. (1997) "The Digital Individual and the Private Realm," *Annals, Association of American Geographers*, 87(4): 681–99.

Dartford River Crossing Limited (1999) "Terms and Conditions of Use of DART-Tag." Online. Available HTTP: <http://www.dartfordrivercrossing.co.uk/dart-tag/terms.htm> (accessed 28 March 2001).

Dingle, J. (1995) "The Federal Highway Administration, IVHS and Privacy," *Santa Clara Computer and High Technology Law Journal*, 11(1): 15–20.

Duncan, J. and Agnew, J. (1990) *The Power of Place*, London: Allen and Unwin.

Electronic Toll Collection (ETC) (1998). Online. Available HTTP: <http://www.ettm.com/etc.html> (accessed 7 December 2001).

European Commission DG XIII C/E (1999) *Telematics Applications Programme, Guide to the 1997–1998 Telematics Applications Projects Sector: Telematics Applications For Transport*. Online. Available HTTP: <http://158.169.50.95:10080/telematics/projectguide/transport.html> (accessed 26 March 2001).

E-ZPass Network (1999) *E-ZPass Regional Consortium Service Center*. Online. Available HTTP: <http://www.ezpass.com/interagency.shtml> (accessed 7 December 2001).

"Flowchart Showing the Dart Tag Checking and Update Process" (2001). Online. Available HTTP: <http://www.school-resources.co.uk/flowchart_showing_the_dart_tag_c.htm> (accessed 28 March 2001).

Frohmann, B. (1994) "Communication Technologies and the Politics of Postmodern Information Science," *Canadian Journal of Information and Library Science*, 19(2): 1–22.

Glancy, D. J. (1995) "Privacy and Intelligent Transportation Technology," *Santa Clara Computer and High Technology Law Journal*, 11(1): 151–203.

Goffman, E. (1959) *The Presentation of Self in Everyday Life*, New York: Anchor Books.

Halpern, S. A. "The Traffic in Souls," *Santa Clara Computer and High Technology Law Journal*, 11(1): 45–73.

HHS Online (1999) "The Dartford Tunnel – Commercial System 2." Online. Available HTTP: <http://atschool.eduweb.co.uk/hatfieldhigh/IT/PT%20 Assignments/Unit %201/case2.htm> (accessed 20 April 2001).

Information and Privacy Commissioner/Ontario (1998) "407 Express Toll Route: How You Can Travel This Road Anonymously." Online. Available HTTP: <http: //www.ipc.on.ca/english/pubpres/papers/407.htm> (accessed 30 January 2002).

ITS America (1998) "MFS Transportation Systems Selected for Electronic Toll Collection in Richmond, VA," *Access ITS*. Online. Available HTTP: <http: //www.itsa.org> (accessed 21 April 1998).

—— (1999) "TransCore Awarded New Toll Collection System Contract for West Virginia," *Access ITS*. Online. Available HTTP: <http://www.itsa.org?ITSNEWS. NSF/a6> (accessed 20 May 1999).

Kerber, R. (2001) "The Privacy Tradeoff," *The Boston Globe*. Online. Available HTTP: <http://digitalmass.boston.com/news/daily/01/010801/privacy_tradeoff. html> (accessed 8 January 2001).

Lyon, D. (1994) *The Electronic Eye: The Rise of Surveillance Society*, Cambridge: Polity Press.

—— (2001) *Surveillance Society: Monitoring Everyday Life*, Philadelphia: Open University Press.

Most, D. (1998) "E-ZPass Rules Proposed," *The Bergen Record*. Online. Available HTTP: <http://www.ettm.com/news/ezpass_privacy.html> (accessed 30 January 1998).

Sipress, A. (2000) "'Big Brother' Could Soon Ride Along in the Back Seat," *Washington Post*, 8 October: A1.

"Smart Tag Statistics" (2000) *Smart Tag News* (Summer).

Smith, B. T. (1993) *VIRGINIA PROGRESS: The Virginia Department of Trans portation's Intelligent Vehicle-Highway Systems Strategic Plan*, Charlottesville, VA: Virginia Transportation Research Council, VTRC 93-TAR6.

Tang, A. (1999a) *Strategic Plan: Northern Virginia District (NOVA) Smart Travel Program*.

—— (1999b) *Executive Summary: Northern Virginia District (NOVA) Smart Travel Program*.

Tuan, Y.-F. (1982) *Segmented Worlds and Self: Group Life and Individual Consciousness*, Minneapolis: University of Minnesota Press.

US Department of Transportation, Federal Highway Administration (1995) *Intelligent Transportation Systems (ITS) Projects*, January.

Voccola, H. (2001) "Commentary: ITS America's Fair Information and Privacy Principles," *ITS America News*, (11)2: 4.

Wright, T. (1995) "Eyes on the Road: Intelligent Transportation Systems and Your Privacy," Toronto: Information and Privacy Commission/Ontario. Online. Available HTTP: <http://www.ipc.on.ca/english/pubpres/sum_pap/papers/ITS-E.H (accessed 20 April 2001).

9 Netscapes of power

Convergence, network design, walled gardens, and other strategies of control in the information age

Dwayne Winseck

Introduction

This chapter challenges the widespread claim that the new media, especially the Internet, are disruptive technologies capable of demolishing "old media" monopolies and ushering in a culture of information abundance. Grounded in an analysis of the North American mediascape, although with broader applications to other regions of the world, I argue that media ownership still matters because of its powerful influence on existing media and the evolution of cyberspace as a whole. Recognizing this, the chapter introduces the idea of "netscapes of power" to capture these realities and the realization that communication networks are powerful entities that raise a host of concerns at the heart of this book: risk management, social inclusion and exclusion, surveillance, and privacy.

Many analysts believe the new media generate an environment of information abundance that will reduce uncertainty, create new sources of economic value, and better approximate the ideals of perfect markets, open societies, and democracy. I suggest, however, that information societies are in fact "risk societies." The idea of risk societies is drawn from Ulrich Beck (1994) and is used to illustrate how technical innovation, the heterogeneous qualities of information, and uncertain demand for ICTs generate more risk, not less. I agree with Beck that risk management is now an axial principle of social organization. I further develop this idea by showing how this imperative is being translated into "netscapes of power": mediascapes designed to buttress market power and to regulate behavior through network architecture, the privatization of cyberlaw, surveillance, and the creation of walled gardens. Overall, these concepts highlight how the growing mediation and extension of surveillance are a result of media conglomerates' attempts to regulate information flows and people's use of the media so that they better conform to the communication industries' preferred visions of cyberspace and the "new economy."

Media ownership matters

A wave of changes swept across the entire American mediascape in the last half of the 1990s during a series of transactions worth over half a trillion (USD). Consequently, only four of the eight regional Bell operating companies (RBOCs) created after the AT&T divestiture of 1984 were left by decade's end. AT&T had reemerged as a dominant force in local communications after taking over TCI and MediaOne in 1998 and 1999 respectively. Through these acquisitions, they owned the networks through which nearly half of all American homes accessed television programs and the World Wide Web. Shortly afterwards, AOL combined with the world's largest "old media" conglomerate, Time Warner, in a bid to gain access to Time Warner's cable networks, film studios and archives, specialty channels, music catalogues and magazines (AT&T 2000; Holson and Schiesel 1999). Microsoft also consolidated its position by leveraging its dominant status in computer operating systems into key interfaces between consumers and media content. They invested several billions of dollars in cable systems throughout North America, Europe, Asia, and Latin America, acquiring WebTV, and new content sources for the Internet such as Slate, iNews, MSBET, MSNBC, and so on (Hickey 1997: 2; Microsoft 2000; Newman 1997: 4–9).

Canadian communication companies scanned this unfolding mediascape and saw a model for their own "convergence dreams." In rapid succession, Canwest took over Western International Communications and a chain of newspapers stretching from Vancouver to Halifax that had previously been owned by Conrad Black's Hollinger Inc. Quebecor absorbed Videotron. Rogers Communications aligned itself with global media titans Microsoft and AT&T and formed an alliance with Shaw Communications and Quebecor to divide Canada's cable industry into Cable Monopoly East, Cable Monopoly West, and Quebec. Shaw Communications-based Corus Entertainment bought Nelvana, the premier creator of animated programs in Canada. And, of course, Bell Canada parlayed its dominance in telecommunications across the vast Canadian mediascape by launching ExpressVu and Sympatico in 1994 and 1995 respectively. They continued this trend in 2001 by acquiring CTV and the *Globe & Mail*.

Many analysts defend these changes on the grounds that vertically integrated multimedia companies are necessary and desirable. Media convergence, so the arguments go, has created a need to fill "new media" channels with content, and eliminated any compelling reason to impede media ownership consolidation. This is especially true given the vast explosion of cyberspace. Proponents also claim that new national champions will build the information infrastructures that will catapult Canada into the information age, ensure that citizens have access to a steady flow of Canadian content, and even guarantee our cultural survival in a "global information age" (CTV 2001b: 15; CRTC

2000: 9). However, as a result of these changes Canadians now have one of the most consolidated media systems in the developed world and an unrivalled scale of cross-media ownership.

These changes ushered in the closure of news bureaus, layoffs, and a greater emphasis on regional and national news and entertainment programs at BCE/CTV and Canwest Global. Many local television stations no longer produce their own programs or news (Marotte 2000a: B3, 2000b: B3; Damsell 2001: M1; Dixon 2001: B7). These are the inexorable results of changes in media ownership, and reflect the fact that resources have been diverted from the production of programming toward financing the costs associated with media acquisitions. Similar trends occurred in the US after a spate of ownership changes at the networks in the last decade and a half led to the elimination of foreign news bureaus; news staffs cut by a third to one-half; and less news overall, especially international news (Aufderheide 1990: 51). The diminution of international news is especially disturbing in light of the trend of globalization.

Many argue that these trends do not matter because of the availability of many alternative sources of information, especially the Internet. However, such claims overlook several realities of the existing media culture. In particular, television and newspapers are still the main source, by a considerable margin, of news and entertainment for most people – even for those who use the Internet. This is because conventional media – in both their "real space" and "online" versions – outstrip the Internet in terms of quality and trustworthiness (Pew 2000).

The Internet-as-alternative-to-media-power argument also neglects the fact that Internet access is far from universal and stubbornly skewed by income, gender, education, and age. Canadians are among the most prolific users of the Internet in the world: just under 30 percent of all households had Internet access *from home* by the end of 1999 (Statistics Canada 2000). Worldwide, the number was 3 percent (Netwizards 1999). The Internet is not universal; cyberspace continues to be divided by class. The link between access and class is direct and unequivocal, as shown in Figure 9.1.

Figure 9.1 also shows that Canadian families in the top income quartile are more than three and half times as likely to have a computer and five times more likely to be connected to the Internet at home than those in the last quartile. In fact, more than 80 percent of households in the bottom half of the income curve do not have access to the Internet *from home*, a factor which undercuts the idea that the Internet is an effective alternative to conventional media. Although this situation will change over time, the gap between "information rich" and "information poor" is expanding. Furthermore, trends in computer ownership, even among high-income households, suggest that access to cyberspace may never be universal, at least not for a long time.

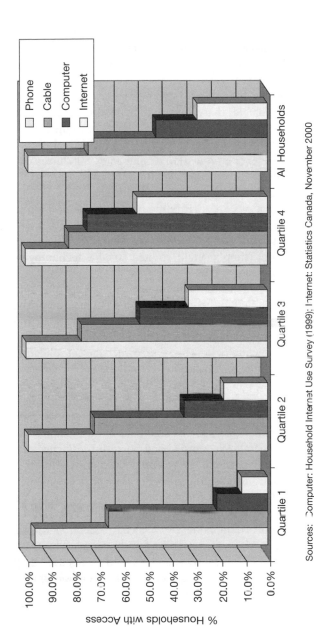

Sources: Computer: Household Internet Use Survey (1999); Internet: Statistics Canada, November 2000 Plugging In: The Increase of Household Internet Use Continues into 1999; Cable & Phone: Household Income and Facilities and Expenditures Survey (1997).

Figure 9.1 Information and Communication Technologies in Canadian Households – 1999 (by quartile)

Even more interesting is the realization that many people – around 25 percent in Canada – do not *want* to use the Internet because of cost, a lack of trust, and the perception that going online is a waste of time (Reddick 2000: 3; Statistics Canada 1999). In the end, the point is that policies governing media evolution should deal with realities – and people – as they *are* rather than as they *might* be in the distant future.

As things currently stand, the Internet and other new media are not so much disruptive technologies as vehicles that allow multimedia firms to reinforce their existing positions and to colonize new mediaspaces with their well-developed "brands." In North America, the most visited websites and portals, for instance, belong to telecommunications companies, broadcasters, newspapers, and Hollywood. The crucial exceptions, of course, are AOL, one of the "new media" stars before it joined the "old media" club in 2000, and Microsoft, whose operations are swiftly moving from the desktop to the network by way of investments in cable systems, set-top boxes, high-speed Internet access and the Internet portal MSN. In short, the "old media" are resilient; they will not simply yield to new media technologies (McChesney 2000; Brethour 2001a: B1).

Generally speaking, new media do not threaten to disrupt the "old media"; they are being recast in their image. This would not have surprised Marshall McLuhan, the early guru of cyberspace, who observed that "old media" typically become the content of "new media." McLuhan saw this as an intrinsic quality of media technologies. However, ownership consolidation is a stronger factor in explaining the absorption of "old media" by the new. This is occurring as familiar patterns of ownership, commercialism, and existing kinds of content are brought into cyberspace. In the process, new technologies are being diverted from a path depicted by uncertainty, risk, and omnidirectional information flows to one that looks more and more like the mass media. Media ownership is a broad and powerful influence that shapes the entire media environment and people's experience of that environment. Of course, BCE's acquisitions spree does not make the Internet. However, couple this with AOL's merger with Time Warner; AT&T's acquisition of nearly half the cable systems in the United States; and the partition of Canada into regional monopolies by Quebecor/Videotron, Rogers and Shaw, as well as the reinforcement of this family compact by these companies' joint and exclusive control over high speed Internet access by cable service – Excite@Home – and the trajectory of media evolution is clear.

Netscapes of power

Significant consequences flow from decisions to allow those who control the medium to own the message. Broadcasters, the press, and cable barons have always done so, but in the case of telecommunications those who owned the medium were prevented from influencing or owning the messages flowing through them in any way. This created an open media system that encouraged those who controlled the pipes to profit by attracting as many content providers and users as possible, rather than by privileging access to their own services. As Janet Abbatte (1999) and Lawrence Lessig (1999) observe, the success of the Internet is due to the fact that it was explicitly designed as an open system where network links between users were kept simple; intelligence and computing power were pushed to the ends of the network; and interfaces between users, content, and networks were kept open and relatively transparent. Media convergence threatens this model as more and more functions are sucked back into the network and as those who own the medium become tightly bound to those who control the content, either through ownership or strategic alliances. As this occurs, the evolution of new media is being biased away from the open systems model of telecommunications and the Internet toward a closed model, where in-house content is favored over other sources. This can be done either in a heavy-handed manner, such as by refusing access to networks altogether (the history of the cable industry and specialty channels), or subtly through network design, acceptable user policies, user menus, search engines, portals, or other ways that give priority access to some sources of content and not others.

This is not a problem if there are multiple gateways to cyberspace and an unconstrained range of information sources. However, the Internet is not immune to consolidation, and this trend is already manifest in the ownership of the Internet backbone linking cities together worldwide. It is emerging among Internet Service Providers. In Canada, there are hundreds of ISPs, but the vast majority are scrambling for survival. The top five – Sympatico, Telus, AOL, the cable companies' @home service, and AT&T – accounted for 75 to 80 percent of all Internet subscribers in 2000. This trend will likely be magnified by the collapse of the dot com bubble, especially among high-speed Internet access providers (Convergence Consulting Group 2000: 12; Brethour 2001b: B1).

These trends would be unremarkable if networks were open and transparent gateways to cyberspace. This is not the case. Networks are not the glassy medium suggested by the fiber-optic cables from which some of them are made. Networks are powerful entities that both include and exclude. Those who control them can exercise a great deal of influence over content providers' access to users, and users' access to content. After neglecting the Internet for years, telecommunication and cable companies are now striving to implement strategies that will help them "attain mind and market share" as well as greater control over the evolution of the Internet as a whole (Cisco 1999a: 6).

Nortel and Cisco, among others, have recognized these needs by designing networks that put intelligence, resources, and capabilities back in the network and under the control of those who own them. Consequently, open network architectures are yielding to network designs that enhance network providers' ability to allocate resources, bandwidth, and speed to varying types of information and services. This is based on their relation to the network owner, revenue potential, class of user served, and judgments regarding the quality of content. According to Cisco, the company's networks put

> absolute control, down to the packet, in your hands. . . . You can identify each traffic type – Web, email, voice, video . . . [and] isolate . . . the type of application, even down to *specific brands*, by the *interface used*, by the *user type and individual user identification* or by the *site address*.
>
> (Cisco 1999b: 3; emphasis added)

While this is marketed as a boon for media companies seeking to cultivate markets, the potential to use these extensive surveillance features to squelch competition, diversity, dissent and freedom of expression are considerable.[1] Their impact on the contours of the Internet and media markets is clearly illuminated in the following passage drawn from Cisco's marketing material:

> The [network's capabilities] allow you to specify the user access speed of any packet by allocating the bandwidth it receives, depending on its IP address, application, precedence, port or even Media Access Control (MAC) address. For example, if a "push" information service that delivers frequent broadcasts to its subscribers is seen as causing a high amount of undesirable network traffic, you can . . . limit subscriber access speed to this service . . . to discourage its use. At the same time, you could promote and offer your own or partners' services with full-speed features to encourage adoption of your services. . . . Further you could specify that video coming from internal servers receive precedence and broader bandwidth over video sourced from external servers.
>
> (Cisco 1999b: 5)

The passage describes a potent netscape of power. Far from being transparent means of channeling information from one point to another, the networks Cisco describes are technologies of discrimination that regulate information flows according to fine-grained criteria set by network owners. In essence, gatekeeping functions have been hardwired into network architectures as part of the communications industries' strategies to cultivate and control markets. These are not abstract potentials. They are the networks used by AOL/Time Warner, AT&T, Bell Canada, Cable & Wireless, Cogeco,

Comcast, Microsoft, Rogers, Shaw, Videotron and "160 of the most successful service providers around the world" (Cisco 2000a: 2, 2000b; Nortel
Networks 2001). These companies now have unprecedented ability to
regulate the Internet, and the extent to which these capabilities will be used
is unclear. However, as AT&T's Internet Services CEO Daniel Somers
exclaimed in defense of his company's refusal to adopt open network policies,
"AT&T didn't spend $56 billion to get into the cable business to have the
blood sucked out of our veins" (cf. Lessig 2000: 995).

The privatization of cyberlaw

As the Canadian government and many others claim to abandon their
attempts to regulate the media (although they are not), media conglomerates
are stepping into the rhetorical breach. They are doing so through four
strategies: network design (as discussed above), acceptable user policies,
surveillance, and "walled gardens." This is most evident with respect to
high-speed Internet services. American and Canadian households only
use such services about 5 percent and 10 percent of the time, respectively
(Convergence Consulting Group 2000: 12; GAO 2000: 6). However, these
ISPs are the pillars of multimedia conglomerates' visions of convergence and
the future of cyberspace. As such, they are worth considering in some detail.

From users' perspectives, communication networks are literally part of the
woodwork. Thus the kinds of design features that enable and constrain
people's use of the media that were referred to above fall beneath the threshold
of perception. Yet, be this as it may, users do confront the realities of a
privately regulated online world through acceptable use policies created and
enforced by telecommunications operators' digital subscriber line (DSL)
services[2] and cable companies' @home service. As such, it is interesting
to interrogate these documents to see their visions of appropriate uses of the
Internet. Generally speaking, the user policies of telecommunications
companies are less restrictive than those of cable companies. However, both
providers see users as mere appendages to the network. Users are destined to
use the Internet mainly as a "read-only" medium and are required to gain
access to additional network functions only on a pay-per basis.

In fact, this "read-only" configuration of the user and commodification
of functionality is hardwired into the architecture of both cable and DSL
networks. Both are asymmetrical networks, meaning that they allow information and images to flood into the home while only offering a narrowband
stream of data to trickle out. Of course, for most users, this design accurately
reflects their usage patterns. However, networks span cities, regions, countries
and even the globe and thus frame communicative action on sociological
and individual levels. Constraints that may be insignificant for millions of

individuals separately sequestered behind closed doors may have large-scale unintended sociological consequences, as thousands of users are deprived of the potential to become creators of media culture in an autonomous, disorganized, and spontaneous way. To think otherwise is to build networks of public life and media culture in ways that saddle those desiring to do more than just read the Internet with the *a priori* constraint of having the inclination and the resources to commodify, professionalize, and register what otherwise might be a commitment to a certain way of life, a hobby, a cause (publishing an environmental or feminist newsletter?), and so on. Such possibilities are not the figment of a deluded imagination. They are integral aspects of "cyberculture" which is widely recognized as a key feature driving innovation on the Net. In that intangible space, unforeseen uses and cultural forms emerge from the margins only to be rapidly transformed into new software packages and technological artifacts that are then propagated through the circuits of cyberspace and/or flogged on the market. The cybernetic features of the Net intensify people's impact on its development, despite attempts to subject it to thoroughgoing commercialization and to turn users into simple appendages of the network.

Some see the power of people to affect the evolution of cyberspace as dangerous. Excite@home adopts this perspective, seeing users as a threat to network security, to viable markets, and to stock holders. Consequently, it has numerous restrictions on what people can and cannot do with its network. This is made abundantly clear in reports filed with the United States Securities and Exchange Commission, in which the company refers to its practice of "limiting users' upstream bandwidth in order to prevent abuse . . . by users, and [its expectation to] continue to limit upstream bandwidth" (@Home 2000b: 13). The company also sees its economic viability as being jeopardized by users who "employ new technology to . . . filter online advertising . . . prevent cookies from being stored on [their] hard drive . . . and shielding e-mail addresses . . . and other electronic means of identification" (@Home 2000b: 22–3). In essence, @Home's view of cyberspace as a thoroughly commercialized, read-only medium clashes with users' expectations, although the latter must yield because, in cyberspace, those who own the networks make the rules.

As mentioned earlier, there are differences between the policies governing the use of the telecommunications companies' DSL services and the cable companies' @home services. There are also parallels. Both sets of policies operate through the following modalities: editorial policies, prohibited uses, surveillance, and enforcement. In both spaces, the network providers reserve a great deal of discretion with respect to monitoring and blocking access to content that contravenes their acceptable use policies or the laws of real space. Their policies often reinforce existing laws by targeting the same types of material – libelous material, child pornography, copyright material, and so on. A bigger problem, however, is the unbound editorial rights that service providers have assumed regarding other types of content. As @Home states, the company "reserves the right to remove or refuse to post any information . . . that they, in *their sole discretion, deem to be offensive, indecent, or otherwise inappropriate regardless of whether such material . . . is unlawful*" (2000b: 5; emphasis added).

This situates service providers as powerful gatekeepers making detailed and arbitrary distinctions between kinds of content that would otherwise be tolerated under freedom of expression rights in North America. This is especially ironic in the United States, where the Supreme Court roundly rejected earlier attempts by Congress to impose the "indecency" standard of content regulation developed in broadcasting to the Internet (ACLU v. Reno 1997). However, in the ensuing years private multimedia conglomerates have usurped the laws of cyberspace and taken to regulating the Internet according to their own standards – standards that are far weaker than those afforded by "real space" laws protecting citizens' freedom of expression rights.

DSL and cable-based high-speed ISPs also prohibit hacking, bulk e-mailing, and cross-posting messages to multiple newsgroups or lists as well as a much longer roster of proscribed uses. Key additional restrictions include a ten-minute limit on the amount of streaming video users can download in a day and another that prevents subscribers from using services that compete with those offered by cable system owners, e.g. Internet telephony (@Home 2000a: 33). Beside such limits, additional restrictions essentially transform the Internet into a read-only medium where access to higher-level capabilities that allow users to become online publishers, broadcasters, and cultural creators are only offered on a pay-per basis. This additional list of proscribed uses includes (@Home 2000b):

- "Bulk mailing of messages, including information announcements, charity requests, petitions for signatures and political or religious messages" (3);
- Maintaining more than two chat connections at the same time (4);
- "Downloading Usenet articles in bulk" (4);
- the operation of a news service, e-mail distribution service or the sending of a news feed (5);
- connecting a server to the network or using a server to operate multi-user interactive forums (5).

Those who disobey these edicts can be banished from cyberspace, at least those spaces under @home and DSL providers' control. Confronted with a context of information abundance and the devolution of media power to the ends of the network and on to users' desktops, the communication industries are striving to pull these powers back into the network where (they think) they belong. The result is a dramatic transformation of cyberspace as we know it, and the resurrection of a model that looks much more like the "old media." Indeed, AT&T now argues that the Internet is an incidental, but integral, part of its basic cable television services, a position that allows it to make editorial decisions regarding the selection of information and services audiences will receive and otherwise "programming the Internet" (AT&T 2000: 11–16). Beyond just redefining the Internet, AT&T has parlayed this conception into at least one decision by US courts recognizing its "first amendment" right to program and control its Internet access services as it sees fit. It wishes to be completely unencumbered by any open network policies or recognition of citizens' rights to freedom of expression (Comcast v. Broward 2000).

Networks of surveillance

The acceptable use policies of Excite@home and others, such as Sympatico and Qwest, are implemented through a sophisticated and automated system of surveillance. Qwest's acceptable use policy, for instance, notes that the company "reserves the right to . . . monitor or exercise editorial control over . . . material created or accessible through [their] networks" (Qwest 2001: 1; see also @Home 2000b: 3; Sympatico 1999: sects 2–7). In essence, surveillance is now a vital part of the communication industries' attempts to anticipate and influence the evolution of all new media and people's communicative behaviors.

The shaky foundations of the so-called new economy are also propelling the surveillance imperative as companies search for new sources of revenue to justify their investments, such as transaction-generated personal information. In addition, the proliferation of information is making it harder, but more advantageous, to "know the audience." This has always been difficult and inaccurate; however, new technologies allow for more detailed audience analysis. This is especially true since agencies such as Neilson's and Arbitron moved into cyberspace in 1995 with the promise of second-by-second analysis of clickstreams and other precise measurements. These options replace cruder methods based on mere exposure to an advertisement, telephone surveys, diaries, and so on. Gandy (1996) and Samarajiva (1997) see these refined attempts to manage consumption as heightening surveillance and augmenting advertisers' ability to discriminate between those audiences they value and those they do not.

At the same time, the potential for new communication networks to offer higher levels of privacy protection are often suppressed because they block the production of a valuable new commodity, personal information, and interfere with efforts to market new services (Samarajiva 1997). Such trends are also reinforced by the proliferation of other surveillance strategies such as discussion group monitoring and cookies. These methods gather information about people's website visits, use of online advertising, and the types of Internet browsers and operating systems, and are used to build up detailed user profiles. In short, uncertainty about the economics of new media, new technological capabilities and fragmentation of the "mass audience" are creating an environment where there can be no expectation of privacy, despite people's desire for "complete control" over personal information (Ekos 1999; Gandy 1996: 105 15; Lyon 1998: 96–8).

These attempts to gain perfect knowledge of users/audiences are often elusive, but they accelerate the momentum of surveillance nonetheless. As Geoff Mulgan explains, "New communication technologies simultaneously bring enormous enhancements of control to governments, corporations, consumers and voters, and a quite new order of chaos and uncontrollability which brings, in turn, a sense that control is unachievable" (1991: 4). Not surprisingly, the intensification of surveillance has increased the sense of risk and, consequently, placed a premium on mechanisms that allow people to deal with the growing loss of control over personal information. In the technical realm, a host of technologies and industry standards are being designed to equip people with tools to control personal information. These include privacy-enhancing technologies (PETs) of encryption and cryptography, secure signatures (VeriSign, Entrust), privacy standards-setting agencies (e.g., WebTrust, Etrust, etc.) and content control measures (Bertelsmann 1999; ICRA 1999).[3]

Reflecting on these developments, many see a major axis in the politics of communication emerging on the frontiers of technology and information service design (Mansell and Silverstone 1996; Agre and Rotenberg 1998). This chapter offers much to reinforce the wisdom of such a view. Indeed, many civil liberties advocates see eliminating controls on PETs as a fundamental human rights and communication policy issue. The Electronic Frontier Foundation and the Electronic Privacy Information Center, for example, have been vocal critics of policies that restrict access to encryption technologies. They have, sometimes successfully, challenged proposals that allow security agencies to intercept private communications over telecommunication networks. From the perspective of these groups, we should distinguish between privacy invasive technologies (PITs) and privacy enhancing technologies (PETs). Simply put, the technological juggernaut driving surveillance must be seen as a double-edged sword. As Bogard observes, computer "screens don't 'watch' people or 'invade' their privacy; increasingly, they are their privacy" (1996: 131). In essence, new information technologies do not just invade privacy, they create it by allowing people to screen themselves off from others mechanically in order to strategically manage who knows what about their communications with others.

While attempts to liberate technologies that enhance people's privacy and efforts to have surveillance capabilities designed *out* of instead of *into* communication networks are laudable, solely focusing on such aims is deeply problematic. For one, PETs are a technological fix to a sociological problem and an example of what Beck (1994) calls "forced individuation." That is, PETs depend on each person making a choice about whether on not to adopt these technologies of personal information protection. This is consistent with the strong libertarian streak that permeates the Internet and creates a real choice that is better than none at all. Yet instead of conceiving of network spaces as social spaces and rationalizing them according to a human rights-based standard of privacy and the socio-cultural conventions that govern everyday interactions, PETs implement a technocratic approach to managing personal information. Under such conditions, privacy negotiation becomes a precondition to communication and to accessing network marketplaces. One can hardly think of a better way to distort communication than by requiring participants to check the technology-enabled privacy status of would-be communicative partners.

In addition, PETs introduce another dimension of social hierarchy into cyberspace, not one that aggravates the divide between the information rich and poor, but between those with the technological savvy to assert their personal preferences and those who do not possess such expertise. Consequently, the human right of privacy becomes dependent on particular technologies and the ability to use them.

Focusing solely on PITs and PETs also fails to grasp how power shapes the agenda and overall context in which struggles over technological design occur. An over-emphasis on PETs leaves the surveillance imperatives being designed into information infrastructures unscathed, while fostering particularistic struggles over the use of technologies. As such they leave the logic of control and closed media systems untouched and, in fact, render communicative spaces more opaque then ever. Rather than focusing exclusively on efforts to liberate technologies of choice, it is more important to address the absence of adequate legal protections for personal information.

Walled gardens

Communication technologies and networks are also being designed and organized in other ways that do more to protect the investment of multimedia conglomerates than to further the goal of creating open and transparent mediaspaces. In the end, netscapes of power and attempts to manage people's relationship to and uses of the Internet reflect these realities and the thrust to change the Internet into an entertainment-driven medium based on advertising, pay-per services, and e-commerce. A key problem, however, for AOL/Time Warner, AT&T, BCE, Excite@home, and Quebecor, among others, is their widely held belief that entertainment-oriented content, especially their own, will turn the Internet into a commercially viable medium. This clashes with current perceptions and uses of the Internet. Yet, literally invested in a specific model of the future, they cling to the belief that, without content, the Internet is "a valueless collection of silent machines with gray screens. . . . It is nothing" (Edgar Bronfman, CEO of Seagram Universal, before being bought by France-based Vivendi, cf. *Economist* 2000a: 24).

The idea that we are living in an age of missing information is a myth. The more urgent concern among these interests is to own specific kinds of content. They believe this will generate revenues enough to finance acquisition binges and a commercially viable Internet: video-on-demand, subscriber-based services, television, and other forms of "old media" content. However, companies such as BCE do not have to own CTV or the *Globe & Mail* to distribute their content. Moreover, they could produce their own content rather than buying that of others, something that would nominally add to the stock of information available to citizens. The conceit of such companies lies in their attempts to superimpose the entertainment-based model of the Internet over top a lengthy list of other activities that are preferred by users, as shown in Figure 9.2.

Figure 9.2 highlights the chasm between views of the Internet as an entertainment-driven medium versus the reality where most people continue to use it extensively as a means of communication, research, to access personally relevant information, and to play games. It is clear that e-commerce, entertainment-oriented uses and pay-per services continue to play a marginal role. Rather than deferring to such realities, however, the major multimedia players at the apex of the "new economy" are seeking to change people's behaviors to conform to their preferred model. Netscapes of power, surveillance and acceptable use policies that regulate people's use of the Net are manifestations of these biases; so too is another strategy: "walled gardens."

This approach was developed by AOL/Time Warner but has subsequently been embraced by many media players, especially in Canada, where BCE and Quebecor explicitly referred to AOL/Time Warner as a model for their own ambitions to create a multimedia giant (Marotte and Damsell 2001: B4; Marotte 2000b: B3). In the walled garden, content, journalism, and all organizational resources strive to cybernetically integrate audiences into a self-referentially enclosed information system governed by the need to defend

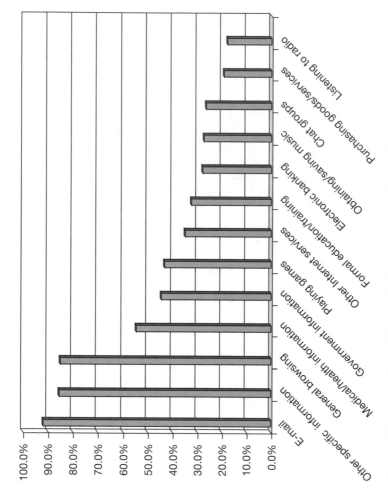

Figure 9.2 Purposes of use within regular home-use households (1999)

Statistics Canada, Nov. 2000 *Plugging In: The Increase of Internet Use continues into 1999*

investments in networks and content. It is a model of media evolution as well that has, at best, weak cultural foundations. The aim is to keep users within specific zones of cyberspace through the creation of content and service menus, the organization of hyperlinks, the bias of search engines, network architecture, the elimination of alternative paths to somewhere else.

Attempts to create enclosed spaces alter the orientation and role of users, media content, and cyberspace altogether, as some possibilities are amputated and others amplified. Content and the organization of network functions and spaces are not driven by quality journalism, creativity, autonomy, or simply pleasure. Instead, they are being turned in on themselves and, in so doing, distorting mediated communication in the interest of preserving the stock market values of highly leveraged multimedia conglomerates. The play of cultural values is stymied. Essentially, as multimedia companies strive to "re-purpose content" and to extend "brand identity" across their media platforms, information, content, and news must be subordinate to the interest in maintaining the organization as a whole.

In this context, innocent theories of language that point merely to its world-disclosing and potential community-constituting roles neglect the burdens of language and media content in an information economy: defending and maintaining economic value, especially in a context where language and words demonstrably move markets. In an information economy, where information is the new wealth of nations, words/messages/content are double-edged swords. On the one hand, they are the anticipated source of great profits and human creativity. Conversely, they can be dangerous threats to the stock market valuations of firms upon which markets as well as national, even global, information economies depend. In a world where information bears such a heavy burden, information, content, and news must be rationalized relative to larger organizational needs and goals. That is the meaning of synergies, cross-purposing, re-purposing and the extension of brand identity.

This is apparent among the leading exemplar of media convergence. At AOL/Time Warner, the function of CNN is no longer just to disclose the news to America and the world, but to deliver audiences to AOL and, in so doing, to prop up its stock prices on Wall Street. As CNN's new Chief Operating Officer, Philip Kent notes,[4] "we hope to be a big content provider to AOL. . . . We are just beginning to conceive of significant cross-promotional opportunities" (cf. Beatty 2001: B9). Moreover, as the *Wall Street Journal* notes, journalists at CNN now worry intensely about the company's stock price and whether or not they will have a job the next day (Anwin and Rose 2001: B1). Examples abound, and the point is clear: journalism, cultural production, and content must serve organizational needs for functional integration and market buoyancy prior to all else.

The role of content, images, and language in creating cybernetically enclosed worlds is also embodied in contracts between AOL/Time Warner and other service providers. For example, AOL's contract with Disney requires Disney to deter users from using Disney's site and related hyperlinks as departure points for larger forays into cyberspace. This is the condition of entry into the "walled garden." Indeed, in this story of the "magic kingdom" meets the "walled garden," AOL can cancel the agreement if more than 25 percent of users visiting Disney's site subsequently leave the AOL "space" (Klein 2000: E1). In essence, Disney assumes the role of immigration officer, policing people's migration in and out of AOL-space. These subtle influences are layered one atop another in ways that imperceptibly encourage people to abandon a nomadic approach to cyberspace. Of course, users do have choices, but the spaces in which such choices are made are explicitly designed to discourage people from exploring a broader universe of information, entertainment, and communication possibilities. This is reflected in the fact that about one-third of all time spent by Americans on the Internet is within AOL/Time Warner-related sites (Walker 2001: E1).

As media merge, organizational cultures collide. This has become particularly evident within AOL/Time Warner as journalists from *Time* magazine or CNN, for example, are forced to give more thought to how their role fits into the larger organization, to learn a broader range of skills, and to consider ways to help AOL meet its aggressive financial goals. The impact on journalism has been considerable in other ways as well, perhaps more dramatically so than in most other areas of the company. Staff and resources at CNN, for instance, were cut by 10 percent, while the rest of the AOL/Time Warner empire received cut-backs that were about one-third that amount (Anwin and Rose 2001: B1; Beatty 2001: B9). If nothing else, such actions reveal the declining priority of news within the overall organization.

These issues are not foreign to Canadian multimedia conglomerates, either. BCE, for example, not only modeled its acquisitions of CTV and the *Globe & Mail* along the lines of the AOL/Time Warner deal; like AOL, it, too, had no experience in journalism, news or entertainment despite taking over Canada's leading players in these fields. Furthermore, its history and organizational culture – again, like the fit between AOL and Time Warner – may pose threats to quality journalism and media freedoms. Bell has a history of a rigid and bureaucratic approach to management; has resisted the formation of labor unions; strictly supervised and intensively surveilled its labor force; and offered little autonomy to its employees. Currently, Bell operators are subject to sixty-five different electronic surveillance measures to assess their work and interaction with customers. This entrenched approach to labor is anathema to the values of autonomy, freedom of expression, and unevenly structured work that are the hallmarks of the entertainment industries and quality journalism.[5]

BCS's threat to journalism is unlikely to be expressed directly. Instead, it will be filtered through the screens of corporate culture and what is not said. Of course, BCE rejects such claims. It strongly defends the ability of CTV and the *Globe & Mail* to continue to report autonomously on all aspects of the organization, as well as to the creation of an elaborate set of measures designed to preserve editorial autonomy within its "units" (CTV 2001a: 9). Canwest Global argues similarly, especially in defense of its extensive cross-media ownership holdings in cities across the country (Canwest 2000: 13). Yet, immediately after invoking these claims, both organizations spurned a CRTC proposal that they adopt a formal code of ethics guaranteeing editorial autonomy in their organizations. However, both companies' Machiavellian approach to language, power, and news reappears time and again in their responses to the regulator's request for information to be placed on the public record. In each instance, the companies cannot quell the impulse to control information. Whatever they throw out the front door is ushered in through the back. Token attempts to demonstrate that media concentration is good for journalism are revoked, as both companies insist that certain information is competitively sensitive and possibly damaging to perceptions of the companies and hence their market valuations (CTV 2001a: 9; Canwest 2000: 13). In the face of such hypocrisy, it is unlikely that journalists in either organization will be either able or willing to engage in the kind of autonomous and critical journalism that Canwest and BCE insist is still possible.

Netscapes of power and bandwidth kings

Despite these attempts to manage almost every aspect of the nascent mediascape – users, networks, markets, content and so on – one of the great ironies is that BCE's embrace of the media convergence bandwagon occurred at precisely the moment when its US counterparts were abandoning key aspects of it. Throughout the last year, telecommunication firms in the US abandoned their content- and television-centric view of the Internet. They now embrace another angle that still has many qualities of the "netscapes of power" discussed above, but with the commitment to content replaced by a focus on data storage, web-hosting, bandwidth, and corporate users. US telecommunication companies jettisoned their plans to get into the television and film industries after recognizing that broadband worldwide continue to report a lack of demand. Also, investments by Microsoft, Rogers, the Canadian maritime telecommunication companies, Aliant,[6] and other web-based television services fail to yield profits. In the mid-1990s all the

US-based Regional Bell Operating Companies had alliances with Hollywood studios and plans to hardwire households to information superhighways. By 2000, however, these initiatives had been junked in favor of more modest projects, such as DSL (Borland 2000; FCC 2001).

Perhaps this was not surprising. Telephone companies have regularly experimented with visions of wired cities and convergence since the 1970s, but none of these efforts have borne fruit. The reasons why have stayed remarkably constant: uncertain demand; the fact that significant numbers do not want to use the new media; and that in a media economy based on the finite resources of time, money, and attention, new media often cannibalize the old media. Telephone companies' entry into video distribution, for instance, would do more to divert people from the corner video shop than expand the market for videos. In Canada, this is interesting in light of the fact that while media expenditures have risen during the last decade and half, the greatest growth has been in telecommunications and computers. It has been slowest in those areas where advocates of full-scale convergence are pinning their hopes, i.e. cable television, video-on-demand, pay-per view, and so on (Statistics Canada 1999). In other words, growth has been concentrated in bandwidth, connectivity, and computers, not content.

These trends suggest that connectivity and bandwidth, not content, might be king (for an extended version of this argument, see Odlyzko 2001). Such possibilities are also borne out by other trends. For example, most websites, with the exception of the *Wall Street Journal* and some porn sites, are unable to sustain a pay-per structure. Also, the prospects for advertising are declining as the holy grail of all measures of value in cyberspace – clickthrough rates – plunge below one-half of 1 percent of users (*Economist* 2000b: 54). The failure of many of the major multimedia conglomerates' portals – Time Warners' late-1990s *Pathfinder* venture, Disney's *Go*, Dreamworks' *Den* – all point in the same direction (Grice and Hu 2001; *Economist* 2000c: 5–27; Marcotte 2001: B3). Other reflections of this appear in the massive cutbacks, layoffs, advertising losses, and stock devaluations at other Internet giants such as Altavista, AOL/Time Warner, Canoe, Excite@home, NBCInteret, and Yahoo.

Conclusion

This chapter has shown that the Internet has underwritten an unprecedented wave of media consolidation, and driven the attempts to manage uncertainty deeper into the design of emerging mediaspaces and the fabric of everyday life. As the fulcrum of the emerging mediascape, communication networks are at the heart of these changes and can thus rightly be called "netscapes of power." In turn, netscapes of power reflect the following modalities of power and control in "risk societies": surveillance, architectural design, risk management, the privatization of (cyber)law, and walled gardens. From a narrow view, these strategies seek to change the Internet into a predominantly "read-only" medium. They integrate audiences, content, and all organizational resources into a cybernetically enclosed information system governed by media conglomerates' need to defend their investments in networks and content. It is a model of media evolution that has, at best, weak cultural foundations. But this is more than just a "media problem." More broadly conceived, these developments stem from the over-burdening of communication with the evolutionary task of building information societies and the "new economy." Groaning under the weight of such projects, and in conjunction with trends in the media economy proper, media spaces are being designed to manage uncertainty and social change through surveillance, control, and pursuit of the information age's illusive holy grail: perfect information.

Notes

1 Also consider these implications in the context of authoritarian and other non-democratic governments. In China, Guatemala, and Singapore, for example, Nortel and Cisco have substantial contracts to provide the networks at the heart of these countries' efforts to modernize their telecommunications systems and Internet capabilities.
2 The following discussion of DSL providers' acceptable use policies is based on those of the US-based RBOC, Qwest, and Bell Canada's Sympatico.
3 Control measures include, for example, SafeSurf, Platform for Information Content Selection (PICS), the Recreational Software Advisory Council and the Internet Content Rating Association standards being promoted by global media conglomerates, such as AOL/Time Warner, Disney/ABC, Bertelsmann, Microsoft, IBM, BT, Bell Canada, etc.
4 Ironically, given the "spectacular" nature of the "information economy," Kent is a former Hollywood talent agent.
5 For more on workplace surveillance, see Kirstie Ball's chapter in this volume.
6 As an example of these failures, the Aliant companies had only 1,500 subscribers to their Imagic web-centric television service after six months in operation and Rogers's comparable service was only able to gain around 5,000 users in Ontario after about the same length of time.

Bibliography

Abbatte, J. (1999) *Inventing the Internet*, Boston, MA: MIT.
Agre, P. and Rotenberg, M. (1998) "Introduction," in P. Agre and M. Rotenberg (eds) *Technology and Privacy: The New Landscape*, Cambridge, MA: MIT.
ACLU (American Civil Liberties Union) *et al.* v. Reno, J., Attorney-General of the United States *et al.*, Appellants, *929 FSupp*, 824.

Anwin, J. and Rose, M. (2001) "Frays, Both Small and Big, Emerge after AOL, Time Warner Merger," *Wall Street Journal*, 9 September: B1.

AT&T (2000) "Comments of AT&T Corp in the Matter of Inquiry Concerning High-speed access to the Internet over Cable and other Facilities (GN Docket No. 00–185)." Online. Available HTTP: <http://www.fcc.gov> (accessed 20 December 2001).

Aufderheide, P. (1990) "After the Fairness Doctrine: Controversial Broadcast Programming and the Public Interest," *Journal of Communication*, 40(3): 47–72.

Beatty, S. (2001) "400 Job Cuts at CNN Units," *Globe & Mail*, 18 January: B9.

Beck, U. (1994) "The Reinvention of Politics: Towards a Theory of Reflexive Modernization," in U. Beck, A. Giddens and S. Lash (eds) *Reflexive Modernization: Politics, Tradition and Aesthetics in the Modern Social Order*, Cambridge: Polity Press.

Bertelsmann (1999) *Self Regulation of Internet Content*. Online. Available HTTP: <www.stiftung.bertelsmann.de/internetcontent/english/frameset_home.htm> (accessed 20 December 2001).

Bogard, W. (1996) *The Simulation of Surveillance*, New York: Cambridge University Press.

Borland, J. (2000) "Phone Companies' TV Ambitions on the Chopping Block," *CNET News.com*. Online. Available HTTP: <http://news.cnet.com> (accessed 30 August 2000).

Brethour, P. (2001a) "PsiNet Crisis Seen as First Shake-out," *Globe & Mail*, 21 March: B1.

—— (2001b) "Bill Comes Due for Web Freebies," *Globe & Mail*, 23 March: B1.

Canadian Radio-television and Telecommunications Commission (CRTC) (2000) "Transfer of Effective Control of CTV Inc. to BCE Inc. (Dec. 2000–747)." Online. Available HTTP: <http://www.crtc.gc.ca/archive/Decisions/2000/DB2000-747e.htm> (accessed 20 December 2001).

Canwest Global (2000) *Station Group License Renewal – Supplementary Brief (Schedule 5A) (Dec. 4)*. Available at: CRTC Public Examination Room, Hull, Quebec.

Cisco Systems (1999a) *New Revenue Opportunities for Cable Operators from Streaming-media Technology*. San Jose, CA: Cisco Systems.

—— (1999b) *Controlling Your Network – A Must for Cable Operators*. San Jose, CA: Cisco Systems.

—— (2000a) *Cisco New World Ecosystem for Cable*, San Jose, CA: Cisco Systems.

—— (2000b) *Company Profiles – @Home*. San Jose, CA: Cisco Systems.

Comcast Cablevision v. Broward County, *No. 99-6934-CIV*. United States District Court, Southern District of Florida.

Convergence Consulting Group (2000) *Strategies and Trends in the Canadian Internet/ISP Market*. Toronto: Convergence Consulting Group.

CTV (2001a) *Station Group License Renewal – Response to Commission's Correspondence of Feb. 8*. Available at: CRTC Public Examination Room, Hull, Quebec.

—— (2001b) *Station Group License Renewal – Deficiency response (Feb. 6)*. Available at: CRTC Public Examination Room, Hull, Quebec.

Damsell, K. (2001) "Canwest Needs a Debt Diet," *Globe & Mail*, 12 January: M1.

Dixon, G. (2001) "Canwest Touts Unit Cross-promotion," *Globe & Mail*, 25 January: B7.

Economist (2000a) "New Media, Old Message," 7 October: 24.

—— (2000b) "The Failure of New Media," 19 August: 53–4.

—— (2000c) "E-entertainment Survey," 7 October.

Ekos (1999) *The Electronic Market Place: The Information Highway and Canadian Communications Household Study*. Online. Available HTTP: <http://www.ekos.ca/> (accessed 20 December 2001).

Federal Communications Commission (FCC) (2001) *Competition in the Market for the Delivery of Video Programming (7th Annual Report)*. Washington, DC: Federal Communications Commission.

Gandy, O. (1996) "Legitimate Business Interest: No End in Sight? An Inquiry into the Status of Privacy in Cyberspace," *University of Chicago Legal Forum*, 77–137.

General Accounting Office, United States (GAO) (2000) *Telecommunications: Technological and Regulatory Factors Affecting Consumer Choice of Internet Providers* (Gao-01-93). Online. Available HTTP: <http://www.gao.gov/> (accessed 20 December 2001).

Grice, C. and Hu, J. (2001) "Write-offs Point to Content Sector Struggles." Online. Available HTTP: <http://news.cnet.com/news/0-1005-202-4653582.html> (accessed 20 December 2001).

Hickey, N. (1997) "The Microsoft Millennium," *Guardian*, 12 December: 2–7.

Holson, L.M. and Schiesel, S. (1999) "Duelling Bids Emerge for Sprint," *New York Times*, 4 October: A1.

@Home (2000a) *1999 10K Report Filed with US Securities and Exchange Commission*. Online. Available HTTP: <http://www.home.com> (accessed 20 December 2001).

—— (2000b) *Acceptable Use Policy*. Online. Available HTTP: <http://www.home.com/suppport/aup> (accessed 8 May 2000).

Internet Content Ratings Association (ICRA) (1999) *An Invitation to Membership*. Online. Available HTTP: <http://www.icra.org> (accessed 20 December 2001).

Klein, A. (2000) "Merger puts AOL's Methods on Trial," *Washington Post*, 3 November: E1.

Lessig, L. (1999) *Code and Other Laws of Cyberspace*, New York: Basic Books.

—— (2000) "Forward to Symposium on Cyberspace and Privacy," *Stanford Law Review*, 52(5): 987–1003.

Lyon, D. (1998) "The World Wide Web of Surveillance," *Information, Communication & Society*, 1(1): 91–105.

McChesney, R. (2000) "The Titanic Sails On: Why the Internet Won't Sink the Media Giants," *Extra*. Online. Available HTTP: <http://www.fair.org/extra/0003/aol-mcchesney.html> (accessed 20 December 2001).

Mansell, R. and Silverstone, R. (eds) (1996) *Communication by Design*, London: Sage Publications.

Marotte, B. (2000a) "BCE Raises Bet on Web Content," *Globe & Mail*, 16 September: B3.

—— (2000b) "Videotron CEO Resigns Post," *Globe & Mail*, 25 November: B3.

Marotte, B. and Damsell, K. (2000) "Content Key to Monty's Plan: BCE Strategy Aimed at being Major Player in Multimedia World," *Globe & Mail*, 12 September: B4.

Microsoft (2000) *Annual Report (1999)*. Online. Available HTTP: <http://www.microsoft.com> (accessed 20 December 2001).

Mulgan, G.J. (1991) *Communication and Control: Networks and the New Economics of Communication*, New York: Guilford Press.

Newman, N. (1997) *From Microsoft Word to Microsoft World: How Microsoft is Building a Global Monopoly*. Online. Available HTTP: <http://netaction.org/msoft/world/> (accessed 20 December 2001).

Netwizards (1999) "Internet User Survey (July 1999)." Online. Available HTTP: <http://www.netwizards.org> (accessed 20 December 2001).

Nortel Networks (2000) *A Policy-based Approach to Application Optimized Networking*, Cambridge, ON: Nortel Networks.

Odlyzko, A. (2001) "Content Is Not King," *First Monday*, 6(2). Online. Available HTTP: <http://firstmonday.org/issues/issue6_2/odlyzko/index.html> (accessed 20 December 2001).

Pew Research Centre (2000) *Media Report – Internet Sapping Broadcast News Audience*. Online. Available HTTP: <http://www.people-press.org/media 00rpt.-htm> (accessed 20 December 2001).

Qwest (2001) *Acceptable Use Policy*. Online. Available HTTP: <http://www.qwest.com/legal/usagePolicy.html> (accessed 20 December 2001).

Reddick, A. (2000) *The Dual Digital Divide: The Information Highway in Canada*. Ottawa: Public Interest Advocacy Centre and Human Resources Development Canada. Online. Available HTTP: <http://olt-bta.hrdc-drhc.gc.ca/download/oltdualdivideen.pdf> (accessed 20 December 2001).

Samarajiva, R. (1997) "Telecom Regulation in the Information Age," in W. Melody (ed.) *Telecommunications Reform*, Denmark: Technical University of Denmark.

Statistics Canada (1999) *Household Internet Use Survey*, Ottawa: Ministry of Supply and Services.

—— (2000) *Plugging In: The Increase of Household Internet Use Continues Into 1999*. Online. Available HTTP: <http://www.statcan.ca: 80/english/research/56F0004MIE/56F0004MIE00001.pdf> (accessed 20 December 2001).

Sympatico (1999) *About Sympatico: Terms and Conditions, Advertising, Services*. Online. Available HTTP: <http://www1.sympatico.ca/> (accessed 20 December 2001).

Walker, L. (2001) "AOL Time Warner Sites Dominate Web Traffic Data," *Washington Post*, 26 February: E1.

Part IV
Targeting trouble
Social divisions

10 Categorizing the workers

Electronic surveillance and social ordering in the call center

Kirstie Ball

Introduction

Surveillance, in one form or another, has always been at the heart of capitalist enterprises, and organizations in general. Within the established business school, knowledge of general management theory and transaction cost economics (TCE), systematic information codification, monitoring and control are argued to be at the center of Western economic activity (and supremacy). In 1916, Henri Fayol's organizational ethnography, described in every standard management text as one of the founding pieces of management theory, identified six management activities. These ranged from planning and forecasting, to organizing, commanding, and coordinating. The final of these activities was "controlling" – the definition of which refers to the monitoring of activities to ensure compliance with existing plans. Similarly, Beniger's (1986) and Yates's (1989) historical studies emphasize the pervasive policing and control elements of large-scale corporate systems which are supported by detailed communication systems (Clark 2000). TCE, in focusing upon the coordination of firms and market mechanisms in the policing of contracts, emphasizes the role of internal firm information in subverting the main market mechanism: price (Coase 1937; Williamson 1975). This is said to decrease risk and increase control over organizational environments by creating internal capital markets.

As with the financial risk associated with capital markets, organizations seek to similarly reduce risk in dealing with the labor market. Extensive data collection about actual and potential employee characteristics, skills, competencies and knowledge, and the electronic storage thereof, is now big business. Fora on E-HRM (Electronic Human Resources Management) are now commonplace, with software vendors selling powerful analytical tools to predict optimum staffing levels, skill and competency combinations. These tools attempt to monitor and assess risks associated with particular staffing strategies, as well as collect, analyze, and categorize existing employee performance and attendance through time. They are often used in tandem with a number of other softer "people management technologies" such as appraisal, 360° feedback (appraisal from subordinates and peers, as well as managers), and various forms of training and development needs assessment.

Recent legislative changes in the UK have simplified the monitoring of workers' computer-mediated activities, establishing legal rights for employers to monitor employee e-mail, telephone calls, and web usage during work time. Nevertheless, other areas of the UK economy have seen industrial action by call center employees (where we see consistent and relentless electronic monitoring of performance) because of "ebullient management tactics" – the unfair application of performance measuring and targets. Between 12 and 25 February 2001, the UK's Trades Union Congress (TUC) conducted a high-profile media campaign which set up a helpline for call center employees. In the first six days of the campaign, 397 workers from all over the UK rang to complain about bullying, impossible sales targets, not receiving wages on time, and hostility to unions (Trades Union Congress 2001).

In this chapter, case material is drawn from one of several studies conducted in UK call centers in the mid-1990s, which examines one particular type of electronic workplace surveillance: computer-based performance monitoring (CBPM). It is argued that the management practices surrounding any employee monitoring system are a system of worker categorization and ordering, and are enmeshed within existing, deeper workplace socio-technical orders and value systems. This is particularly significant since the majority of existing research conducted in North America in the mid-1980s to early 1990s strove to identify how managers might monitor their staff in an effective and fair way. This same research, however, only attended to task and feedback design rather than broader social factors in the workplace. Whilst job and feedback design factors can certainly be a vehicle for fair monitoring practice, the manner in which feedback is given is also set within a social context of management–worker relations and ordering which is more deeply embedded in the fabric of social interaction at work. I begin the chapter with a review of the North American literature, which establishes and summarizes best-practice guidelines. Then, using Marx's (1998) framework, I introduce the proposition that attention to procedural and distributive justice in monitoring processes brings the need to examine deeper social orders, which are not included in existing best-practice frameworks. An investigation of such orders requires a methodology sensitive to their negotiation and construction, which is then used to analyze some interview data from a UK call center in Norco (a pseudonym).

Electronic surveillance in the call center:
"the technological whip of the electronic age?"[1]

Electronic surveillance, in the form of CBPM, is one of the main management tools used in the call center. CBPM monitors workers' performance over a predefined time period, and uses the statistics and voice recordings it generates to categorize and evaluate them according to certain performance criteria which are usually defined by the organization (see Higgins and Grant 1989). It has been referred to as a "technological whip," because of the strong implication that its application in this context is unquestionable, and is essentially one of control. At the time of writing, current estimates range from there being between two to five thousand call centers in the United Kingdom, employing up to 400,000 people. Datamonitor provides a more conservative prediction that 247,000 (2 percent of the UK's working population) will be employed in a call center by the end of 2002. The UK's Call Center Association (CCA) currently has 420 members, facilitating many smaller non-member operations behind the scenes.

The rise of the call center is symbolic of other industry and policy moves to promote, at both regional and national levels, competitiveness on the basis of "knowledge capital." North American business analyst Peter Drucker (2000) portrays this phenomenon as an epochal shift in business organiza-tion. Since the early 1990s, the call center has been promoted as a means of employment regeneration in economically depressed areas of the UK (particularly with customers' reported preferences for northern regional accents). This has dovetailed with the current UK government's emphasis on lifelong learning and its North American-influenced reconceptualization of service sector work as "knowledge work" (Blackler 1995).

Other critical management writers and I acknowledge the slipperiness and problematic nature of "knowledge" as a concept (Alvesson 1993, 2001). However, leading business writers such as Nonaka and Takeuchi (1995) and Drucker (1993) argue that those in boundary-spanning roles who work with information and communication technologies (which include the customer-facing call center worker), and who employ and share organizationally and individually idiosyncratic knowledge are "knowledge workers." There is scant evidence, however, to support any resultant worker upskilling at a general level (Graham 2000), and only the occasional anecdote suggests that call center work experience adds value for the worker. Plenty, however, exists to claim knowledge worker status for highly paid problem-solving roles within merchant banks, and management, IT, and engineering consultancies (Sveiby and Lloyd 1987). Indeed, it is more frequently noted that the distinguishing feature of knowledge work is the deft ability of organizations to engage their workers in elaborate forms of social process management, and rhetorical and identity-related control (Alvesson 2001).

Call center workers are likely to be poorly paid, working with computer and information technologies that contain all "required" knowledge about products and customers. They often read from a quality-controlled script, working to a set of predefined targets, leaving little margin for innovation or the application of one's own "knowledge." The frequent customer interaction in call centers also feeds into marketing-based surveillance systems which further aggregate customer information before it is sold on in the "knowledge economy." Similarly, proponents of "knowledge capital" frequently overlook questions of power. The constant monitoring of calls and performance means call center workers are exposed to intense surveillance by the organization which makes them the more likely target of knowledge creation, categorization, and use, than its source.

Before knowledge work hit the headlines, literature about call centers in the UK and US concerned worker surveillance and performance monitoring. It dates from the mid-1980s (OTA 1987), and addresses a number of areas: its impact on worker stress levels (Nebeker 1987; OTA 1987; Smith *et al.* 1986), its consequences for workplace social relations (Aiello 1996; Attewell 1987; Ball 1996; Deutsch 1986; Smith and Amick 1989) and how this varies across cases (Ball 1996; George 1996). Drawing on Willmott (1999), I argue that the way in which CBPM is conducted in organizations is laden with double-edged organizational "value orientations."

First, there is the distributive justice of reward (material or otherwise) for effort and punishment for non-effort. In CBPM terms this refers to the accuracy of feedback and representation of employee effort. Second, the procedural justice of employee voice in the monitoring process: communication, trust, involvement and mutual responsibility between management and workers for performance (Alder 1998). It is clear from the content of pieces about CBPM, and from personal experience as an author in this area for a number of years, that authors share similar concerns about these aspects of CBPM-related practice. To elaborate, whilst management and some pro-management writers present it as a necessity, the academic literature suggests that it be applied in a manner that is considerate both to workers' psychological and physical health, and well-being, as well as to organizational concerns for efficiency. Furthermore, if such considerations are not met, workers should have a way of resisting or challenging unfair monitoring practice. These research concerns also inform a neat range of dilemmas (Introna 2000) for practitioners and academics to consider: the extent to which workers are entitled to a degree of privacy under surveillance (Sipior *et al.* 1998); the extent to which workers are expected to sacrifice aspects of their mental and physical health when they come to work (Lund 1992); the extent to which workers have the reasonable expectation of a meaningful and satisfying job (Chalykoff and Kochan 1989); and the extent to which workers have the reasonable expectation of a level of "normal" human interaction during the course of the working day, rather than being treated like machines (Alder 1998; Westin 1986).

To understand how procedural and distributive justice may work in practice, it is important to explore the legacy of past research into CBPM, which is split in two. First, some research attempts to measure monitoring practice in terms of specific identifiable guidelines and organizational structural contingencies which have been argued elsewhere to determine workplace level "outcomes: for *inter alia* job design, worker health, and so on (e.g., Attewell 1987; Higgins and Grant 1989; Kulik and Ambrose 1993; Westin 1986, 1988). These are typically expressed in a series of "should be" (Parker 1999) statements about CBPM. The assumption behind these statements is that there is such a thing as objectively "good" and "bad" monitoring practices which have measurable direct effects for the employee in terms of job satisfaction, stress, turnover, and productivity (Chalykoff and Kochan 1989). This creates a yardstick against which different configurations of CBPM practice can be measured.

Second, some research examines management–worker relations from a Foucaultian perspective. This research particularly examines the local, discontinuous, socially constructed nature of relations surrounding monitoring practice, which afford it different meanings in different contexts. These in turn reflect the power relations within that context (e.g., Ball and Wilson 2000; Sewell and Wilkinson 1992). CBPM's embeddedness within social relations leads a research agenda away from performing a simple "checklist"-based evaluation. Instead, researchers examine how individual organizations and their members socially construct the use of their monitoring technologies, and how the socio-technical relation between technologies, workers, supervisors, management, and organization emerges. This leads us to question how CBPM and its outcomes might be known other than as a predefined element of organizational structure with measurable effects, and how these value-laden best-practice guidelines become subject to and the subject of social practice.

Thus, the latter research moves away from the structured ontologies of best-practice frameworks, and towards a reputation as a set of emergent socio-technical practices constructed during the everyday speech and social interaction of the research act (Alvesson and Karremann 2000; Ball and Hodgson forthcoming). Ball and Wilson (2000) argued that a fine-grained discourse analytic approach to interview analysis has much to reveal about the nature of socio-technical workplace relations wherein CBPM is embedded. Details of both these streams of work are described next.

Best-practice guidelines: Structures and outcomes

This section considers the work of Westin (1986, 1988), Smith and Amick (1989), Kulik and Ambrose (1993), Higgins and Grant (1989) and DeTienne and Abbott (1993). Westin (1986) surveyed 147 US-based organizations and developed a model of possible uses of CBPM based on the Taylorism–Labor relations control dialectic found in labor process theory. "Taylorist" approaches to CBPM emphasize restricted communication and participation between management and workers, employee compliance and obedience, individual quotas and piecework. The "Labor Relations" model emphasizes open communication, participation and discussion between management and workers, employee autonomy, team-based quotas, and fair pay. In naming the latter the "fairness" model of monitoring, and the former the "Taylorist" model, Westin's (1986) model is heavily laden with notions of how procedural and distributive justice in CBPM processes might translate into identifiable practices (such as the abolition of piecework, team-based bonuses, intermittent rather than constant monitoring, etc.). He also investigated broader contextual issues (Westin 1988) and concluded that comprehensive training on computer applications, good ergonomic arrangements, the choice to move away from one's workstation, and social aspects such as trust, good formal and informal communication with management and peers, and staff involvement in relevant decisions were also significant.

Smith and Amick (1989) conducted extensive survey work throughout the 1980s, and found CBPM to be a major determinant of job satisfaction and stress. They produced several recommendations on how to deliver feedback. Their recommendations concerned designing the feedback's timeliness and credibility according to worker need, thus maximizing its value to the worker and its elicitation of their effort. "Timeliness" also featured in the work of Higgins and Grant (1989) and Grant *et al.* (1988), who also advised managers about the choice of monitoring measures. According to their empirical work, each measure sent a value-laden message to employees about what the organization expected of them in terms of service and quality. Privacy issues also inform this work, as Irving *et al.* (1986) warned against the wide broadcasting of feedback and the close individual monitoring of the employee.

Finally, DeTienne and Abbott (1993) suggest that the "value-laden message" inherent in the delivery of feedback is also inherent within the design and implementation of a particular CBPM system from the start. As such, they suggest that an "employee-centered" design would be best. Such a design would encourage the system's performance-related parameters to be specifically constructed around the abilities, aptitudes and skills of a given workforce, rather than expecting the workforce to fit a predefined set of machine-performance criteria which may not be contextually appropriate. All of these authors provide case examples of how some of these recommendations have been achieved and they are summarized as "best practice" guidelines in Table 10.1.

Table 10.1 Summary of guidelines concerning the implementation and use of CBPM derived from previous research

Technology implementation

1 Positive aspects of the system should be emphasized.
2 Good reasons for the implementation of CBM should be demonstrated to staff (e.g. performance-related pay).
3 Employees should feel that there is much to gain from having CBM.

Technology use

1 Quantitative monitoring should be appropriate for the tasks being measured.
2 The monitoring should not attempt to measure non-quantitative aspects of the job.
3 The system should adequately represent employee performance.
4 The measuring process should be foolproof: everyone should know how it's done.
5 Feedback should be given on a meaningful timescale to employees.
6 Feedback should be delivered personally, not via the machine.
7 A computer which monitors the process as well as the results of the work is more likely to be seen as spying by those subject to it.
8 Management should be sensitive to the fact that some employees may not want their productivity rates broadcast.
9 The feedback should reinforce to employees what is considered to be "good" performance.
10 The performance information should be readily and easily accessible to employees.
11 The employees should feel able to challenge information generated by the system.
12 Standards should be flexible and allow for employee error.
13 A production shortfall should lead to discussion, not discipline.

Social orders under surveillance: the use of repertoires

Alternative accounts of CBPM practice focus on the way feedback processes and management–worker relations are constructed in interview talk. These accounts depict versions of CBPM situations that examine individuals' experiences as subjects of CBPM, and surrounding social systems, in more detail. Since the focus is on talk, a number of different conversation analytic or discourse analytic strategies can be employed to this end (see Alvesson and Karreman 2000 for a useful classification of modes of discourse analysis).

Interpretive repertoires is one such method, which attempts to identify the different lexicons of themes, concepts, and ideas individuals use when they describe something, and the interplay between them (Potter and Wetherell 1987; Wetherell 1998). In effect, they focus upon how individuals construct and identify social relations within their worlds, observing the identity work and ideological practice through which this is achieved (Wetherell 1998). They advocate a reading of interview texts which emphasizes the constructed nature of accounts. In other words, what interviewees say should not be read as indicative of some external, measurable context. Individuals use their battery of repertoires to make their reality seem real to the researcher, placing emphasis on the accounting function in the context of the research interview. In addition, variation rather than congruity is sought between accounts. The idea is, therefore, that individuals use their interpretive repertoires to position themselves and others in relation to a subject of conversation (in this case, the departmental context of computer-based monitoring practice). The interpretive-repertoires approach seeks to analyze this positioning.

In an organizational study, positioning of self in relation to one's colleagues, department, and organization is central to the understanding of social relations in context both within and between organizational sites. Positions are classified as either troubled or untroubled. The notion of the troubled and untroubled subject position refers to how a subject position may be sitting comfortably within the action orientation of a conversation at one point in an account, and become uncomfortable and troubled when the action orientation changes. A troubled position can occupy either a dominant (when an important speaker claims an untroubled position) or subordinate (used either to support or oppose the dominant repertoire) repertoire, either reciprocally or alternatively. Reciprocal positioning occurs when individuals position themselves or others as troubled in a dominant repertoire by virtue of its terms, but in inverse relation to that repertoire. Alternative positioning describes where one is positioned as troubled in an alternative repertoire to that which is dominant (Ball and Wilson 2000).

This method has attracted criticism from a number of conversation analysts. Schegloff (1997), for example, argues that a much closer reading of the interview text reveals the "actual" positions of speakers. Other users of discourse analysis (e.g., Michael 1996) note that the application of interpretive repertoires may involve too great an abstraction of the individual and hence has an "elitist" tendency. In her defense of the method, Wetherell (1998) draws on Foucault's genealogical method to assert that the focus is on interaction and construction of context, rather than the individual. Thus interplay of repertoires in any particular conversational context is reflective of local social relations, with an emphasis on power and resistance (Henriques

1998). In the study of CBPM in context, therefore, the identification of interpretive repertoires and subjects' positions within them will show the qualitative bases of power and resistance within that context, allowing the identification of social orders. It also shows how access to the procedural and distributive justice associated with this best practice might differ between groups of workers.

Studying surveillance through multiple perspectives

This bifurcation in research approaches to CBPM in the workplace resonates with Marx's (1998) analysis of the ethics of any surveillance-based practice. Marx advances twenty-nine questions which identify criteria concerning the means of data collection, the context and conditions under which it is collected, and the uses or goals thereof, as a way of judging the fairness of surveillance activity in relation to its context of application. He uses the notions of social and physical border violation, procedural and distributive justice, and communication and sharing of goals, described above, to construct the relevant aspects of surveillance. Marx highlights criteria to judge practice, and also stresses the importance of contextualizing any analysis of surveillance-based practice. Specifically, he is at pains to highlight the symbolic meaning attached to surveillance practice, and the capacity of surveillance to distort forms of social equality. In effect, Marx is suggesting that, to fully investigate surveillance, it is necessary to examine both technological and practice configurations as well as its meaning in context.

If we apply this argument to CBPM, multiple analytical strategies can be applied which are sensitive to both factors. In my discipline, organization studies, combining methods in this manner is problematic,[2] although situated knowledges and the material semiotic approach[3] (Haraway 1991) as analytical strategies have been suggested as one potential solution (Ball 2001). In this chapter, case-study material from an organization, Norco, demonstrates that a combination of two methods (use of an *a priori* classification and interpretive repertoires) reveals more about the social ordering and value systems inherent in a case of CBPM in practice than would an application of either strategy on its own.

CBPM in Norco's collections department

Norco is a large financial services organization operating in the north of England. In the early 1990s they launched a hugely successful personal loans product. The collections department was responsible for collecting arrears pertaining to customers' personal loans. In the department, six teams of six employees (two senior clerks and four clerks) were at work, each with a supervisor, and the whole department was run by a management team of three: one manager and two assistants. All had been working in the department since its inception in 1990. Work in the department was entirely computer-based, and the computer monitored everything. The teams dealt with two areas: four handled accounts that were up to five payments in arrears (called "collections"), and two handled accounts that were over five payments in arrears (called "recoveries"). A total of eleven employees from this department were interviewed: the manager, an assistant manager, two supervisors, two senior clerks, and five clerks. These were drawn from two of the teams in the department. The interview asked all employees their views about monitoring and appraisal practice, management–worker relations, and their views on the organization as a whole. Collectors and their supervisors were also observed for several periods of time.

CBPM in Norco

CBPM in Norco has a history that is recognizable as one of "office automation." At its inception in 1990, the department used a paper-based filing system, which, according to the interviewees, became unwieldy, inefficient, and frustrating with the growth of the personal loans product. Accordingly, alongside a change in management, the department was transformed into its present computerized format. Management promised staff that their work would be easier to manage with the new system, and all were required to work very hard to reduce the backlog that had mounted with its predecessor. Because of the increased responsibility taken on by staff to reduce the backlog, and development in their roles more generally, their jobs were regraded. Each staff member was automatically awarded a pay raise and promotion during the system implementation. Whether this was coincidence or the result of attitude engineering, management had successfully emphasized positive aspects of the CBPM system to render it more acceptable to their staff.

The overall performance management process formed an elaborate worker categorization exercise, integrating both electronic (CBPM) and paper-based (appraisal) modes of assessment, effectively covering every aspect of collectors' behavior: towards the customers, their peers, their supervisors and their managers. Day-to-day monitoring practice was all-encompassing. The department worked the accounts on the *Debt Collection System (DCS)*, which logged all the calls and entries made to the individual accounts. The task of each collector was to telephone debtors and arrange payment promises on their respective personal loans, entering the details of their call onto the debt collection system. The workers were monitored on the number of accounts worked, the amount of money arranged to be collected, the amount of money actually collected, number of broken promises for payment, and the amount of talking and typing time per case. Management emphasized that the most important statistic was the number of broken promises over a given time period, as this reflected the quality of the arrangements made by the collectors and how well they had understood the customer's needs. The same performance criteria also applied to short-term (typically three-hour) "collection campaigns" using a power dialler. The dialler would be set to select cases on the basis of geographical area or amount in arrears. It would then automatically dial the debtors, and only link to the collector's headset when a connection was made, thereby machine-pacing the calls. Thus the collector had the difficult task of speaking to different debtors, one after another without a break, and being subject to constant monitoring.

Collectors reported that perceptions of the overall performance management process encouraged them to be more quality-aware, and not to fiddle their performance figures. Some discretionary fiddling took place, however, which involved collectors leaving their telephone lines open after the customer had gone, so that they could type the details into the machine and appear to have reduced their typing time (for which the collectors were only allowed one minute). According to one informant, this happened very infrequently. Furthermore, as monitoring concerned only performance outcomes rather than processes, informants explained that there was no "big brother" feeling in the department. Information about the statistics was readily available to the collectors, but they were not always aware of this. Despite this, every collector interviewed felt that they could challenge or query any aspect of performance statistics at any time. Examples of the official monitoring criteria can be found in Appendix 1.

A unique aspect of the department was the widespread broadcasting of performance statistics – although it was not the official figures that mattered. Far more important was the staff's own system of performance feedback broadcast. Every two or three months, a group of collectors would get together and organize an informal collections competition based on a humorous theme (such as "pub crawl," or "the pop charts"). Individual collectors formed teams of three with anyone from the department, and the amount of money collected by each person represented their team's score. This was an interesting incidence of electronically mediated worker surveillance, as referred to by Sewell (1998). The competition scoreboards were usually drawn on the back of wallpaper measuring two or three meters in length, featuring cartoon-like depictions of each team engaged in a race to the top of the charts, the most elite nightclub, etc., which was based on the amount of money collected. Prizes for each team were sourced from various collectors' lofts, garages, and sheds. This was widely referred to as symbolic of the department's self-reported "work hard–play hard" culture. They even awarded me a prize (an old Sex Pistols 7-inch single) during my time there, for "being a laid-back researcher"!

The ultimate collector achievement was to collect one million pounds for the organization, rewarded by membership in the organization's "million-aires' club" which offered them various perks and privileges. In addition, the department had a football team which played on a Wednesday evening, and a tradition of the majority heading down to the local pub after work on a Friday for a drink. All informants reported positive management–worker relations, and management and supervisors noted few disciplinary problems, with a low annual staff turnover rate (5 percent). High levels of trust, a high level of information communication up and down the hierarchy, and a strong mutual appreciation of each other's position were reported to dominate social relations in this department.

The supervisors and assistant managers were key in the management of the whole process. All had come through the collector ranks to their current positions. Both clerks and supervisors argued that this in itself was responsible for the smooth running of the department, and its largely developmental culture. Whilst there were no formal targets set, there was an informal understanding between all parties that the collectors should aim to work ten cases an hour. When I reviewed some confidential performance data on site, all but a few collectors regularly attained this goal. Supervisors delivered this information to their teams on a weekly and monthly basis, but all supervisors were informally in contact with their teams every day, and so performance feedback, coaching, advice, and encouragement was always at hand. When I asked the supervisors how they managed the underachieving staff, it appeared that individual shortfalls did not lead to any punishment. Rather, they were classified by the appraisal system as having a developmental need in that particular performance area. Further, they reported that staff members were categorized as "problematic" if they had misbehaved in any inter-personal manner (such as verbally abusing another member of staff, or having an "attitude problem," which referred to their slow adaptation to new ideas). Appraisals took place every quarter, and there were many skill areas in which collectors were assessed: communication, teamwork, information use, planning, accuracy, initiative, learning capacity, and analytical skills. Each pay grade (there were four, from clerk to supervisor) had different standards in each area, and work study had determined the amount of time they should spend doing each. Collectors were ranked on a scale of one to five for each skill area. I was only able to view a few appraisals (they were confidential documents), but I noted a central tendency in the scoring. The outcomes were either that workers received more formal training and development, or were informally required to at least maintain their status quo until the next quarterly appraisal, when they would be reviewed again. It is clear from this brief description that the vertical (by management) and horizontal (through staff competitions) electronic surveillance practices in Norco were situated in a complex network of non-electronic surveillance (appraisal), and long-standing social relations, which, as we shall see, also performed a crucial categorizing role.

Assessment of monitoring practice according to best-practice guidelines

So, how did Norco fare in relation to published "best-practice" guidelines? An aggregated and interpreted summary of the responses is presented in Table 10.2.

Table 10.2 Norco's CBPM practices, compared to previous research

Table 1 number	Finding
1	Implementation which led to pay rises through job regrading and an ease on workload.
2	Acceptance of both the quality and quantity measures by the staff. A widespread acknowledgement of quality being more important than speed.
3	Employee performance statistics a small part of broader competency-based appraisal system
4	Low occurrence of figure fiddling because of quality awareness, but an acknowledgement of its potential.
5	Delivery of feedback using a variety of timescales and methods.
6	Supervisors delivering feedback, informal, staff-led humorous feedback system.
7	Work outcomes (i.e., money collected) monitored, no listening in on calls.
8	A degree of sensitivity in the way in which feedback is delivered to different operators.
9	"Work hard, play hard" ethic reflected in informal feedback mechanisms to balance money collecting, and feedback always delivered constructively.
10	Not complete awareness of accessibility of performance statistics.
11	All employees felt able to challenge the information generated by the system.
12	Flexible approach taken to the achievement of targets.
13	Developmental, not punitive, approach to feedback delivery.

Table 10.2 shows that, in terms of the normative guidelines, the practice of CBPM in Norco seems to fare quite well. Tenets of implementation and feedback style were met with the exception of staff awareness of monitoring statistics. Distributive justice concerns, relating to the perceived accuracy, timeliness, critical focus, and balance of performance data in relation to statistics were being met. Similarly, in terms of procedural justice, employees' rights to challenge and discuss statistics seemed to be securely in place. But what happens when we take a more fine-grained look at the data? Are the employees all healthy, happy, and equally represented in departmental power relations given this proximity to normative "best practice"? Whose voices in the workplace get heard and acknowledged by management in the everyday work situation? Do some workers have a greater "right" to challenge management than others? Do others miss out on developmental opportunities? These questions have a bearing on how fine-grained attention to deeper social ordering, which is invisible in a best-practice account, may reveal more about this case than initially meets the eye.

Interpretive repertoires in Norco

On closely examining extracts of talk from the interviews, two interpretive repertoires emerged, which operated in tandem:

- The "empowerment" repertoire drew upon ideas of proactivity, choice and freedom in worker and manager performance and conduct in social relations.
- The "life in work" repertoire brought other aspects of workers' personal identities (e.g., gender, age, pastimes, personal preferences) to bear on their conduct in social relations.

The following paragraphs contain extracts from interviews that show the repertoires in action. Because of space limitations, not many extracts could be exhibited, but I consider these to be good representations of a significant number of the speech fragments classified using the interpretive repertoires analytical method.

The empowerment repertoire

The title "empowerment" is drawn directly from the language of the senior manager in this case, and is a label for the many interrelated themes arising in his talk. These are crucial to the operation of this repertoire and the following extracts present evidence of some of subject positions occupied within it. In extract 1, the manager describes his approach to management, positioning himself and the types of staff he would want working for him. His self-positioning as "he who empowers staff to self-manage" and "he who oversees" in effect achieves the status of one who is most powerful in terms of people management, using visual terminology to denote this. He positions his preferred employee using the empowerment repertoire: "They who should try to better themselves."

1

You empower people, people start throwing out ideas and actually manage themselves, and that's worked, we think, quite well in our area, but I don't see it in any other areas of [the company] . . . I'd rather have someone that's always trying to be one level above . . . to have a blend of people who do that job and are happy doing the job, but I like to see people trying to actually go outside of their job description and try to impress.

This extract illustrates how the empowerment repertoire is constitutive of the most powerful person in this regime. Comments from staff underpin and augment these positions. Extract 2 represents the views of the majority of the clerks, about the current management style and its implications:

2

. . . the people that came in actually, because they were prepared to let you have a laugh and you felt as if you really wanted to work hard for them which people did which is why we've performed really well.

In extract 2, the individual speaker positions herself alongside her colleagues as imaginary group spokespeople, and as members of their department with its particular ethos of "having a laugh and working hard." The powerful and benevolent position of the manager is shown by his positioning as "being prepared" to let the staff "have a laugh," for the return of hard work. Essentially, these individuals construct the element of choice and proactivity in wanting to work hard for their bosses, which places these positions within the empowerment repertoire.

Certain types of resistant positions were evident in the accounts from managerial, supervisory, and clerical levels and the empowerment repertoire was mobilized to this effect. In particular, it was used by a young, male senior clerk, who was describing resistant behavior in the department as a group of older women who met at coffee-time to "moan." In doing so, he self-positions as "technically astute" and positions these older women as "other," in not being "geared up to technology and targets." Extract 3 illustrates this:

3

. . .shall we say the more mature ladies of the section; shall we say the younger ones who have come in and know no different are fine. The others, well it used to be files and they preferred files because it was easier. Maybe they're scared of the technology – I don't know if they used the remote controls at home, but . . . that's the gripe . . . maybe there's some of the older end that aren't as geared up to computers, and technology and targets and all that.

There are many contingencies to the mobilization of this repertoire, which bring not only subject positions, but also social ordering into the picture. Position in this social order is contingent upon proficiency with information technologies that produce monitoring practices, which is reinforced by other management evaluation practices (such as appraisal). "Being able to do the job" as outlined by the manager (who empowers), will necessarily involve a degree of technical affinity and competence which will necessarily lead to an appraisal which will reinforce these (and other) skills. Unfortunately, none of the resistant women in this department were interviewed, as senior management scheduled the research interviews and prevented them from participating. Another repertoire, "life-in-work" in use in Norco explains these resistant processes further.

The "life-in-work" repertoire

The "life-in-work" repertoire comprises another set of patterns – positions of gender, age, pastimes, and personal preference – which bring them into the realm of work. Reciprocally, work – and the manager's position in particular – is constructed as "objective," "neutral," and "egalitarian" in this repertoire. The "life-in-work" repertoire therefore is seen to trouble or reinforce these egalitarian positions (for example, the manager's position), through linguistic construction. It can, in certain respects, be used to bolster, through an "othering device," the equanimity of organizational disciplinary practices, such as dismissal, promotion, and appraisal. Examples of this are given below.

This repertoire appears to operate in tandem with the empowerment repertoire. Comments from a clerk help to construct a dynamic between them. In extract 4 the senior clerk positions some employees as "wronged" in relation to the manager's intentionally egalitarian position. Note, it is their practices and positions after work which seem to count:

4

He treats in his own way everybody equal, but he's got his own way of running things, and his way of running things is that he's one of the lads

. . . the people that don't like going out don't think that they're getting a fair crack of the whip.

Individuals who are deemed to not like going out (or playing football, which is mentioned later) are positioned as "feeling discriminated against" within the workplace, thereby occupying "othered," potentially resistant positions. Similarly, the manager is positioned as "one of the lads," rooted within the "life-in-work" repertoire. The manager's need to work "in his own way" is troubled by that of being egalitarian, as would be expected within the workplace. The basis of the "empowering" position occupied by the manager in an earlier account is now challenged by this new position afforded to him by one of his "favored" clerks as "one of the lads." This is also clear from the following two extracts, both of which use positions in "life-in-work."

5
He has a lot more to do with the staff. And fortunately he has a lot more to do with the blokes as well . . . we play football every Wednesday so that is looked at in a different light by other members of staff. For me personally he's fine . . . for some it's a case of "Well, I won't get anywhere in here."

6
The people that do tend to get on – the team leaders – you tend to find that they're all the same, they're all fairly outgoing, bubbly . . . anything that's out of work, they'll always join in when it's possible for them to do and yeah it's – he goes for the people who are like him to be honest.

In these extracts, "life-in-work" replaces the empowerment repertoire in positioning resistant workers, and bolsters it in the power positioning of the manager. The empowerment and life-in-work repertoires are thus aligned. Claiming a position in the empowerment repertoire appears contingent on adopting this manager's personal practices. These data are summarized in Table 10.3.

Discussion

This chapter makes two points about the study of CBPM, in particular when we pay attention to procedural and distributive justice. The first, and most obvious, is that when we apply two contrasting analyses with different epistemological underpinnings, we are bound to reveal findings which at first, appear to be contradictory. In the case of Norco, analysis using "best-practice"

Table 10.3 Repertoires: Extract 1

Positioning	Management	Management → Staff	Staff → Management	Staff ↔ Staff
Repertoire *empowerment* *(Extract 1)* *Life-in-work* *(Extract 1)*	*Empowering Overseeing	Hardworking and happy Try to impress	Powerful Benevolent Allow humour *Manages as "one of the lads"	Hardworking *Enjoy humour *Technologically astute/**not astute** *Young male/**older female** *Beer drinking/**coffee drinking** *Sporty/**domestic**

guidelines told us that the organization appeared to be practicing CBPM in a "fair" way, whereas closer scrutiny revealed that departmental social relations had a discriminatory topography which favored the younger, most likely male, members of the department. This directly reflects upon distributive justice of performance evaluation and appraisal, since those less technologically "apt" were likely to be categorized as less competent in face-to-face performance evaluations, and were more likely to be regarded as resistant by managers and supervisors.

It also reflects upon the procedural justice of voice and communication surrounding monitoring statistics. Those constructed as having a negative attitude to technology, as part of a resistant group, are more likely to have their concerns dismissed as "moans" rather than any more arguably legitimate problems raised by workers to management, but on management's terms.

These arguments become even more pervasive when we examine the second point. The discourse analysis found a subtle link between CBPM practice and social relations. Within the case there was a dominant repertoire (empowerment) and subordinate repertoire (life-in-work). The empowerment repertoire relied upon themes of democracy, proactivity, choice, and freedom, and displayed a strong thematic feature in its mobilization of positions of both management and staff which involved proficiency with or control over CBPM output, outcomes, and the technology through which CBPM was operational. "Technical ability" was positioned in the empowerment repertoire, thus mastery over technology, good CBPM practice and empowerment in management–worker relations went hand in hand.

The subordinate repertoire referred to aspects of individual identities, which were brought to bear on the work situation (e.g., their gender, position, age, pastimes, and social preferences, etc.). The empowerment repertoire normalizes behavior which goes "beyond the job." Empowered positions thus draw on resources from within the life-in-work repertoire to identify with management, particularly socially. "Life-in-work" colludes with "empowered" to further distinguish empowered groups and thus disempower other groups (older, female in this case). Similarly, the life-in-work repertoire's dismissal of the manager as an "egalitarian," and presentation of him as "one of the lads" suggests that the position he claimed as a dispenser of "empowerment" was one which was heavily qualified and skewed towards the staff with whom he most identified.

Those unfavorably positioned in the life-in-work repertoire are so positioned because they did not fit social norms. These "othered" positions have also had experience of other regimes. Therefore they are able to compare the current management strategies with their other experiences. The manager's and "favored" clerks' positions as those who produce procedurally and distributively just performance evaluations and social relations are intensely troubled by this analysis. The message for the consideration of questions concerning distributive and procedural justice under monitoring is quite clear: any such discussion must examine fine-grain social processes with an eye to incorporating broader patterns of discrimination which may affect equity of treatment and equality of voice under computer-based performance monitoring in the workplace.

Conclusion

Using Marx (1998), and referring to Parker (1999) and Haraway (1997) (see notes), I have addressed the question of how we could use complementary research strategies to examine how we might come to understand practical configurations of CBPM as value-laden. This was analytically fruitful. Because of the connection revealed between technical ability and (historically negotiated) position within social relations, it is argued that there are practices which can be seen to be more or less fair according to previous research examining stress, ergonomics, and performance management. Crucially, however, this was subject of and to organizationally specific historical and cultural practices which accomplish social ordering and worker classification, both formally and informally, in a negotiated and ongoing fashion. Workers' positions as regards these practices are by no means fixed, and subject to claim upon claim for legitimacy and positioning within the sphere of monitoring application. It is argued that this has shed fresh light on the evaluation of employees' access to distributive and procedural justice under monitoring. In future, I recommend that if these ethical questions are to be examined at any depth, an analysis according to "best-practice" guidelines is insufficient if a more responsible account of practice is to be gained.

Table 10.4 An example of CBPM statistics in Norco

Name	Hours worked	Cases worked	Total contacts	Total promises	Broken promises	Dialler conn/hr	Talk time	Type time	£ coll. (000)
Op 1	69.15	933	192	145	23	21	2.02	0.07	53
Op 2	67.38	905	162	98	14	20.3	1.26	0.5	46
Op 3	86.57	1338	173	79	12	17.5	1.32	1.19	49
Op 4	119.5	1475	304	170	27	17.6	1.52	1.02	76
Op 5	89.03	1269	272	184	35	20.8	1.48	0.32	58
Total	431.6	5920	1103	676	111	19.44	1.52	0.62	279

Notes

1 This is the term used to describe CBM by "Nine to Five: The National Association of Working Women" in North America. The organization has conducted a number of surveys and studies on monitoring practice in North America, and commonly reports accounts of monitored women which feature images of rape, sexual abuse, harassment, degradation, and humiliation in their rhetoric. Its ethical message is clear: the use of CBM in this way is morally reprehensible.

2 Parker (1999) outlines the two main areas of organization studies currently embroiled in this discussion: labor process analysis and organizational analysis. In summarizing the debate, he pitches social realists such as Smith and Thompson (1992) and Thompson and Ackroyd (1995) against post-structuralists such as Knights and Willmott (1995), highlighting the "fundamental antagonism" (Parker 1999: 35) between the two groups of writers. The root of this antagonism is embedded in the various commitments to which each position is bound in the research process. Whilst emergent post-structuralists such as Knights, Willmott, Parker, and others were arguing for an organizational microsociology focused on the context-specific subject, or agent, as constructing reality through speech as social action, structural realists such as Smith, Thompson, Ackroyd, and Reed fundamentally oppose such ontological and epistemological positioning. The former critique the latter accounts as the product of the white, heterosexual and phallogocentric, dualistic systems that we (*sic*) aim to critique, which "place a constraining hierarchy around knowledge" (Knights 1997: 3). Instead, the former approach advocates a dynamic conceptualization of the power/resistance relation which calls the material, structural "givens," such as class, gender, and resistance, into question. Most notably, Knights and Willmott (1992) argue for a problematization of the position of "the subject," "subjectivity," and "subjection" in capitalist relations of power. This subject becomes the center of empirical and epistemological interest and speaks *per se*, constituting identity, culture, and power by speaking about their working lives. The speaking subject was, in theory at least, able to introduce many different, clashing, incongruous identities into its account of workplace *assujetissement*, which is socially constructed, and hence problematized the aforementioned structural "givens," and needed to be investigated in a theoretically grounded and methodologically consistent way. Thompson, Ackroyd, Smith, and others, on the other hand, prefer to categorize (for example) the study of resistance in organizations in a deep, detailed, and structured way, drawing on texts from across the range of social sciences to provide a detailed *a priori* categorization of what to expect in the process of empirical investigation. This is the basis of the realist critique of post-structural work. Writers such as Reed (1997) attack anti-realist positions for failing to "confront" and "conveniently forgetting" structure, instead opting for radically subjective, one-level, relativist, and process-dominated social ontologies. Thus for Reed, the essence of this opposition is the unconscionable dismissal of structure and its implications, such as the inadequate engagement with politics and ethics.

3 Situated knowledges is Haraway's (1991) feminist response to the realist/relativist stalemate, which she characterizes as defining

> how to have *simultaneously* an account of radical historical contingency for all knowledge claims and knowing subjects . . . *and* a no nonsense commitment to faithful accounts of a "real" world, one that can be partially shared and friendly to earth-wide projects of finite freedom, adequate material abundance, modest meaning in suffering, and limited happiness.
>
> (Haraway 1991: 187)

Her alternative, entitled "situated knowledges," is based on a recasting of the nature of vision – the gaze of the theorist which produces knowledge – as embodied, and necessarily situated within what can only ever be a partial translation of what is "out there." She argues that what we observe as natural scientists, human scientists, and social scientists is simultaneously material and solid, and constructed semiotically by the technologies and techniques that we use to observe them, and hence they are also observer-dependent but not unequivocally relativized. They are at the same time material and semiotic. Most importantly, material-semiotic artifacts themselves are to be understood as being in a mutually constitutive relation with the agentic network (both non-human and human) that produces them. This has two implications for this work. Among other things, this supports the notion that a conceptualization of CBPM as having a material-semiotic ontology necessitates a dual analytic methodology which is sensitive to the contrasting subtleties of this simultaneous conception: as something which is measurable and socially constructed.

Bibliography

Aiello, J. R. (1993) "Computer Based Work Monitoring: Electronic Surveillance and its Effects," *Journal of Applied Social Psychology*, 23: 499–507.

Alder, G. S. (1998) "Ethical Issues in Electronic Performance Monitoring: A Consideration of Deontological and Teleological Perspectives," *Journal of Business Ethics*, 17(7): 729–43.

Alvesson, M. (1993) "Organization as Rhetoric: Knowledge-Intensive Firms and the Struggle with Ambiguity," *Journal of Management Studies*, 30: 997–1016.

—— (2001) "Knowledge Work: Ambiguity, Image and Identity," *Human Relations*, 54(7): 863–86.

Alvesson, M. and Karreman, D. (2000) "Varieties of Discourse: On the Study of Organizations through Discourse Analysis," *Human Relations*, 53(9): 1125–49.

Attewell, P. (1987) "Big Brother and the Sweatshop: Computer Surveillance in the Automatic Office," *Sociological Theory*, 5: 87.

Ball, K. (1996) *Computer Based Monitoring in UK Service Organizations: A Comparative Study*, Aston University: Unpublished doctoral thesis.

—— (2001) "Situating Surveillance: Representation, Meaning, Movement and Manipulation," *Birmingham Business School Working Paper Series No 2000–07*.

Ball, K. and Hodgson, D. (forthcoming) "Can We Talk about Discourses of American Management Knowledge?" *Journal of Managerial Psychology*.

Ball, K. and Wilson, D. (2000) "Power, Control and Computer Based Performance Monitoring: Subjectivity, Repertoires and Resistance," *Organization Studies*, 21(4): 539–66.

Blackler, F. (1995) "Knowledge, Knowledge Work and Organizations: An Overview and Interpretation," *Organization Studies*, 16(6): 1021–39.

Beniger, J.R. (1986) *The Control Revolution: Technological and Economic Origins of the Information Society*, Cambridge, MA: Harvard University Press.

Chalykoff, T. and Kochan, R. (1989) "Computer Aided Monitoring: Its Influence on Employee Job Satisfaction and Turnover," *Personnel Psychology*, 42(4): 807.

Clark, P. A. (2000) *Organizations in Action: Competition Between Contexts*, London: Routledge.

Coase, R. (1937) "The Nature of the Firm," *Economica*, 4: 386–405.

DeTienne, K. and Abbott, N. T. (1993) "Developing an Employee Centered Electronic Monitoring System," *Journal of Systems Management*, 44: 12.

Deutsch, S. (1986) "The Context for Exploring Workplace Monitoring," in *Contractor Report for OTA (1987)*, Washington: United States Office of Technology Assessment.

Drucker, P. (1993) *Post-Capitalist Society*, Oxford: Butterworth-Heinemann.

—— (2000) "Knowledge Work," *Executive Excellence*, 17(4): 11–12.

George, J. F. (1996) "Computer Based Monitoring: Common Perceptions and Empirical Results," *Management Information Systems Quarterly*, 20(4): 459–80.

Graham, N. (2000) "Information Society as Theory or Ideology: A Critical Perspective on Technology, Education and Employment in the Information Age," *Information, Communication and Society*, 3(2): 139–52.

Grant, R. A., Higgins, C. A., and Irving, R. G. (1988) "Computerised Performance Monitors: Are They Costing You Customers?" *Sloan Management Review*, 30: 39.

Haraway, D. (1991) *Simians, Cyborgs, and Women: The Reinvention of Nature*, New York: Routledge.

—— (1997) *Modest_Witness@Second_Millennium.Femaleman©_Meets_Oncomouse*, NewYork: Routledge.

Henriques, J. (1998) *Changing the Subject: Psychology, Social Regulation and Subjectivity*, London, Routledge.

Higgins, C. A. and Grant, R. A. (1989) "Monitoring Service Workers via Computer: The Effect on Employees, Productivity and Service," *National Productivity Review*, 8(2): 101.

Introna, L. "Workplace Surveillance and Organizational Justice," paper presented at ESRC Virtual Society Surveillance Seminar, Edinburgh, March 2000.

Irving, R. H., Higgins, C. A., and Safayeni, F. R. (1986) "Computer Performance Monitoring Systems: Use and Abuse," *Communications of the ACM*, 29(8): 794–800.

Knights, D. (1997) "Organization Theory in the Age of Deconstruction: Dualism, Gender and Postmodernism Revisited," *Organization Studies*, 18(1): 1–20.

Knights, D. and Willmott, H. (1993) "It's a Very Foreign Discipline: The Genesis of Expenses Control in a Mutual Life Assurance Company," *British Journal of Management*, 4: 1–18.

Kulik, C. T. and Ambrose, M. L. (1993) "The Impact of Computerised Performance Monitoring Design Features on the Performance Appraisal Process," *Journal of Managerial Issues*, 5: 182–97.

Lund, J. (1992) "Electronic Performance Monitoring: A Review of the Research Issues," *Applied Ergonomics*, 23(1): 54–8.

Marx, G. T. (1998) "An Ethics for the New Surveillance." Online. Available HTTP: <http://web.mit.edu/gtmarx/www/ncolin5.html> (accessed 19 December 2001).

Michael, M. (1996) *Constructing Identities*, London: Sage.

Nebeker, D. M. (1987) "Automated Monitoring, Feedback and Rewards: Effects on Workstation Operator's Performance, Satisfaction and Stress," in H.J. Bullinger and B. Shackel (eds) *HCI Interact '87*, Amsterdam: Elsevier.

Nonaka, I. and Takeuchi, H. (1995) *The Knowledge Creating Company*, New York: Oxford University Press.

Office of Technology Assessment (OTA) (1987) *The Electronic Supervisor: New Technologies, New Tensions*, Washington: United States Office of Technology Assessment.

Parker, M. (1999) "Capitalism, Subjectivity and Ethics: Debating Labour Process Analysis," *Organization Studies*, 20(1): 25–46.

Potter, J. and Wetherell, M. (1987) *Discourse and Social Psychology: Beyond Attitudes and Behaviour*, London: Sage Publications.

Reed, M. (1997) "In Praise of Duality and Dualism: Rethinking Agency and Structure in Organizational Analysis," *Organization Studies*, 18(1): 21–42.

Schegloff, E. (1997) "Whose Text? Whose Context?" *Discourse and Society*, 8(2): 165–87.

Sewell, G. (1998) "The Discipline of Teams: The Control of Team-Based Industrial Work through Electronic and Peer Surveillance," *Administrative Science Quarterly*, 43(2): 397–429.

Sewell, G. and Wilkinson, B. (1992) "Someone to Watch Over Me: Surveillance, Discipline and the JIT Labour Process," *Sociology*, 26(2): 271–89.

Sipior, J. C., Ward, B. T., and Rainone, S. M. (1998) "Ethical Management of Employee Email Privacy," *Information Systems Management*, 15(1): 41–7.

Smith, M. J. and Amick, B. J. (1989) "Electronic Monitoring in the Workplace: Implications for Employee Control and Job Stress," in S. L. Sauter, J. J. Hurrell, Jr., and C. L. Cooper (eds) *Job Control and Worker Health*, Chichester: John Wiley and Sons.

Smith, M., Carayon, P., and Meizio, K. (1986) *Motivational, Behavioral and Psychological Implications of Electronic Monitoring of Worker Performance*, Washington: United States Office of Technology Assessment.

Sveiby, K. and Lloyd, T. (1987) *Managing Know-How: Add Value by Valuing Creativity*, London: Bloomsbury.

Thompson, P. and Ackroyd, S. (1995) "All Quiet on the Workplace Front? A Critique of Recent Trends in British Industrial Sociology," *Sociology*, 29(4): 610–33.

Trades Union Congress (2001) "Web Site of the Trades Union Congress." Online. Available HTTP: <http://www.tuc.org.uk> (accessed 18 December 2001).

Westin, A. (1986) "Privacy and Quality of Work Life Issues in Employee Monitoring" in *Contractor Report for OTA (1987)*, Washington: United States Office of Technology Assessment.

—— (1988) "Electronic Monitoring or Clerical Work on Video Display Terminals: The Organizational Climate Factor and Models of Good Employee Practice," in *Contractor Report for OTA (1987)*, Washington: United States Office of Technology Assessment.

Wetherell, M (1998) "Positioning and Interpretive Repertoires: Conversation Analysis and Post Structuralism in Dialogue," *Discourse and Society*, 9(3): 387–412.

Williamson, O. E. (1975) *Markets and Hierarchies: Analyst and Antitrust Implications*, New York: Free Press.

Willmott, H. (1999) "Towards a New Ethics? The Contributions of Post Structuralism and Post Humanism," in M. Parker (ed.) *Ethics and Organizations*, London: Sage Publications.

Yates, J. (1989) *Control Through Communication: The Rise of American Management*, Baltimore: Johns Hopkins University Press.

11 Private security and surveillance

From the "dossier society" to database networks

Greg Marquis

A casual reading of the literature on police history confirms a basic fact: surveillance was not invented in the age of computers, digitization, and the Internet. For more than 150 years, police in Western society have operated through "reading" and categorizing persons, places and situations on the basis of risk.[1] In this sense, patrol and detective police have always been involved in risk management and policing has always been targeted or discriminatory. The same is true of private security, which has competed with and complemented the police since the nineteenth century. Policing seeks to maintain order and enforce criminal law. Private security is about predicting and preventing actions that cause economic loss (Carroll 1975: 2; Lyon 1994: 110–13).

This chapter reviews the development of North American private security, both in-house and contract, since 1960, its use of technology and information, and its relationship to public police. Drawing on themes in policing history, it assesses the significance of private security categorization of potential and actual offenders against criminal and administrative law; of employees and prospective employees; of residential dwellers; of customers in the marketplace and of the public in general (Hunt 1990; Marquis 2000a; Morn 1982; Rigakos 1999; Williams 1998). In the broadest sense, private security consists of not only the classic in-house and proprietary guard, investigation, cash transit and alarm services, but also the broader "police-industrial complex" that includes industry-protective associations, credit bureaus, and human resource management experts that administer "integrity" testing (O'Toole 1978: ch. 8; Reynolds 1991).

My basic argument is that North American private security, like public policing, developed historically through ordering space and categorizing individuals. Yet since the 1960s heightened anxieties over personal security, business and insurance concerns over property, profits, and liability, the proliferation of inexpensive new technologies for gathering, storing, sorting, and transmitting information, and a drift towards privatization in the security "marketplace" has given new meaning to the old Pinkerton slogan "We Never Sleep." The "Eye That Never Sleeps" was an evocative image for the private investigator or undercover operative who served client needs through physical surveillance (Morn 1982). In the surveillance society that has evolved since the 1960s, a multitude of private eyes manage risk not for a political ideology, the state nor the "public interest," but for profit. And although physical surveillance, such as Closed Circuit Television (CCTV) remains important and will no doubt grow in intensity, physical surveillance has been surpassed by data surveillance.

Communications and information technology (CIT) has broadened the scope of surveillance of individuals, and raised important questions pertaining to privacy, accuracy, accountability, and uses of information held in state and private data banks. By way of example, consider the detailed files kept by the Ministry of State Security or Stasi on more than sixteen million East Germans prior to the 1990s. Through a network of hundreds of thousands of citizen informers, state agents, and surveillance equipment, the Stasi amassed security files that took up two hundred kilometres of shelf space. Each kilometer of dossiers contained ten million sheets of paper. This unwieldy system, which spread fear and suspicion among the population, was searched manually. Computerization would have made this huge security apparatus even more oppressive, but file cards were sufficient. When the communist regime crumbled starting in 1989, Stasi offices and records were among the first targets of protestors (Koehler 1999: 8–9, 20–1).

North American police, since their inception in the early 1800s, have never monopolized surveillance and social categorization as they relate to law enforcement. In recent years, academic, professional and governmental studies of and conferences on policing have paid greater attention to the growth of private security, which provides guard, cash transit, alarm, and investigative services. In 1970, there were one and a half private security employees for every American police officer; by the mid-1990s the ratio was three and a half to one. By 1996, Canada had more than 12,000 private investigators and greater numbers of guards (Gerden 1998; Nye 1999: 5; Statistics Canada 1999).[2] The rank-and-file unions represented by the Canadian Police Association have reacted with suspicion and hostility towards their private sector counterparts. Police managers have been more open (Kinnear 2000: 108–16; Marquis 1993). According to late twentieth-century commentators, who include private security spokespersons, an overburdened public sector, taxpayer fatigue, public perceptions of rising crime rates, and business dissatisfaction with the performance of police agencies has led to a proliferation of private policing. Murphy postulates that postmodernity, "declining cultural and social homogeneity and lack of political consensus" are feeding demands for increased security and order (KPMG 1998: iii–iv; Murphy 2000: 35–7; Murray and McKim 2000: 4–14).[3]

Most security textbooks and company advertisements begin with the assumption of "an unprecedented rise in crime" that justifies more robust security. The web site for the Ontario company Intelligarde, for example, states that "crimes like car jacking and home invasion are becoming commonplace" and that Canadian society is increasingly threatened by "disorderly conduct and drug culture" (Intelligarde; Oliver and Wilson 1978: ix). Other allegations have to do with the alleged ineffectiveness of the police, or even the failure of the courts and corrections system to deter or rehabilitate violent and repeat offenders. While the latter has little to do with policing, it does contribute to a political climate that is less resistant to an expansion of surveillance.

Such assertions clash with crime statistics gathered by the state. Aside from specific locales, where official crime rates can fluctuate from year to year, for the past several years Canada has experienced a decline in rates of serious crime (offences covered by the Criminal Code). Throughout the 1990s for example, national rates of youth crime, property crime, violent crime, and homicide fell (Statistics Canada 1996; Tremblay 1998).[4]

Public perceptions of crime, as framed by the media, count more than criminological expertise in the politics of policing and security. Cost is another important factor. In an era of falling or stagnating worker productivity, corporations, governments, even police agencies, have hired or contracted out to security firms to protect assets, investor profits, and the public treasury. According to the Solicitor General's 1990 discussion paper *Police-Challenge 2000*, Canada's "new blue line" would be shaped by economic factors:

> Private policing will become even more established as the dominant mode of policing in Canada. As a result, public police will serve, in part, a coordinating role for private policing, providing backup when "real" crime occurs. Alternatives will be sought to high quality but expensive public policing, such as passive, technologically-enhanced surveillance, and the use of parallel policing.
>
> (Normandeau and Leighton 1990: 15, 20)

Another theme is technology: by the 1970s and 1980s, public bureaucracies and corporations were making greater use of technology to regulate inter-personal relationships and market transactions. According to private security advocates, their industry is better able than the police to respond to the security and crime challenges of the Information Age. Private security, for example, popularized the use of CCTV, a form of surveillance that many police departments have adopted or will adopt (Barney 2000; Hunt 2000:

137–41; Marquis 2000b). In Britain the expansion of CCTV to monitor public space has little to do with official rates of crime (Norris and Armstrong 1999). A variation on this theme is the "national security" argument, put forward by President Clinton in a speech in 1999: foreign terrorists are imperilling American military and economic interests through not only violence but also the threat of "cyber attacks." Although this rhetoric is meant to justify national and military security efforts, it also serves as a marketing tool for private security consultants in the post-Cold War world (Clinton 1999; Marquis 2000b).[5]

According to a host of social science commentators, North American society after the Second World War evolved from the industrial to the post-industrial or Information Age (Beniger 1986; Galbraith 1968). The most obvious change was in the structure of the workforce. In 1880, only 6.5 percent of the American civilian workforce belonged to the "information" sector; one century later the figure was 42 percent. Agricultural employment had declined from 43.7 to 2.1 percent and industrial from 43.7 to 22.5 percent. By the early 1960s, an estimated 29 percent of the American GNP was linked to the "production and distribution of knowledge" (Beniger 1986: 19–24). By the mid-1980s, one Canadian worker in seven used CIT; a decade later the proportion had climbed to two out of five (Betcherman and McMullen 1999: 110).

The storage and distribution of information were increasingly facilitated not simply by bureaucracy, but by CIT. In the mid-1950s, for example, the United States government maintained 45 computers. A decade later, federal departments and agencies operated close to 2,000 mainframes. Computer applications were adopted for administrative, licensing, regulatory, and criminal justice purposes (Relyea 1996; Rule 1974). In the 1960s, the aerospace company Space-General, utilizing computers and system analysis, studied the California criminal justice system and made recommendations on police data processing, tracking the results of sentencing and predicting outbreaks such as the Watts riot of 1965 through a series of socioeconomic indicators (Brown 1971).

The growth of computerized data banks within the governmental and corporate sector, recording the activities of millions of North American workers, citizens, and consumers, gave rise in the 1960s to a political concern over privacy that was evident in both academic and popular culture (Bennett 1995; Gellman 1999; Lester 2000). Much of the ensuing literature was journalistic and anecdotal. Brenton, in *The Privacy Invaders*, warned that the increasing use of computers to store and sort data on individuals was a potential "death blow not only for privacy, but for the very democracy upon which it nourishes" (Brenton 1964: 232). The allegedly invasive and dehumanizing power of surveillance technology employed by private detectives, corporations and public investigative agencies and revelations of domestic spying by the Nixon White House, the FBI, the CIA, the IRS, US military intelligence, and the Canadian RCMP also fueled concerns (Dash 1959; Halifax *Chronicle Herald* 13 April 1964; Lapidius 1971; Packard 1964; Westin 1970, 1971; Wise 1976). One result in the United States, which affected private investigators, was the banning of private eavesdropping under the American Omnibus Crime Control and Safe Streets Act of 1968 (Lapidius 1971: 43–8). In 1969, Canada's minister of justice pronounced "data surveillance" a serious threat to individual privacy (*Globe & Mail* 15 July 1969).

The resulting discourse on protection of privacy tended to focus on the dangers of government acting as Big Brother. The chief reason was that public officials, departments and agencies could be monitored and controlled through the courts, the political process and media exposure. There was a lively debate on the socially acceptable uses of information. One result of the privacy discourse of the late 1960s was the American Privacy Act of 1974, which affected federal government records (Hare, 1976: 4; Long 1967; Packard 1964; Westin 1971). Citizens' right to examine their government file was enshrined in national and state freedom of information laws, an innovation that caused the FBI and other American police agencies to warn that criminal intelligence information would "dry up." Canada's federal government passed protection of privacy legislation in 1974, although its safeguards were weaker than that of the American law. A number of provinces also passed consumer protection laws to regulate credit reporting agencies. In Canada the public occasionally expresses concerns over the growth of personal information in government records (witness the recent controversy over the secret Longitudinal Labour Force Databank).[6] As political issues, the gathering, lending, and selling of personal data by the private sector are not well understood by the public, but lobbying by privacy advocates has resulted in federal legislation, Bill C-6, that will phase in a regulatory framework for businesses that attempt to share personal data (Statistics Canada 1981, vol. 2: 85–93; Thibodeau 2000).[7]

Although the record-keeping systems were rudimentary by twentieth-century standards, when the "new" police appeared in the nineteenth century, its activities were built around notions of social categorization. The immediate targets in the 1840s and 1850s were urban working-class neighborhoods. Patrol officers placed specific locales under surveillance and detectives kept track of individuals and organizations through observation and informants. The police station blotter was an intimate record of the quarrels and conflicts of the urban neighborhood. In addition to petty offenders, the police maintained informal records on the local "underworld" and, as a result of statutory provisions, formal records on pawnbrokers, peddlers and cab drivers

(Ericson and Haggerty 1997; Harring 1983; Marquis 1993, 1994; Monkkonen 1981).

The roots of private security categorization also date from this era. Private policing, far from being a twentieth century invention, was a creature of the Commercial and Industrial Revolutions. Modern "police for hire" in the United States emerged at the same time as railroad networks, mass production and distribution, communications technology such as the telegraph and telephone and the industrial corporation. Business historian Alfred Chandler describes American railroads as the first modern business enterprises. They also were the first major private sector clients of private police agencies (Beniger: ch. 6; Chandler 1977: ch. 3).

By the late 1800s, urban police in North America had developed a work culture based not only on patrolling the beat, the public interface of law enforcement, but also on predicting behavior by creating, updating, and exchanging records on suspected and convicted offenders. Central to police lore, for both patrol officers and detectives, was the ability to "read" individuals and situations (Johnson 1976). Each successive technological innovation in police operations, from typewriters to automobiles and two-way radios to laptop computers, has reinforced a professional culture based on observing and tracking individuals who seem "out of place" (Ericson 1992; Marx 1988). The historical literature suggests that the purpose of technological adaptation was not simply to "fight crime" but also to manage and control police workers (a similar case can be made for private security technology) (Marquis 2000b).

Criminal intelligence techniques developed from basic municipal and private police record gathering (Morgan 1980: ch. 2). Following the Civil War municipal police departments exchanged telegraphic bulletins, written physical descriptions, and photographs. Later, records of anthropometric Bertillon measurements and fingerprints of arrested and convicted individuals were added to municipal, state, provincial, and national police bureaucracies. Starting in the 1920s and 1930s, police agencies could communicate via teletype. Police departments maintained "just in case" information on individuals who had never been arrested, charged or convicted, but who were suspected of criminal activity. Private agencies, such as the railway police and Pinkerton's National Detective Agency, urged the public police to coordinate criminal intelligence better in the face of rapid technological change, divided political jurisdiction, and increasingly sophisticated economic crime (Marquis 1994; Morn 1982; Nadelmann 1993: 55–99).

The private police, in addition to protecting physical assets such as mines, factories, railways, warehouses, banks, and hotels, virtually invented mass surveillance in North America through their infiltration of the labor movement. The Pinkerton, Thiel, and Burns agencies, contracted by both industrial corporations and national, state and provincial governments across North America, targeted organized labor through the infiltration of spies and agents provocateurs, the compilation of blacklists and the provision and safeguarding of strikebreakers (Hunt 1990; Marquis 2000a; Morgan 1980: ch. 2; Williams 1998).[8] "Private detectives flourished," one historian has written, "because they were the more reliable servants of class interests than the established police who had to answer to elected officials" (Hunt 1990: 196–7). Pinkerton's, other branch plant security operations, and Canadian-owned companies continued to monitor and infiltrate unions and workplaces into the 1970s if not later. A number of organizations of the far political right in the United States between the 1920s and the 1960s, such as the American Defense Society, the American Vigilant Intelligence Foundation, and the American Security Council, were associated with private police and industrial security (Donner 1980: 414–18).

The popular literature on private security from the 1950s and 1960s tends to stress violations of privacy by undercover agents and intrusive surveillance technology. The first technological challenges to privacy came not after the Second World War, but starting in the 1880s: private detectives and police had recourse to tapping telephone lines, listening to conversations through microphones, recording conversations on dictographs and documenting activity with low-cost, instantaneous photography (Dash 1959: ch. 1; Westin 1970: 338–39).[9] By the mid-twentieth century, surveillance of places and persons was enhanced by tape recorders, miniature microphones, and cameras, infrared "night vision" photography and motion picture cameras.[10] For controlling access and monitoring employees, customers, the public, and spaces such as factory gates, shop floors, doors, and lobbies, companies and institutions later installed CCTV, video cameras, and locks activated by punch codes (Wilson 1978: ch. 3).[11]

Far more important than audio and visual monitoring devices to the evolution of the surveillance society were advances in data surveillance: creating, storing, sorting, and accessing files on individuals and organizations. Prior to the mid-twentieth century, the basic dossier was a file containing typewritten sheets. Police agencies, in amassing both criminal and national security intelligence, added fingerprints, *modus operandi* information, mug shots, and newspaper clippings (Hannant 1995; Marquis 1994). Large police agencies, like government agencies and corporations, next adopted key-punch machines and machine-readable punch cards. With computerization in the 1960s and early 1970s, records were transferred to magnetic tape and eventually to magnetic disk. Storage capacity and search time improved tremendously with each advance (Beniger 1986; Carroll 1975; Westin 1971). The basic police records identified by mid-century experts such as O. W. Wilson were complaint, arrest, and identification records (Wilson 1973). The growth of police record keeping reflects the classic rules of bureaucracy, and has been influenced by external institutions such as the insurance industry, provincial and state motor vehicle departments, and the courts (Ericson and Haggerty 1997: 23–34, 209–47, 310–15).

The use of private policing in industry prior to the 1940s was not accompanied by major professional or theoretical discussions other than property protection and efficiency.[12] A self-conscious industrial security sector was launched during the Second World War, when more than 100,000 American war production plants were in operation. Cold War imperatives, which maintained a large defense research, development, and production sector into the 1990s, also fed demands for security experts, investigators, employee screening, surveillance techniques, security barriers and guards. The American Security for Industrial Security, which publishes the trade journal *Security Management*, reflects the institutionalization of large-scale private security. On the contract investigation side, most work was specific to individual client needs, such as evidence of infidelity in divorce cases. By the early 1960s, millions of Americans were employed by aerospace and other industries bidding for defense contracts and subcontracts. Cold War and anti-radical concerns, according to Donner, rehabilitated private security following the excesses of the 1930s, creating a market worth billions a year. Polygraph testing subjected prospective and actual employees, and even executives considered for promotion, to "moral vaccination." By the 1970s, one in five of America's top one thousand corporations made regular use of polygraphs, often contracting firms such as Reid Associates. Pinkerton's advertised the importance of monitoring sensitive employees not only at work, but also in their extracurricular activities. By the 1960s, management consultant firms such as Bishop's Service were maintaining files on millions of business managers and administrators. Polygraphy in the private sector in theory was ended by a privacy law of 1988, but the public sector and defense employers were exempt, and loopholes allow the private sector to test employees in cases of economic loss ("American Report" 1978; Brenton 1964: ch. 6; Dash 1959: 8–14; Donner 1980: 425–26; Lipson 1975; Packard 1964: 51–52, 76–77; Westin 1970: ch. 9).

A striking recruitment pattern of twentieth-century North American security is the easy movement of retired police, national security and military personnel into private policing at the lower, middle, and upper levels. Ex-police officers, in addition to knowing basic investigation techniques, supposedly are effective at acquiring information from police and other public agencies. In 1961 the Bank of Nova Scotia proudly announced that it had hired L. H. Nicholson, former Commissioner of the RCMP, to head a new protection and investigation department. Fifteen years later, the Canadian Press noted a firm formed by ex-military intelligence officers that specialized in analyzing business security systems. The president of KPMG Investigation and Security Inc., Norman Inkster, is a former commissioner of the RCMP who advocates an increased private sector role in the social control marketplace.[13] The head of Intelligarde is an exception in security management: he is a former sociology professor (Halifax *Chronicle Herald*, 5 September 1961; *Industrial Canada*, January/February 1972: 20–2; Saint John *Evening Times Globe*, 4 May 1976). In the early 1970s, the "Americanization" of Canadian private security, like the larger problem of foreign control of the economy, was an issue discussed within the security sector (Jeffries 1973: 65–8). Many American insurance investigators in the 1960s were FBI veterans. Packard, in *The Naked Society*, described the predilection of former investigators from the FBI, CIA, Secret Service, Treasury Department, and the US Post Office for work in industrial security. Although few of its employees were recruited from state intelligence and security, the giant Wackenhutt firm was founded by former FBI personnel (Brenton 1964: ch. 3; Packard 1964: 24–9, 57, 74–7).

Security textbooks and training manuals in the 1960s and 1970s were surprisingly "non technological," reflecting the reality that most workers in the industry, either in-house or contract security, were low-paid, minimally trained stationary or ambulatory guards with basic technological skills.[14] Hemphill's 1971 manual, aimed at managers and administrators, discussed such mundane topics as time locks, shipping and deliveries, and warehousing and stockroom controls as well as CCTV, vehicle tachographs, wire taps, homing devices, hidden microphones, telephone scramblers, polygraphs, and "the undercover man" (Hemphill 1971). Other texts stressed classic "police"-type activities, such as the importance of maintaining individual notebooks, communal occurrence books and incident and accident reports in preparing cases for criminal prosecution or civil actions (Oliver and Wilson 1978: 82–90).

In terms of overall volumes of personal information generated by national security, criminal justice and the private sector, private security's activities are insignificant. Carroll's 1975 text *Confidential Information Sources* provided the following breakdown on volumes of personal information:

state governments – 25 percent;
federal government – 20 percent;
banks/financial sector – 15 percent;
local governments – 13 percent;
insurance companies – 12 percent;
other businesses – 10 percent;
employee files – 5 percent.

Police and criminal justice information is included in the state, federal, and local government categories[15] (Carroll 1975: 40–7). Given the expansion of consumer credit since the mid-1970s, the relative percentage of private sector information has probably increased (Branscomb 1994: 168–9). But as in the 1970s, private security is more like to buy or borrow information than to create it. Most of its social categorization data, therefore, is derived from that of the police, insurance companies, other private investigators, credit rating firms, social welfare agencies, and regulatory bodies. By the early 1980s, a study conducted for the Office of Technology Assessment indicated that criminal justice records, largely because of computerization, were increasingly employed for non-justice purposes (Bennett 1995; Gerden 1998: 150–60; Marchand 1980). Recently the FBI reported that information requests for non criminal justice purposes such as licensing now exceed those for justice purposes. Information may be sought for civil law cases, insurance purposes, or to discredit an individual or group (IACP 2001).

Have the police acknowledged the role of private security in fighting or preventing crime? Police management literature at the height of the professional model ignored the practice of information sharing with the private sector (Wilson 1973). And a major survey of Philadelphia security firms in the 1970s suggested that a large minority of criminal incidents were never reported to the police (National Advisory Committee 1976). Yet private security by the 1970s, according to Carroll, was a major provider of information to the police (for example, a security firm patrolling public housing projects). It has been to the advantage of the police to share information on outstanding warrants and wanted and missing persons. Crime control advocates suggest that the dissemination of arrest and conviction records through private security and other non-criminal justice channels is an effective crime prevention tactic. As Ericson and Haggerty argue, the brokering of information suggests a mutually supportive relationship between the public and private police, and an expansion of police information categories. Brokering information also has been a source of revenue (Ericson and Haggerty 1997: 29–30, 167–72, 340–2, 436–7; Marchand 1980: 103–4; Thurston 1973: 31–40).

By the 1970s, both Canada and the United States had computerized national criminal records systems. By 1979 the National Crime Information Center (NCIC) maintained by the FBI included more than six million active records, including records on wanted persons, more than one million criminal histories and reports on stolen vehicles, securities, and property. The debate surrounding its establishment included concerns over confidentiality and what we would now term "computer matching." Individual states such as New York and Massachusetts and large metropolitan police forces maintained their own computerized criminal justice information systems. By the late 1990s, the NCIC database contained 56 percent of total criminal records in the United States. Uniformity and easier transfer of data on offenders convicted under state law was advanced by the Law Enforcement Assistance Administration (LEAA), which provided grants for computerization. In an attempt to integrate criminal justice information from police, courts and corrections, the LEAA supported state offender-based transactions statistics. By 1972, most states had automated one or more of their criminal justice record systems. The Canadian Police Information Centre (CPIC), maintained by the RCMP, allowed 250 member police forces to access a sixty-year-old collection of fingerprints, convictions, arrest records, and photos of persons charged with indictable offences. By 1998 and the advent of laptop computers and wireless transmission, CPIC had more than 15,000 points of access and was handling more than 110 million transactions a year. Running background checks through the more centralized CPIC system was much easier than similar activities in the United States (Carroll 1975: 90–1, 117–21, 241; Gallati 1971: 40–6; Lyon 1994: 110–12; Marchand 1980: 66–71; "Standardization" 2000).[16]

Information and communications technology has not altered the goals or objectives of policing or private security, but it does expand the capabilities of record gathering and dissemination. In the late nineteenth-century United States, prior to the creation of a national criminal identification collection based on written descriptions, aliases, photographs, Bertillon measurements and fingerprints, the records of a private company, Pinkerton's National Detective Agency, filled the gap (Morn 1982). The exact scale and nature of information held by private security are unknown, as is the statistical impact of private security information or evidence on insurance, property recovery or administrative and civil law.

This information is considered private and sensitive by the private sector (Statistics Canada 1981, vol. 2: ii). In the early 1970s, one of the major contract firms in the United States boasted of having records on six million individuals. Wackenhutt, which led the "counter subversive private detective industry" in the 1960s, and whose founder was associated with the far right, maintained files on more than two million Americans. Unlike the police, security tends not to share its information with competitors, although there has been cooperation amongst the in-house security sector (two examples being railway police and campus security) (Donner 1980: 424–5; Thurston 1973: 36). Contract and in-house security, plus private investigators, traditionally have guarded their records and sensitive information from the public gaze (Wilson 1978: 205). Thus it is difficult to generalize about the number of "transactions" made through private security's information network, or even if a network exists.

The security sector relies heavily upon public or quasi-public information such as criminal, licensing, and credit records. Like the police, it "siphons off" information from private and public bureaucracies (Lyon 2001: 121). By the mid-1970s, Associated Credit Bureaus (ACB), a network of 2000 bureaus operating in 50 states and 10 Canadian provinces, employed 30,000 workers who processed 50 million credit requests each year. In the early 1960s ACB's records were described as an intelligence network more vast than that of the FBI and CIA combined (Brenton 1964: 28; Carroll 1975: 128–33). And although consumer legislation did address a number of abuses in credit reporting, these records continue to allow financial institutions a powerful and often hidden influence over the lives over tens of millions of North Americans. And studies indicate that credit files often contain inaccurate information (Brin 1998: 58–9; Sykes 1999: 6, 30–1).

State records (criminal justice, health, education) have been a key source of private security intelligence. According to Haggerty, "extra-state forms of governance are still bound to the state to the extent that they rely on knowledge that only state agencies can produce" (2001: 189). A survey revealed that almost one-third of the members of the American Society for Industrial Security made daily and weekly use of public criminal justice records (National Advisory Committee 1976: 209). In the words of Marchand, the dissemination of criminal justice information to security companies and prospective employers, combined with discriminatory record-keeping laws and personnel practices, represents a serious social cost to disadvantaged elements in American society. He points out that because most arrests are of a summary nature, they are simply records of "suspicion," not records of guilt. Yet a record of arrest, obtained through a background check, is sufficient to deny employment in most private sector situations (Marchand 1980: 93–9).

Private security sales pitches stress the ability to "get the facts," not having them in the first place. In the information market, the sector is a net user of data, not a net provider. And the focus often is not mass surveillance but targeted individuals such as job applicants, suspected shoplifters, dishonest employees, persons suspected of insurance fraud or individuals who have launched litigation against a client or employer. Yet computerization has decided benefits for companies and organizations that collect and transfer risk assessment data, often without the intermediary role of the private investigator. One CIT application is the pre-employment check based not on personal interviews but accessing services such as Avert and Infotel. In a sense, CIT potentially undercuts the traditional role of the private investigator in routine background checks, much as cybercrime is undermining the role of both police and private security by creating a new class of IT security managers and operatives. A number of web-based risk-assessment services include information on personal credit, arrests and criminal convictions, workers' compensation claims, and bankruptcies. Crimcheck Inc. "through the miracle of the Internet," will provide a criminal report on "that potential partner, employee, child care giver, or any number of people that may become important in your life or business." In addition, screening companies specialize in vetting workers in specific industries, a practice which has echoes of the blacklisting practices of the early twentieth century, and the insurance industry maintains an electronic data bank on individuals suspected of insurance fraud (Berstein 1997; Crimcheck; Infotel; Privacy Rights Clearinghouse).[17]

The increased use of private security was first noticed by the media and academic community in the 1960s (Kakalik and Wildhorn 1977). By the early 1970s, in an urbanized and industrialized society such as Ontario, private security employees outnumbered the police by between two and three to one. By 1973 Ontario, which passed a Private Investigators Act in 1965, had more than 200 licensed investigation firms. Given that the police experienced significant growth in the 1960s and 1970s, the expansion of private security is even more remarkable. In Canada the largest component was the in-house sector, which included the Canadian National Railways and Canadian Pacific Railway Police and the National Harbours Board Police. Between 1961 and 1971, expenditures on contract security in Canada grew by more than 800 percent. In 1971 the Canadian Corps of Commissionaires, which employs military veterans, supplied several thousand guards to government facilities and to the private sector. As in the United States, guards tended to be low-paid older white males, with low levels of education. Many worked part time. Investigators were younger, better educated and better paid. Companies such as Dominion Electric Protection Co., Chubb Industries, Diebold of Canada, and Ampex manufactured safes, vaults, alarm systems and recording equipment. Security industry statistics also included business and institutional fire alarm and suppression systems. By the mid-1970s, the estimated market for security goods and services in Canada was estimated as: 46 percent in industry and transportation; 32 percent in institutions; 11 percent in the financial, commercial and retail sectors and 11 percent in the consumer sector (Farnell and Shearing 1977; Warren 1973: 53).

With police patrolling North America "from behind closed doors, on wheels, in communication with the outside world through a windshield and a radio frequency," citizens were more likely to come into contact, or be monitored by, a private security guard than a police officer (Murphy and Plate 1977: 262). Police also were becoming more rule-bound and formalistic, following a professional model that made them more distant from neighborhoods and communities (Skogan 1995: 108–9). Changes in urban planning, the proliferation of large-scale office complexes, shopping malls, public housing, apartment buildings, college campuses, industrial and business parks, and other forms of mass property gave a boost to a private security industry that had been previously confined to the manufacturing and transportation sectors. Most businesses, financial institutions, and retail outlets installed CCTV or video monitoring for high traffic areas and exits and entrances and many contracted private security for alarm responses (Marquis 2000a).

In the 1970s and 1980s the increasing privatization of social control fitted in with the new strategy of community policing, which was to shift part of the burden away from the police onto the "community," including citizens' groups such as Neighborhood Watch, business groups, and the private sector. While many dismiss community policing as a public relations ploy or worse, it paved the way for an expansion of private security, including the outsourcing of second-level police duties (Ericson and Haggerty 1997: 29–30, 70–2). By the 1980s, research had seriously compromised many of the key assumptions on which post-1945 policing had been built, such as placing most officers in random motorized patrols and improving response times to citizen calls for assistance. Increased numbers of police in an area, or "saturation" policing, had no impact on crime rates (Skolnick and Bayley 1986: 4–5).[18]

Despite the supposed importance of the "new economy," the North American security industry, in terms of personnel, is dominated by the traditional sector, guard and cash transit services. Rather than a "hired gun" as in the nineteenth century, the private guard acts as the eyes and ears of the employer, either business or government. He also controls access to private, semi-public and even public space (government buildings). The security market, although still focused on territory and "mass public property," and employing mainly blue-collar workers, is decentralized and diversified (Shearing and Stenning 1981, 1983). According to the Securitas web site, Canada's guard market, like the American market, is fragmented and operates on slim profit margins. The European security giant Securitas, by gaining control over Pinkerton's in 1999 and Burns International in 2000, secured an important foothold in Canada. On the guard side, the competitors of Securitas include Group 4, the Canadian Veterans' Organization and the Canadian Corps of Commissionaires. The cash transit is dominated by Loomis Canada and Brinks. Securitas estimates that it controls only 5 percent of the Canadian security market and 5 percent of the world market (Securitas).

Second-level police services, such as monitoring CCTV systems deployed in central urban districts, are a form of para-policing that private security firms can deliver at low cost (Norris and Armstrong 1999: ch. 6). Companies such as Intelligarde are striving to become more involved in para-police activities. In the mid-1990s, for example, Intelligarde was hired by the Toronto Transit Commission to keep known pimps away from underage females at the Bay Street bus station. The security company, also involved in patrolling public housing projects in Toronto, cooperated with police in exchanging information. When banned individuals persisted, police laid trespassing charges. Intelligarde K-9 units deployed police dogs in more than a dozen public housing buildings in order to root out trespassers suspected of drug activity (Lynas 1999; Toronto *Sun*, 11 August 1993, 30 May 1996). Rigakos has described how Intelligarde patrols "electronic checkpoints" in Toronto public housing. Essentially, the use of bar-coded "deister" strips to monitor the rounds of security officers is an updated version of a major urban police management and communications tool of the late nineteenth century: the electric call box system. For the most part, the guard sector resembles the police of the nineteenth and early twentieth century, whose work was based on "mere observation and presence" as opposed to "data gathering and data analysis." In North America, the industry is moving away from in-house security towards alarm installation and contract security (Manning 2000; Rigakos 1999: 6–7).[19]

Surveillance of the workplace is increasingly bypassing traditional security approaches. For example, in addition to physical surveillance, employers eavesdrop on millions of employee telephone calls each year, track the destination/origin and length of calls, count computer keystrokes and have access to e-mail, voice mail, and computer files. The physical location of workers can be traced not only by CCTV, but also by "active badges" that track their movements. By the mid-1990s, an estimated two-thirds of major American corporations were resorting to one or more of the above security measures. In the digital age, the IT manager, not the security guard or investigator, implements and oversees the surveillance of the workplace (American Civil Liberties Union 1996; Barney 2000: ch. 5; Marquis 2000b).

Surveillance is not inherently detrimental to privacy, civil liberties or social and economic equality. Policing and private security, like CIT, have a capacity for good and bad (Lyon 1994; 201). Yet the open-ended nature of surveillance, particularly as conducted by the private sector, is a cause for concern. As the economy, workplace, role of the public sector, and nature of surveillance change, both policing and private security are bound to be affected. Policing is becoming more decentralized and information-based (Ericson and Haggerty 1997; Marquis 2000b; Shearing 1997). Unlike the "dossier society" visions of the 1960s, contemporary technology-mediated surveillance is not based on centralized social control. Yet the objectives of social control are little different from those of a century ago. Private security is concerned with risk. It watches, classifies, and orders the same groups that have been the historic targets of police surveillance and ordering: the poor, the young, minorities, certain types of workers, and those with arrest and conviction records. Like police, the private security complex creates "a certain type of knowledge about facts, people and behaviour" (Nogala

1995: 193) and increasingly that knowledge is derived from data banks, not physical surveillance. Because of the importance of mass private property as public space, and surveillance of the workplace, "private eyes" are now more pervasive than the actual or virtual gaze of the police. The police in Britain have turned to CCTV, pioneered by private security, to watch the inner city. If replicated in North America, this has the capacity to expand not only visual surveillance but also the role of private security (Lyon 2001a: 59–64; Norris 2001; Norris and Armstrong 1999). Both police and private security will make greater use of digital technology, video and biometrics for forecasting, identifying, and tracking, and these technologies, in the absence of a political debate and response, will strengthen the discriminatory aspects of social control (Lyon 2001b). Industry hyperbole, such as the following Intelligarde sales pitch, evokes visions of the public policing withering away: "an increasingly concerned and frustrated public is turning to private security companies for the security services they so desperately need" (Intelligarde). In reality, the two sectors cooperate in social control; the police could no more manage without private security than security could exist without the police.

Notes

1 For the definitive work on policing and risk, see Ericson and Haggerty (1997). In contrast to academics who focus on technology and utilize concepts such as the risk society, techno policing and privacy in analyzing social control, the professional culture of both policing and private security continues to stress that investigation is an "art" that is merely enhanced by technology and information brokerage.
2 The statistics can include part-time crosswalk guards and bouncers and doormen at pubs and nightclubs.
3 Commentary emanating from KPMG and other providers of private security and forensic accoutings services reflects the vested interests of this sector.
4 For Canadian crime statistics, see Haggerty (2001). The most commonly cited statistics are from the Uniform Crime Reports, based on incidents reported to the police.
5 In December 2001, in light of the 11 September terrorist attacks on Washington and New York, and subsequent scares over anthrax, the American Society for Industrial Security staged, at Pentagon City, Arlington, Virginia, a conference entitled "Target America: The New Reality of Terrorism." (Available online at <http://asisonline.org/pdf/terror.pdf>).
6 The Longitudinal Labour Force Databank controversy erupted in the late 1990s when it was revealed that Human Resources Development Canada (HRDC), through computer data banks, had the ability to create detailed master files on 33.7 million Canadians, living and dead. Each file contained up to 2,000 items of personal information. In 2000, following media and political controversy, the HRDC minister announced that the computer program that linked employment, social benefit, and tax information had been eliminated (Human Resources Development Canada, 29 May 2000).

7 The full title of Bill C-6, which at first applies only to federally regulated businesses, is the Personal Information and Electronics Documents Act. For proposed changes to the province of New Brunswick's Privacy Act that would have affected both private security work and news gathering, see Saint John *Telegraph Journal*, 3 March 2001.

8 Williams, who is not an academic, offers an unusually sympathetic portrayal of Pinkerton's operations in early twentieth-century Canada.

9 As Dash noted, both private individuals and the police engaged in tapping into telephone lines prior to the invention and commercial adaptation of the telephone.

10 In 1963, the Ontario courts accepted as evidence a 18 mm film, made by a Pinkerton's of Canada operative, in a civil action involving a Toronto transit worker who claimed to have been injured in an accident (Saint John *Evening Times Globe*, 21 December 1963).

11 In domestic intelligence and criminal intelligence investigation, informers, not high-tech equipment, remained the most important source of information.

12 Industrial security in a sense was an outgrowth of Taylorism, scientific management to increase productivity.

13 In the early 1970s, the Canadian subsidiary of Intertel, a security consulting firm, included a number of former high-ranking RCMP officers. Its clients were banks, hotels, airlines, transportation companies, and manufacturing firms.

14 In the wake of the 11 September 2001 terrorist attacks in the United States, the issue of low-paid private-sector operatives providing security at airports has become a media and political issue.

15 Carroll cited no sources for his statistics on information holdings.

16 For the role of CPIC in screening paid and unpaid childcare workers and amateur sports volunteers, see Royal Canadian Mounted Police (1996).

17 At present the degree to which data marketers have taken business away from private investigators is unknown. For a discussion of the issue, see Berstein (1997).

18 On the other hand, the controversial aggressive policies of the New York Police Department in the 1990s suggest that targeted policing can diminish street crime, but at considerable cost to civil liberties and police–minority relations.

19 Manning possibly overstates his case by suggesting that the nineteenth-century police did not gather data. According to Monkkonen (1981), the police following the 1860s were the pre-eminent urban bureaucracy.

Bibliography

American Civil Liberties Association (ACLU) (1996a) "Privacy in America: Electronic Monitoring." Online. Available HTTP: <http://www.aclu.org/issues/ privacy/hmprivacy.html> (accessed 1 March 2001).

—— (1996b) "Surveillance Incorporated: American Workers Forfeit Privacy for a Paycheck." Online. Available HTTP: <http://www.aclu.org/issues/ privacy/ hmprivacy.html> (accessed 1 March 2001).

"American Report" (1978) *Canadian Business*, 51(4): 30.

Anonymous (2000) "Standardization of Large Technological Systems in Canada-Renewing Policing," M.-E. Lebeuf (ed.) *Police and Information Technology: Understanding, Sharing and Succeeding, May 28–30, 2000*, Ottawa: Canadian Police College CD-ROM.

Barney, D. (2000) *Prometheus Wired: The Hope for Democracy in the Age of Network Technology*, Vancouver: University of British Columbia Press.

Beniger, J. (1986) *The Control Revolution: Technological and Economic Origins of the Information Society*, Cambridge: Harvard University Press.

Bennett, C. J. (1995) "The Political Economy of Privacy: A Review of the Literature," paper prepared for the Center for Social and Legal Research, DOE Human Genome Project. Online. Available HTTP: <http://sitka.dcf.uvic.ca/poli/bennett/research/gnom.htm> (accessed 20 February 1997).

Berstein, N. (1997) "OnLine High-Tech Sleuths Find Private Facts," *New York Times*, 15 September: A1–20.

Betcherman, G. and McMullen, K. (1999) "Impact of Information and Communications Technologies on Work and Employment in Canada," in R. Boyce (ed) *The Communications Revolution at Work: The Social, Economic and Political Impact*, Kingston: McGill-Queen's University Press.

Branscomb, A.W. (1994) *Who Owns Information? From Privacy to Public Access*, New York: Basic Books.

Brenton, M. (1964) *The Privacy Invaders*, New York: Coward-McCann Inc.

Brin, D. (1998) *The Transparent Society: Will Technology Force us to Choose Between Privacy and Freedom?* Reading, MA: Perseus Books.

Brown, E. (1971) "California Hires the Aerospace Companies," in A. F. Westin (ed.) *Information Technology in a Democracy*, Cambridge, MA: Harvard University Press.

Carroll, J. M. (1975) *Confidential Information Sources: Public and Private*, Los Angeles: Security World Publishing Co.

Chandler, A. D. Jr (1977) *The Visible Hand: The Managerial Revolution in American Business*, Cambridge, MA: The Belknap Press.

Clinton, President W. J. (1999) "Remarks on Keeping American Secure for the 21st century," Washington: National Academy of Sciences, 22 January. Online. Available HTTP: <http://www.cybercrime.gov/nas9901.htm> (accessed 28 February 2001).

Crimcheck Inc. Online. Available HTTP:<http://www.crimcheckinc.com/ crime-prices.htm> (accessed 26 February 2001).

Dash, S., Schwartz, R., and Knowlton, R. (1959) *The Eavesdroppers*, New Brunswick, NJ: Rutgers University Press.

Donner, F. J. (1980) *The Age of Surveillance: The Aims and Methods of America's Political Intelligence*, New York: Alfred Knopf.

Ericson, R. V. (1982) *Reproducing Order: A Study of Police Patrol Work*, Toronto: University of Toronto Press.

Ericson, R. V. and Haggerty, K. D. (1997) *Policing the Risk Society*, Toronto: University of Toronto Press.

Farnell, M. B. and Shearing, C. D. (1977) *Private Security: An Examination of Canadian Statistics, 1961–1971*, Toronto: Centre of Criminology, University of Toronto.

Galbraith, J. K. (1968) *The Affluent Society*, Scarborough: New American Library.

Gallati, R. R. J. (1971) "The New York State Identification and Intelligence System," in A. F. Westin (ed.) *Information Technology in a Democracy*, Cambridge, MA: Harvard University Press.

Gellman, R. (1996) "Privacy," in Hernon, P., McClure, C. R., and Relyea, H. (1996) (eds) *Federal Information Policies in the 1990s: Views and Perspectives*, Norwood, NJ: Ablex Publishing Corporation.

Gerden, R. J. (1998) *Private Security: A Canadian Perspective*, Scarborough, ON: Prentice Hall.

Gordon, D. (1987) "The Electronic Panopticon: A Case Study of the Development of the National Criminal Justice Records System," *Politics and Society*, 15(4): 483–512.

Haggerty, K. D. (2001) *Making Crime Count*, Toronto: University of Toronto Press.

Halifax Chronicle Herald.

Hannant, L. (1995) *The Infernal Machine: Investigating the Loyalty of Canada's Citizens*, Toronto: University of Toronto Press.

Hare, W. H. (1976) *Privacy Issues in the Private Sector*, Santa Monica: The Rand Corporation.

Harring, S. L. (1983) *Policing a Class Society: The Experience of American Cities, 1865–1915*, New Brunswick, NJ: Rutgers University Press.

Hemphill, C. Jr (1971) *Security for Business and Industry*, Hollywood, IL: Dow Jones-Irwin.

Hernon, P., McClure, C.R., and Relyea, H. (eds) (1996) *Federal Information Policies in the 1990s: Views and Perspectives*, Norwood, NJ: Ablex Publishing Corporation.

Human Resources Development Canada (2000) "News Release: HRDC Dismantles Longitudinal Labour Force File Databank." Online. Available HTTP: <http://www.hrdc-drhc.gc.ca/common/news/dept/00-39.shtml> (accessed 7 December 2001).

Hunt, D. (2000) "Private Investigation: An Effective Response to the National Crime Challenge," in J. Richardson (ed.) *Police and Private Security: What the Future Holds*, Ottawa: Police Futures Group, Canadian Association of Chiefs of Police.

Hunt, W. R. (1990) *Front-Page Detective: William J. Burns and the Detective Profession, 1880–1930*, Bowling Green: Bowling Green State University Popular Press.

Hyde, D. M. (2000) "A Theory of Evolution: A Look at the Factors That Are Contributing to the Revival of Private Policing and Whether the Industry is Up to the Task," paper submitted in partial fulfilment of an M.Sc. (Security and Risk Management), University of Leicester.

Industrial Canada.

Infotel Corp. Online. Available HTTP: <http://www.infotel.net/> (accessed 2 March 2001).

Intelligarde. Online. Available at HTTP: <http://www.intelligarde.org/> (accessed 2 March 2001).

International Association of Chiefs of Police (2000) "Towards Improved Criminal Justice Information Sharing: An Information Integration Planning Model." Online. Available HTTP: <http://www.theiacp.org/> (accessed 15 January 2001).

Jeffries, F. (ed.) (1973) *Private Policing and Security in Canada: A Workshop*, Toronto: University of Toronto Press.

Johnson, D. R. (1979) *Policing the Urban Underworld*, Philadelphia: Temple University Press.

Kakalik, J. and Wildhorn, S. (1977) *The Private Police Industry: Its Nature and Extent*, New York: Crave Russell.

Kinnear, D. (2000) "Privatization – A Threat to Public Police and the Public Good," in J. Richardson (ed.) *Policing and Private Security: What the Future Holds*, Ottawa: Police Futures Group, Canadian Association of Chiefs of Police.

Koehler, J. O. (1999) *Stasi: The Untold Story of the East German Secret Police*, Boulder: Westview Press.

KPMG (1998) *Project Report: Strategic Study of RCMP Economic Crime Program*, Ottawa: KPMG.

Lapidus, E. J. (1971) *Eavesdropping on Trial*, Rochelle Park, NJ: Hayden Book Co.

Lester, T. (2001) "The Reinvention of Privacy," *The Atlantic Monthly*, 287(3): 27–39.

Lipson, M. (1975) *On Guard: The Business of Private Security*, New York: Quadrangle/New York Times Book Co.

Long, E. W. (1967) *The Intruders: The Invasion of Privacy by Government and Industry*, New York: Frederick A. Praeger.

Lynas, M. (1999) "Cry Freedom," *Corporate Watch*, 8. Online. Available HTTP: <http://www.corporatewatch.org/magazine/issue8/cw8g4.html> (accessed 14 March 2001).

Lyon, D. (1994) *The Electronic Eye: The Rise of Surveillance Society*, Minneapolis: University of Minnesota Press.

—— (2001a) *Surveillance Society: Monitoring Everyday Life*, Philadelphia: Open University Press.

—— (2001b) "Surveillance as Social Sorting: Computer Codes and Mobile Bodies," paper presented at Surveillance, Risk, and Social Categorization Workshop, Kingston, ON, May 2001.

Manning, P. (2000) "Technology Revealed," in M. -E. Lebeuf (ed.) *Police and Information Technology: Understanding, Sharing and Succeeding, May 28–30, 2000*, Ottawa: Canadian Police College CD-ROM.

Marchand, D. (1993) *The Politics of Privacy: Computers and Criminal Justice Records*, Arlington: Information Resources Press.

Marquis, G. (1993) *Policing Canada's Century: A History of the Canadian Association of Chiefs of Police*, Toronto: University of Toronto Press.

—— (1994) "The Technology of Professionalism: Criminal Identification in Early Twentieth Century Canada," *Criminal Justice History*, 14: 165–87.

—— (2000a) "Social Contract/Private Contract: The Evolution of Policing and Private Security," in J. Richardson (ed.) *Policing and Private Security: What the Future Holds*, Ottawa: Police Futures Group, Canadian Association of Chiefs of Police.

—— (2000b) "The Evolution of Information Technology in Private Security: Recent History" in M. -E. Lebeuf (ed.) *Police and Information Technology: Understanding, Sharing and Succeeding, May 28–30, 2000*, Ottawa: Canadian Police College CD-ROM.

Marx, G. (1988) *Undercover: Police Surveillance in America*, Berkeley: University of California Press.

Monkkonen, E. (1981) *Police in Urban America, 1820–1920*, New York: Cambridge University Press.

Morgan, R. E. (1980) *Domestic Intelligence Monitoring Dissent in the United States*, Austin: University of Texas Press.

Morn, F. (1982) *The Eye that Never Sleeps: A History of the Pinkerton National Detective Agency*, Bloomington: University of Indiana Press.

Murphy, C. (2000) "Public Policing and Private Security in Postmodern Canada," in J. Richardson (ed.) *Policing and Private Security: What the Future Holds*, Ottawa: Police Futures Group, Canadian Association of Chiefs of Police.

Murphy, P. V. and Plate, T. (1977) *Commissioner: A View from the Top of American Law Enforcement*, New York: Simon and Schuster.

Murray, T. and McKim, E. (2000) "Introduction: The Policy Issues in Policing and Private Security," in J. Richardson (ed.) *Policing and Private Security: What the Future Holds*, Ottawa: Police Futures Group, Canadian Association of Chiefs of Police.

Nadelmann, E. A. (1993) *Cops Across Borders: The Internationalization of U.S. Criminal Law Enforcement*, University Park: Pennsylvania State University Press.

National Advisory Committee on Criminal Justice Standards and Goals (1976) *Private Security: Report of the Task Force on Private Security*, Washington: Department of Justice, Law Enforcement Assistance Administration.

Nemeth, C. P. (1989) *Private Security and Law*, Cincinnati: Anderson Publishing Co.

Nogala, D. (1995) "The Future Role of Technology in Policing," in J. -P. Brodeur (ed.) *Comparisons in Policing: An International Perspective*, Brookfield: Avebury.

Normandeau, A. and Leighton, B. (1990) *A Vision of the Future: Police-Challenge 2000*, Ottawa: Solicitor General.

Norris, C. (2001) "CCTV: Surveillance and the Social Construction of Suspicion," paper presented at Surveillance, Risk, and Social Categorization Workshop, Kingston, ON, May 2001.

Norris, C. and Armstrong, G. (1999) *The Maximum Surveillance Society: The Rise of CCTV*, New York: Berg.

Nye, J. (1999) "Information Technology and Democratic Governance," in E. Karmarck and J. S. Nye Sr (eds) *Democracy.com? Governance in a Networked World*, Hollis, NH: Hollis Publishing.

Oliver, E. and Wilson, J. (1978) *Practical Security in Commerce and Industry*, 3rd edn, Epping, Essex: Gower Press.

O'Toole, G. (1978) *The Private Sector: Private Spies, Rent-a-Cops and the Police-Industrial Complex*, New York: W. W. Norton.

Packard, V. (1964) *The Naked Society*, New York: David McKay Company Inc.

Payne, R. (1967) *Private Spies*, London: Arthur Barker Ltd.

Privacy Rights Clearinghouse. Online. Available HTTP: <http://ww.privacyrights. org/fs/fs16-bck.htm> (accessed 22 January 2001).

Relyea, H. C. (1996) "National Security Information Policy After the End of the Cold War," in P. Hernon, C. R. McClure, and H. Relyea (eds) *Federal Information*

Policies in the 1990s: Views and Perspectives, Norwood, NJ: Ablex Publishing Corporation.

Reynolds, L. (1991) "Truth or Consequences," *Personnel*, 68(1): 5.

Rigakos, G. S. (1999) "On Securing Risk Markets: Police as Commodity in Late Capitalism," paper presented at the British Society of Criminology Conference, Liverpool, July.

Royal Canadian Mounted Police (1996) "Screening Volunteers and Employees to Prevent Sexual Abuse." Online. Available HTTP: <http://www.citytel.net/rcmp/screen.htm> (accessed 10 December 2001).

Rule, J. (1974) *Private Lives and Public Surveillance: Social Control in the Computer Age*, New York: Schocken Books.

Saint John *Evening Times Globe*.

Saint John *Telegraph Journal*.

Securitas. Online. Available HTTP: <http://www.securitasgroup.com/www/> (accessed 2 February 2001).

—— (1983) "Private Security: Implications for Social Control," *Social Problems*, 30: 493–506.

Shearing, C. (1997) "Unrecognized Origins of the New Policing: Linkages Between Private and Public Policing," in M. Felson and R. V. Clarke (eds) *Business and Crime Prevention, Monsey*, NY: Criminal Justice Press.

Shearing, C. and Stenning, P. (1981) "Modern Private Security: Its Growth and Implications," in M. Tonry and N. Morris (eds) *Crime and Justice: An Annual Review of Research 3*, Chicago: University of Chicago Press.

—— (1983) "Private Security: Implications for Social Control," *Social Problems*, 30: 493–506.

Skogan, W. (1995) "Community Policing in the United States," in J. -P. Brodeur (ed.) *Comparisons in Policing: An International Perspective*, Brookfield: Avebury.

Skolnick, J. and Bayley, D. H. (1986) *The New Blue Wall: Police Innovation in Six American Cities*, New York: The Free Press.

Statistics Canada (1991) *The Future of National Justice Statistics and Information Canada: Report of the National Project on Resource Coordination for Justice Statistics and Information*, 2 vols, Ottawa: Supply and Services.

—— (1999) *Perspectives*, Spring.

Statistics Canada, Canadian Centre for Justice Statistics (1996) *A Graphical Overview of Crime and the Administration of Criminal Law in Canada*.

Stead, J. P. (ed.) (1977) *Pioneers in Policing*, Montclair, NJ: Patterson Smith.

Swol, K. (1998) "Private Security and Public Policing in Canada," *Juristat*, 18(13): 1–11.

Sykes, C. J. (1999) *The End of Privacy*, New York: St. Martin's Press.

Taylor, F. W. (1967) *The Principles of Scientific Management*, Toronto: George J. McLeod.

Thibodeau, P. (2000) "Canadian Privacy Law Raises Ante," *Computerworld*, 4. Online. Available HTTP: <http://www.computerworld.com/cwi/s...7> (accessed July 9 2001).

Thurston, J. E. (1973) "Relations Between Public Police and Private Security Forces,"

248 *Targeting trouble*

in F. Jeffries F. (ed.) *Private Policing and Security in Canada: A Workshop*, Toronto: University of Toronto Press.

Toronto *Globe & Mail*.

Toronto *Sun*.

Tremblay, S. (1998) "Crime Statistics in Canada, 1998," *Juristat*, 19(9): 1.

Warren, M. R. (1973) "Address," in F. Jeffries (ed.) *Private Policing and Security in Canada: A Workshop*, Toronto: University of Toronto Press.

Westin, A. F. (1970) *Privacy and Freedom*, New York: Athenaeum.

—— (1971) "Civil Liberties in Public Databanks," in A. F. Westin (ed.) *Information Technology in a Democracy*, Cambridge, MA: Harvard University Press.

Williams, D. R. (1998) *Call in Pinkerton's: American Detectives at Work for Canada*, Toronto: Dundurn Press.

Wilson, J. Q. (1978) *The Investigators: Managing FBI and Narcotics Agents*, New York: Basic Books.

Wilson, O. W. (1973) *Police Planning*, 2nd edn, Springfield, IL: Charles C. Thomas.

12 From personal to digital

CCTV, the panopticon, and the technological mediation of suspicion and social control

Clive Norris

Introduction

The image of the panopticon has been one the most powerful metaphors in locating the theoretical and social significance of CCTV in contemporary society. For Davis (1990), the design and operation of the urban shopping mall, with its centralized security control room, CCTV cameras, and private security guards, "plagiarizes brazenly from Jeremy Bentham's renowned nineteenth-century design for the 'panopticon prison'" (1990: 245). Fyfe and Bannister have argued that the spread of CCTV across British streets represents a dispersal of an "electronic panopticon" (1996). Similarly, Reeve has noted that in the commercial centers of towns and cities the use of CCTV is "clearly reminiscent of what Foucault has described as the disciplinary society, in his use of the metaphor of the panopticon as a device of total surveillance in a rationally ordered society" (Reeve 1998: 71).

The similarities of CCTV with the panoptic principles embodied in Bentham's model prison with its central observation tower, staffed by an unseen observer, watching over the minutiae of a prisoner's behaviour, housed in transparent cells, is of course, highly resonant. The spread of CCTV over city-center streets represents the most visible sign of the "dispersal of discipline" from the prison to the factory and the school, to encompass all of the urban landscape. Moreover, since it is impossible to know whether one is being monitored, CCTV, like the panopticon, has the potential, as Foucault observed, "to induce in the inmate a state of conscious and permanent visibility that assures the automatic functioning of power" (1977: 201). This is because:

> He who is subject to a field of visibility, and knows it, assumes responsibility for the constraints of power, he makes them play spontaneously upon himself; he inscribes in himself the power relations in which he simultaneously plays both roles, he becomes the principle of his own subjection.
>
> (1977: 202–3)

However, we must be careful not to over-privilege the visual aspects of the panopticon: the panopticon implies far more than the power to watch. Significantly, Foucault's analysis of the panopticon does not start with a discussion of Bentham's design of the model prison but with a description and analysis of the measures taken to combat an outbreak of plague in one French town in the seventeenth century. This is then contrasted with the older, more traditional, method of dealing with another highly contagious disease, leprosy.

The regulation of the plague started with a "lock-down" where all citizens except the "intendants, syndics and guards," were confined to their own residences and prohibited from going outside. Once this was in place the populace became subject to a formidable regime of surveillance:

> based on a system of permanent registration . . . the role of each of the inhabitants present in the town is laid down one by one, this document bears the "name, age and sex" of everyone not withstanding his condition. . . . Everything that may be observed during the course of the visits – deaths, illnesses, complaints, irregularities – is noted down and transmitted to intendants and magistrates. . . . It lays down for each individual his place, his body, his disease and his death, his well being, by means of an omnipresent and omniscient power.
>
> (Foucault 1977: 196)

This power is not simply maintained through surveillance but includes the potential for coercion, as there are "guards at the gate, at the town hall and in every quarter to ensure the prompt obedience of the people and the most absolute authority of the magistrates" (Foucault 1977: 196). We can see that power is being exercised through much more than observation; it also involves the individualization of pathology through bureaucratic codification, decision-making based on the power of classificatory categories, and all this is backed up by force should resistance or non-compliance result.

Power over the plague victims is exercised by "differentiation," "segmentation," and "training." In contrast, power over the leper is managed by enforced "segregation," "separation," "confinement," and "exile." One involves branding and exile, the other identification and discipline. Leprosy is managed by exclusion, the plague through inclusion. For Foucault the history of social control is composed of the interplay of these two forms of power and the "panopticon is the architectural figure of this composition" (1977: 198–200). It is exclusionary in that it segregates the deviant from the wider community, but inclusionary because segregation is aimed not merely at warehousing deviants but transforming them into "docile bodies" to be returned to the fold.

The panopticon is then far more than an architectural form of visualization. It is also the social, political, and technical infrastructure that renders visualization meaningful for the basis of disciplinary social control. At the heart of the panoptic project is the collection of individualized codified information, and this provides the rationale for classification and subsequent authoritative intervention.

It is in this context that this chapter seeks to explore the extent to which the pervasive spread of CCTV represents the panopticonization of predominately urban space in contemporary Britain. To do so, we want to contrast contemporary CCTV-mediated surveillance with traditional surveillance practices achieved through co-presence and face-to-face interaction Finally, we will examine the implications of the introduction of the next generation of digital, computer-based, CCTV systems which herald the promise of automated visual surveillance.

Face-to-face knowledge and social control

As Lyn Lofland (1973) pointed out nearly thirty years ago, it is only in the modern world that being in the company of strangers becomes the dominant mode of interaction. Throughout the majority of human history people lived their lives in close proximity to intimates and acquaintances. To draw on John Lofland's analysis, for most of human history we have had knowledge *of* and not just knowledge *about* people: we *knew* them, not *about* them. The basis of knowing *of*, rather than *about* people, is face-to-face interaction. When we only know *about* people our knowledge is secondhand, based on media accounts, official reports, gossip, rumor, and hearsay, and there is the danger that our judgment falls prey to stereotypical prejudice and results in the dehumanization of the "other" (Lofland 1971: 1–2). Face-to-face interaction has the capacity to undermine such processes because face-to-face interaction requires, to some degree at least, putting oneself in the position of the other. It requires, in Goffman's (1972) terms, the mutual coordination of co-presence. Even in the modern world, inhabited more and more by strangers, it is still this mutual coordination of co-presence that largely underpins public order. As Jane Jacobs observed:

> The first thing to understand is that public peace – the sidewalk and street peace – of cities . . . is kept primarily by an intricate, almost unconscious, network of voluntary controls and standards among people themselves, and enforced by the people themselves.
>
> (Jacobs 1961, quoted in Bannister *et al.* 1998: 23)

Public order is highly localized, informal, and personalized. It is based on face-to-face knowledge. Moreover, order is maintained not primarily through the intervention of police or security – indeed their intervention is often a sign of disorder – but by the ordinary mass of citizenry, interacting to reproduce order (Ericson 1982). However, where disorder does occur and the police are called, order is still restored through face-to-face interaction. And while the police may be thought of as a primarily coercive institution involved in the enforcement of laws, studies of routine patrol have shown that the primary mandate of the patrol officer is the restitution of order. This is achieved predominately by means of face-to-face negotiation, often with a highly tuned awareness of situational norms and interpersonal dynamics.

As numerous studies of everyday policing have shown, policing cannot be reduced to a simple application of legal or even cultural norms. Rather, the process of policing has to be understood as a result of the complex interplay of legal, organizational, occupational, situational, and interactional rules (cf. Kemp *et al.* 1992; Hoyle 1998). And what is true of police work in general is also true of police suspicion in particular. Nothing is inherently suspicious, it only becomes so when it is interpreted though the lens of police relevancies and seen through the light of local situated knowledge. As Dixon *et al.* (1989) have rightly argued, suspicion is less an event than a process. Thus while the contours of police suspicion may begin to take shape at a distance, before face-to-face interaction has taken place, it becomes substantiated through interaction, through face-to-face evaluation of the moral worthiness of the person under scrutiny. One of the main consequences of this is that policing is highly discretionary and this discretion results in both differentiation and discrimination (Reiner 1992).

CCTV mediated social control

The introduction of CCTV fundamentally changes the nature of the surveillance gaze both quantitatively and qualitatively. As McCahill has argued:

> One of the most significant impacts of the electronic revolution has been the remarkable capacity of the new surveillance technologies, such as CCTV to transcend both spatial and temporal barriers. . . . Surveillance is no longer confined to controlled and arranged spaces and longer requires the physical co-presence of the observer.
>
> (1998: 41–2)

Furthermore, as he goes on to note:

> The information (i.e. images) produced by CCTV is "controllable, and not subject to the messiness or unruliness of time" (Simpson, 1995: 158).

This allows deviant identities to be "stored" in electronic spaces (on a computer file or a video tape) ready to be "lifted out" at some future, as yet unspecified, time and place.

(1998: 44)

This time–space distanciation has another effect: it allows for the separation of monitoring from intervention functions. Whereas patrol officers on the street use surveillance as the basis for action and direct intervention, security guards in the control room cannot operate in the same way. They watch but have to deploy someone else to intervene.

But it is not just the organization and scope of surveillance that is affected by the mediation of the cameras. As Marx has noted, for some, the electronic surveillance technologies can be viewed as democratizing the surveillance gaze:

> Fixed physical responses that eliminate discretion also eliminate the potential for corruption and discrimination. The video surveillance camera . . . [does] not differentiate between social classes. Data are gathered democratically from all within their purview.
>
> (Marx 1995: 238)

Finally, the spread of CCTV heralds a massive expansion of the disciplinary – and inclusionary – social control. That is, the ever-present threat of authoritative intervention to any acts of deviancy creates anticipatory conformity on a scale unthinkable on the basis of mere co-presence.

Put simply with the introduction of CCTV:

- the surveillance gaze has been expanded to a level unimaginable on the basis of co-presence;
- the surveillance gaze becomes removed from spatial constraints implicit in face-to-face surveillance;
- the surveillance gaze becomes freed from the temporal constraints of face-to-face interaction and co-presence;
- surveillance and authoritative intervention become functionally separate;
- the act of surveillance becomes more democratic: all become equally subject to the surveillance gaze;
- the disciplinary project of the panopticon is expanded as inclusionary social control is promoted over exclusion.

In the following analysis we wish to explore in greater detail the implications of these six contrasts between suspicion and social control based on co-presence compared with CCTV-mediated control. We will also consider the extent to which the operation of CCTV can be said to lead to the panopticonization of urban space.

The introduction of CCTV represents an expansion of the surveillance gaze unimaginable on the basis of human face-face monitoring based on co-presence – however it does not signal the arrival of panoptic control.

The limitations of face-to-face police surveillance have long been recognized. In their review of the literature on police effectiveness, conducted for the British Home Office in 1984, Clarke and Hough demonstrated that:

> Given the present burglary rate and an evenly distributed patrol coverage, a patrolling policeman in London could expect to pass within 100 yards of a burglary in progress once every eight years and even then not realise that the crime was taking place.
>
> (Clarke and Hough 1984: 7)

The promise of CCTV changes all this as Michael Howard, the home secretary responsible for initiating the program of central government funding, eulogized:

> CCTV catches criminals. It spots crimes, identifies lawbreakers and helps convict the guilty. The spread of this technology means that more town centres, shopping precincts, business centres and car parks around the country will become no-go areas for the criminal. . . . CCTV is a wonderful technological supplement to the police . . . One police officer in Liverpool likened the 20-camera system as having 20 officers on duty 24 hours a day, constantly taking notes.
>
> (*CCTV Today*, May 1995: 4)

It is this panoptic appeal that helps explain the enthusiastic take up of CCTV across the UK. In 1985 there was only one open-street system, in the south-coast town of Bournemouth. Over the next decade there was gradual diffusion of the technology to other towns and cities. Even so, by 1991 there were no more than ten city-center/high-street systems in operation. Among these were systems in King's Lynn, Coventry, Wolverhampton, and Plymouth. They were all financed at the local level. Over the next four years the rate of diffusion increased, and by 1994 the Home Office reported that seventy-nine towns or cities had some form of open-street CCTV systems although many of them were small-scale systems, financed predominantly at the local level, either by police, local authorities, private business, or some combination of all three (Home Office 1990, 1994).

In 1994 the uptake of CCTV was to increase from a trickle to a rush. In the wake of successive rises in recorded crime rates, and public anxieties unleashed by the tragic killing of Jamie Bulger by two ten-year-old boys, the Conservative Government announced that the Home Office was setting aside £2 million to support open-street city-center CCTV through a City Challenge Competition. This competition would pay for up to 50 percent of the capital costs of a scheme, the remainder being found from partnership funding from business, local authorities, police or other government departments (*CCTV Today*, January 1995: 7). Over 480 bids were received from towns throughout the country and, although funding was increased to £5 million, only 106 schemes were allocated grants. In light of this strong demand, between 1995 and 1998 three further competitions were held, the last under the New Labour administration, which had ousted the Tories in the 1997 general election. These later schemes also expanded the criteria for inclusion to include schools, hospitals, and residential areas as eligible for funding. In total, the four competitions raised £85 million to secure the capital funding of 580 CCTV schemes, £31 million from Home Office funding and £54 million from the partnerships (*CCTV Today*, November 1995: 4; Hansard, written answers for 2 November 1999 [pt 10]; Home Office 1996).

For some commentators the change in government signalled the end of the CCTV boom with the final competition under New Labour taking two years to put in place and only allocating an additional £1 million above previously agreed Tory spending plans (Webster 1998). However, in 1999 the New Labour Government announced an ambitious crime-reduction program. At its heart was the continuing expansion of CCTV, and £153 million of Home Office money was set aside to support expansion over the next three years. In the first round of the competition some 750 bids were received and by November 2000, 339 new schemes had been granted capital funding at a total cost of £59 million. The results of the second round of the competition were announced in July 2001 and from the 800 bids received 108 schemes were awarded a total of £79 million (Home Office 2002).

In the decade 1992–2002 central government, through its City Challenge Competition and Crime Reduction Programmes, will have committed over a quarter of a billion pounds of predominantly public money to the expansion of CCTV. And this only represents a fraction of the overall investment in CCTV.

On the roads, railways, metro systems, in schools and hospitals, in retail shops, department stores, and shopping malls the cameras have proliferated. During the early part of the 1990s the total value of the equipment market for CCTV products in the UK was around £100 million per annum (Evans 1998: 20). Between 1996 and 2000 the average annual value of the total UK CCTV market including equipment, installation, and maintenance costs was £361 million. According to Drury, such trends are predicted to continue for the next five years (2001b: 6). On the basis of these figures, over the decade 1992–2002 we would estimate that around three billion pounds has been spent on the installation of CCTV and maintenance of CCTV systems, and this excludes the monitoring costs associated with these systems.

Precisely how many cameras this represents in the UK is unclear. As the Home Office minister, Charles Clarke, told Parliament in November 1999, "Information on the number of police, public sector and private operators of CCTV systems currently in operation and the number of cameras in use is not held centrally" (Hansard, written answers for 2 November 1999 [pt 10]). Suffice it to say, in the first decade of the new millennium, when average Britons leave their homes what will be remarkable is if their presence is not seen, their behavior not monitored and their movements not recorded by the omni-presence of the cameras, CCTV operators, and video recorders.

While this clearly represents a massive expansion of surveillance capacity compared with that based on co-presence, this cannot simply be seen as an increase in panopticonization. The power of the panopticon is not just embodied in its ability to subject all to a surveillance gaze, but in the ability to link observation to a named subject through an individualized record, which can then be used for the purposes of identification, bureaucratic codification, and eventual classification. This secondary element, which in the Foucauldian sense transforms mere surveillance into discipline, is largely absent in the routine operation of CCTV systems. The images produced by the multiplicity of cameras are generally anonymous. Just as the majority of people who pass into police view in busy urban environments are unknown to the patrol officer so too are the majority of images that are fleetingly captured on the video monitor. Without the capacity to put a name to a face, and the bureaucratic apparatus to link the events captured on video to a named dossier, the mere expansion of the cameras does little more than quantitatively increase the surveillance gaze. With the introduction of CCTV the spatial limitations of co-presence as the basis surveillance are removed – but such distancing facilitates anonymity undermining its panoptic power.

From the vantage point of the CCTV control room with its bank of monitors, displaying images from multiple cameras, many fitted with pan, tilt, and zoom functions, so much more becomes visible than with the "eyes on the street" of the patrol officer or security guard. However, while more may be seen, less may be known. As distance increases, situated knowledge is lost. The control rooms where images are monitored are necessarily distanced from the specific locale. In spatial and cultural terms this distancing may be relatively limited, with the control room situated at the heart of the area under surveillance, and face-to-face knowledge still the main basis for suspicion.

For instance, in Airdrie, site of one of the UK's first CCTV systems, the control room is located in the police station in the heart of the town center. Thus, while surveillance no longer requires co-presence, it is still largely based on face-to-face knowledge. In the small town of Airdrie the local police are highly likely to know, based on previous face-to-face interaction, the identity of those that come under the cameras' gaze (Ditton and Short 1999). This is confirmed by McCahill's study of the operation of three CCTV systems in a northern town (McCahill 1999). In one of his systems, based in the shopping center of a large run-down public housing estate on the outskirts of town, the operators personally knew nearly eight out of ten of those whom they targeted for extensive surveillance. Their knowledge was based on the face-to-face interaction, a consequence of their mutual membership in a tight-knit community, being schooled in the area, and still residing in it. By contrast, in the city-center system, only 16 percent of targeted surveillances were based on personalized knowledge. Although the city-center control room was also located in the heart of the mall, because of the volume of people who visited the mall every day, drawn from all over the city and region, the vast majority were largely unknown to the camera operatives (McCahill 1999).

So while distanciation results from the introduction of the cameras, the extent to which it replaces knowledge based on face-to-face interaction depends on the local cultural and environmental contexts not just spatial distances. However, with advances in fiber-optics and digitized Internet-based systems, a control room may now be tens or even hundreds of kilometers away from the area being monitored. This of course intensifies the anonymity of those subject to the surveillance gaze.

Distancing is intensified by the shift from localized, discrete control rooms to centralized, multiple monitoring stations responsible for watching a number of separate systems. This is largely driven by the huge operational costs of monitoring. Central government funding, which has fueled the growth of CCTV, has only been available to finance the capital costs of installations. As a result, the financial burden of running and monitoring the systems has fallen on local providers – most often local authorities. These costs are not negligible. In 1996 Norris *et al.* calculated that the average running costs of open-street systems was £72,000 and the total cost of monitoring the 400 systems then in operation was in the region of £23 million. By 2002 these costs will have increased substantially as the number of public systems has increased to around 800 and the effects of the minimum wage legislation have affected pay rates in a notoriously low wage industry. For instance, the four-town, forty-seven-camera system installed by Swale Borough Council has annual running costs of £300,000 per year, and a number of local authorities are "dealing with operating budgets in excess of

£500,000 per year" (Wade 2000: 28). Indeed, some local authorities have been talking about a revenue crisis threatening to undermine existing systems and place a limit on expansion (*CCTV Today*, January 2001: 5). One of the main solutions to this problem has been to advocate the centralization of monitoring functions so that the costs of monitoring are shared between a number of systems that can then benefit from the resultant economies of scale. The effect, however, is to distance the control room further from the locus of control and to further increase the chances that those who are being monitored are unknown to the CCTV operatives.

For example, the West Yorkshire Passenger Transport Executive has installed an 118-camera system to surveille the main bus terminals covering Bradford, Calderdale, Kirkless, Leeds, and Wakefield council districts. The central control room in Leeds is manned for twenty-four hours and covers bus stations located in an area spanning 324 square kilometers (Drury 2001a: 50–1). Similarly, in Hertfordshire the cameras in Hitchin, Stevenage, and Letchworth town centers and two retail parks are monitored from a centralized control room based in Stevenage. The control-room operators are therefore responsible for monitoring five CCTV systems located in an area of over 100 square kilometers. However, the control room had been deliberately designed with the capacity to expand the number of sites so that the monitoring costs of around of £150,000 could be shared between more systems (Drury 1997: 23). This distancing is perhaps at its greatest in the South Eastern Railways Management Information Communications Centre. Located in Central London, this network monitors and controls 1,500 cameras covering stations from the south coast of England to the northern shores of East Anglia: from Brighton to Sheringham, some 260 kilometers apart (Hook 1997: 12).

While centralization represents one solution to the problem of the costs associated with monitoring, it simultaneously decreases the panoptic power of surveillance since the chance that the identity of those monitored is known is simultaneously decreased. Put simply, the chances of CCTV operatives in London having a personal knowledge of a person whose image is displayed on their video monitors from Sheringham some 190 kilometers away is, for most practical purposes, zero.

With the introduction of CCTV the surveillance gaze becomes freed from the temporal constraints of face-to-face interaction and co-presence – however, the archive of the past is often incomplete and inaccessible.

With the introduction of CCTV surveillance, evidence based on co-presence, chiefly witness testimony relying on human memory, can be substituted with images of the past that have been captured and stored by the CCTV system.

Therefore, panopticonization is further enhanced as the surveillance gaze is no longer limited to the here and now; tapes may be searched retrospectively for evidence of infraction.

The lifting-out of surveillance from the temporal fixity implied by co-presence greatly enhances its panoptic appeal. Not only can more and more be seen in real time but the tapes can be searched retrospectively to find evidence of previously unnoticed infractions. Locations can also be searched for the identity of the culprits after the event has taken place. This logic has underpinned the establishment of the London stations' CCTV system run by Railtrack and British Transport Police. Prompted primarily by the threat of further terrorist attacks on the capital's mainline interchanges, 1,800 cameras were installed across 16 stations, the aim being to enable

> total coverage of the areas at risk. This effectively meant the use of cameras with a dedicated field of view, carefully chosen to ensure an overlapping line of sight with those of neighbouring units. It was important, for the purposes of any criminal enquiry that the investigating officer should be able to establish who had entered a particular area, whether or not he had left, and the date and time at which he did so. That level of information could only be guaranteed if there was a total and continuous CCTV coverage of the area in question.
>
> (Hook 1997: 11)

In this system, given the sheer number of cameras, a policy decision was taken not to routinely monitor the cameras in real time, but to regard the tapes as a purely historical record, to be used only when incidents came to light. However, the lifting out of surveillance from the here and now of face-to-face interactions does not magically provide a silver bullet solution to the problem of criminal investigation. One reason for this is that the archive of images held on the tapes comprises only a fraction of the original video signal. In order to cope with the huge quantity of frames generated by, for example, a twenty-five-camera system, rather than having twenty-five video recorders taping the images from each camera, most systems have opted to only have the primary monitor recorded in real time at twenty-five frames per second. The images from all the other cameras are multiplexed, with only one frame per second being recorded on a single videotape. As we will see, this makes the retrospective tracking and identification of suspects a very time-consuming task. Indeed, in some respects it may merely represent an alternative yet equally resource-intensive tool as other investigative strategies. For example, when two men robbed twenty-five people on a single compartment of a mainline train in October 1996 it was disclosed at their trial that they had been:

Caught on CCTV from the moment they entered the rail system at Holloway Road to travel to Waterloo East. They were again filmed as they boarded the 2012 Charing Cross to Deptford train by some of the 4000 cameras that cover the main line, Docklands Light Railway and London Underground network.

(Hook 1997: 12)

However, to identify them and make a case that was evidentially strong enough to stand up in court required that the police searched through videotape from over 500 cameras as the two men travelled across the rail network. We can only guess at how long this took, but it probably amounted to thousands of hours of detective time.

This is confirmed from details of the arrest of the London nail bomber, David Copeland, who set off his first bomb in Brixton, south London, on 17 April 1999. He was eventually arrested for the offence thirteen days later, but only after detonating two other bombs. The last bombing took place on 30 April 1999 in the Admiral Duncan public house in central London, killing three people and injuring seventy-six others. Despite the availability of video footage from the first bombing, in order to identify him the Metropolitan Police had to examine "1097 videotapes containing an estimated 26,000 hours of recorded material, much of it multiplexed, often on a frame-by-frame basis. Some 4000-man hours of video analysis was involved" (Fassbender 2000: 34). It was not until 29 April 1999 that an image of sufficient quality to enable identification was released to the media. In effect, the identification of the suspect took a team of fifty detectives over ten days work, but as the senior officer leading the investigation noted "the excellent detective work, that had carried on in parallel with that of the video identification team meant we would have tracked him down even if the CCTV lead had failed" (*CCTV Today*, September 2001: 3).

Thus the panoptic potential for CCTV to render the past visible by facilitating the retrospective searching of tapes becomes, in reality, very limited. The archive is only partial and because of this requires major resources to identify a suspect.

With introduction of CCTV, the act of surveillance and authoritative intervention become functionally separate – such separation undermines the certainty of authoritative intervention.

This functional separation means that the CCTV operative is in a very different position to a patrol officer on the street. CCTV operatives do not have the ability to intervene on their own account when they see something or someone suspicious. Patrol officers, on noticing something they deem suspicious, have both the legal and organizational mandate for intervention.

This may involve anything from "having a word" with a group of youths, to a full adversarial stop and search. But in these matters officers are acting as their own agents. Under the Police and Criminal Evidence Act the police have the power to stop and search based on the concept of "reasonable suspicion." As various commentators have noted, this concept of reasonable suspicion is remarkably slippery and contestable. Furthermore, as Dixon *et al.* (1989) have convincingly argued, stop and search is a process rather than an event. As such, the police often do not have reasonable suspicion to stop and then search a person before a stop is underway; the justification for a search is generated in the process of the encounter. If a stop does not result in a search or a search is deemed consensual, then the officer is under no obligation to make an official record of the event. Officers can, therefore, act on their suspicions in the knowledge that they are of low visibility and are unlikely to be called to account for their actions. Put simply, if the officer decides to intervene with someone on the street, in the main they do not have to provide any official justificatory account as to what warranted it. When they do have to provide an account these are constructed in the light of what was found during, not before, the interaction.

CCTV operatives are not in such an autonomous position. They do have to involve others, and are therefore always accountable to justify the request for intervention and, unlike the patrol officer, do not have the benefit of hindsight. This very process of accounting serves to limit requests for deployment to only those events that can generate the most concrete and strongest justifications.

The effect of this functional separation appears to be quite stark. In Norris and Armstrong's study (1999b) in over 600 hours of observation of CCTV control rooms there were only 45 deployments – on average less than one per eight-hour shift. Moreover, there was considerable variation in deployment rates between their three sites: 71 percent in Metro City, 22 percent in County Town, and only 7 percent in Inner City. In Inner City during 200 hours of observation only three deployments occurred.

Norris and Armstrong (1999b) found that deployment practice could not simply be determined by the nature of what the CCTV operatives observed. In some cases the operatives ignored unambiguously illegal actions but responded to relatively trivial events. The crucial factor determining deployment practice was the level of system integration between the operators and the police, which in turn depended on spatial distancing, technological linkages, and social interaction. As Norris and Armstrong observed:

> In Metro City, the CCTV control room was housed in the operational control room of the local police station. The police controller who activated deployment from a variety of sources was in close proximity

to the operators, no more than ten feet, with no physical barriers between them. They, therefore, shared the same working space and the police controller could view the bank of monitors from his or her desk independently of any specific request. This close and sustained proximity between operators and police controller/dispatchers facilitated the development of a set of informal understandings as to what may warrant deployment and what would at least warrant a further look. Operators could simply ask the controller to "take a look at this" either on the banks of monitors or by relaying it to the dedicated monitor on their desk. Similarly on receipt of a call from the public, the controller could relay the information to the CCTV operator to place the cameras at such and such a location. Often, even this was not necessary because the operators could easily overhear the controller's conversation.

This integration was enhanced by the constant flow of visitors into the control room, on average seven per shift, as patrol officers would regularly come in to see if an incident had been captured on tape, or just for a general chat, and at night some would take their meal breaks while watching, and at times playing with, the cameras. . . . In this way the formal and informal aspects of the system facilitated the development of a set of shared understandings, which encouraged the sharing of information, and led to a high level of integration with police deployment practice.

(1999b: 170–1)

The Inner City site contrasted markedly with the Metro City experience:

The system was housed in a purpose-built control room in the grounds of a local authority car park, a few hundred yards from the main area under surveillance. There were few visitors, less than one per twelve-hour shift. If police did try to visit, they had to ring the bell, be formally admitted and were always made to sign the visitors' book, a fact that may have discouraged them from using it as an unofficial "tea-hole" when out on patrol. Although they could relay the pictures to a dedicated police monitor in the police station some 500 yards away, this would involve a telephone call on a line that was prone to be engaged and, when they did get through they would be talking to an unknown voice at the end of the line. Moreover, police rarely sought the CCTV operator's assistance when they had received information. Instead, they would ring up and ask for the system to be turned over to them and would offer no explanation as to what they were looking for. The operators often merely became passive spectators as cameras moved at the hands of the police.

(1999b: 173)

Thus it is not possible to infer that the mere presence of cameras and observers will lead to automatic intervention. Indeed, as the surveillance gaze is further spatially and culturally distanced from a locale, its impact is likely to be progressively diminished.

With the introduction of CCTV, the act of surveillance becomes more democratic: all become equally subject to the surveillance gaze – but in reality categorical suspicion is intensified.

CCTV has been portrayed, to use the words of one Home Office minister, as a "Friendly Eye in the Sky" benignly and impartially watching over the whole population and targeting only those deemed as acting suspiciously (Norris and Armstrong 1999a: 158). As one code of practice for a northern city-center system states, "CCTV is not a 'spy system'. There will be no interest shown or deliberate monitoring of people going about their daily business." Similarly Graham, writing of the North Shields system, states that the CCTV operators "have strict guidelines for the operation of the system. For example, guards are not permitted to 'track' people around the town unless they are acting suspiciously" (Graham 1998a: 99). However, what constitutes "suspicious behavior" is not addressed by codes of conduct or by training. As Bulos and Sarno note: "the most neglected area of training consists of how to identify suspicious behaviour, when to track individuals or groups and when to take close-up views of incidents or people. This was either assumed to be self-evident or common sense" (1996: 24).

The issue of selectivity is central to any discussion of CCTV operational practice because the sheer volume of information entering a CCTV system threatens to swamp the operators with information overload. Consider how much incoming information there is in a medium-sized, twenty-four-hour, city-center system with eighty cameras. The answer, as we can see from Table 12.1, is a staggering 172 million "pictures" per day. Inevitably, operators cannot focus their attention on every image from every camera – somehow they must narrow down the range of images to concentrate on. This problem could, of course, be solved entirely randomly, so that each person on the street has an equal chance of being selected for initial surveillance but only a small proportion is actually sampled. However, this would still leave operators with the problem of whom to pay prolonged attention to once initial selection had taken place. For some the answer is obvious: those behaving suspiciously. But this begs the question as to what, in practice, constitutes suspicious behavior.

It is instructive here to draw on the writings of Harvey Sacks on the police construction of suspicion. For Sacks, one key problem for police patrol officers is how they could use a person's appearance as an indicator of his or

Table 12.1 Incoming information as measured by individual frames of video
footage in an eighty camera, twenty-four-hour city-center system

25 frames per second per camera		25
× 80 cameras in systems	total number of frames entering the system per second	2000
× 60 frames per minute	total number of frames entering the system per minute	120,000
× 60 frames per hour	total number of frames entering the system per hour	7,200,000
× 24 frames per day	total number of frames entering the system per day	172,800,000

her moral character and thus, "maximise the likelihood that those who turn out to be criminal and pass into view are selected, while minimising the likelihood that those who do not turn out to be criminal and pass into view are not selected." (1978: 190). In essence, Sacks is asking: when the police have no other information to go on as to a person's moral identity, when they do not know the person's identity or history, and before they engage in face-to-face interaction, what criteria can they use to focus their observations?

The problem is identical for CCTV operators. Bombarded by a myriad of images from dozens of cameras and faced with the possibility of tracking and zooming in on literally thousands of individuals, by what criteria can they try and maximize the chance of choosing those with criminal intent? Compared to a street patrol officer, they are at both an advantage and a disadvantage. Because their "presence" is remote and unobtrusive, there is less likelihood that people will orientate their behavior in the knowledge that they are being watched and, by virtue of the elevated position and telescopic capacity of the camera, they have a greater range of vision than the street level patrol officer. However, these advantages must be offset against their remoteness which means they are denied other sensory input, particularly sound, which can be essential in giving context to visual images. Unlike patrol officers, CCTV operatives are both deaf and dumb. They cannot simply ask citizens on the street for information, nor can they hear what is being said.

Faced with such an avalanche of images, and a limited range of sensory data, how then does the CCTV operator selectively filter these images to decide what is worthy of more detailed attention? The problem is that the operatives do not have prior knowledge that would enable them to determine which persons are going to engage in criminal activity. It is therefore an occupational necessity that they develop a set of working rules to narrow down the general population to the suspect population.

As Norris and Armstrong have shown in their study of the operation of three CCTV control rooms, selection for targeted surveillance is, at the outset, differentiated by the classic sociological variables of age, race, and gender. Nine out of ten target surveillances were on men (93 percent), four out of ten on teenagers (39 percent) and three out of ten on black people (32 percent) (1999b: 167).

In terms of the general population, men were nearly twice as likely to be targeted than their presence in the population would suggest; similarly teenagers, who accounted for less than 20 percent of the population, made up 40 percent of targeted surveillances. Moreover, they calculated that black people were between one and a half and two and a half times more likely to be targeted for surveillance than their presence in the population would suggest. (For further details see Norris and Armstrong 1999b.)

It could, of course be argued that such differentiation merely reflected the distribution of suspicious behavior displayed by different peoples. But for those monitoring the screens, selecting which behaviors are indicative of deviant identity and malign intent is highly problematic. Fighting is an obvious candidate for targeted surveillance as it is represents a clear and visible indication of normative, if not, legal infraction. But what behaviors signal the presence of a potential car thief, mugger, or shoplifter? Given that they want to mask their intentions and try and "pass" as normal, identifying them before they act is unlikely. Instead, operatives rely on a set of normatively based, contextual rules to draw their attention to any behavior that disrupts the "normal." Put simply, behaviors are suspicious if they are unusual. Thus on busy urban streets people who were running, rather than walking, standing still rather than moving, sitting down rather than standing were all subject to targeted surveillance. Similarly those who appeared "out of place" through dress or appearance and those who appeared "out of time" by being present when most others were absent, were also deemed suspicious and subject to targeting. Finally, those who orientated their behavior to the camera through avoidance (by trying to keep away from the camera's gaze), through confrontation (by abusive gestures towards the cameras), or through masking (by obscuring their face with articles of clothing), were also subject to intensive surveillance (see Norris and Armstrong 1999b: ch. 7).

But given that most people who are running are merely trying to catch a bus, those obscuring their face merely trying to mitigate the effects of a biting northerly wind, and those loitering, waiting for their friends, it is hardly surprising that such strategies are largely unproductive in identifying the deviant. Nor is it surprising that, although Norris and Armstrong found that displays of "suspicious behaviour" played a part in determining who was surveilled, it was not the most important reason. Their study found that 36 percent of people who were subject to prolonged targeting were surveilled for "no obvious reason." Only one-quarter (24 percent) of people were targeted for surveillance because of their behavior, but 34 percent of people were surveilled merely on the basis of belonging to a particular social or subcultural group (1999b: 112–13).

Moreover, unwarranted suspicion did not fall equally on all social groups. Two-thirds (65 percent) of teenagers were surveilled for no obvious reason compared with only one in five (21 percent) of those aged over thirty. Similarly black people were twice as likely (68 percent) to be surveilled for "no obvious reason" than white people (35 percent), and men three times (47 percent) more likely than women (16 percent). The young, the male and the black were systematically and disproportionately targeted, not because of their involvement in crime or disorder, but for "no obvious reason" and on the basis of categorical suspicion alone. As Norris and Armstrong concluded, "As this differentiation is not based on objective behavioural and individualised criteria, but merely on being categorised as part of a particular social group, such practices are discriminatory" (Norris and Armstrong 1999b: 150). Thus rather than promoting a democratic gaze, the reliance on categorical suspicion intensifies the surveillance of those already marginalized and further increases their chance of official stigmatization.

With the introduction of CCTV the disciplinary project of the panopticon is expanded as inclusionary social control is promoted over exclusion – however, in operation it appears that exclusionary strategies are intensified.

As von Hirsch and Shearing have noted, exclusion is frequently at the heart of situational crime prevention strategies and it is "now being extensively used in privately owned spaces that have public functions, such as shopping malls" (2000: 77). Moreover, in the UK, as Reeve has shown, with the development of the Town Centre Management movement in the mid-1990s city-center space was also increasingly subject to new bylaws and prohibitions aimed at eliminating certain behaviors and, ultimately, classes of people from disrupting the proper commercial image of the high street. These predominately local measures have been given national substance with the passing of the Crime and Disorder Act 1998 and its introduction of Anti-Social Behaviour Orders so that, according to von Hirsch and Shearing, "exclusionary strategies are being extended further, to publicly owned spaces" (2000: 77).

Two recent studies of the operation of CCTV in private shopping malls, Wakefield (2000) and McCahill (1999), document the extensive use of exclusionary-based control. Wakefield's study was of three security systems in publicly accessible commercial facilities, Arts Plaza (an arts center), Quayside Centre (a shopping center), and City Mall (a retail and leisure complex). As she explains during the five-week observation period at each site:

> One or more people were excluded on 12 occasions at the Arts Plaza, and the total number of excludees was 34 (allowing for the multiple counting of persons repeatedly excluded). At Quayside Centre exclusions were made on 234 occasions, and a total of 578 persons were excluded. At City Mall exclusions were used 45 times, and the total number of excludees was 63.
>
> (Wakefield 2000: 133)

The main reasons for the exclusions were for: being a known "regular offender" (65 percent); drunkenness and vagrancy (11 percent); children or youths playing/loitering (5 percent); or being the associate of known offenders (4 percent).

McCahill's study also found strong evidence of exclusion. In his city-center shopping mall, teenagers were not only most likely to be targeted for extended surveillance, but most likely to be involved in incidents that resulted in a deployment, and most likely to be excluded from the shopping centre. Indeed, over "four out of ten teenagers who were deployed against were evicted from the shopping centre" (1999: 211). As he goes on to note:

> The main preoccupation of the security personnel at the city centre mall was with behaviour that disrupted the commercial image and in particular with the behaviour of groups of youths who were not shopping. More than four out of ten (43%) of teenagers who were deployed against were ejected from the shopping centre, and the influence of age was shown to be compounded by being part of a group. Thus, when a guard was deployed to deal with a group of teenagers there was a fifty–fifty chance that someone would be ejected.
>
> (McCahill 1999: 219–20)

In McCahill's mall these exclusions then were not based on infractions of the criminal law but on commercial considerations that saw youth as "flawed consumers" and this was part of the official policy of management. One written instruction of management read: "If you see any groups of youths hanging around you can ask them to move along. If you have to tell them more than twice could you please ask them to leave the centre?" (McCahill 1999: 211). Rather than facilitating inclusionary social control, CCTV significantly becomes a powerful tool in managing and enforcing exclusion.

We have seen that the shift from suspicion based on co-presence and the possibility of face-to-face interaction to CCTV-mediated suspicion, has both quantitatively and qualitatively shifted the nature of the surveillance gaze. The widespread introduction of CCTV only represents one element of panopticonization. Notably, it increases the amount of surveillance. But even then, the volume of information entering the system threatens to overwhelm the system through information overload. This results in an over-reliance on stereotypical categorization as the basis for determining whom to target, and a set of simplistic and rather unproductive working rules as to what behaviors are indicative of criminal intent. The surveillance gaze is still partial and is still discretionary and discriminatory.

As an instrument of disciplinary power it is also partial. The effect of spatial distancing means that there is a functional separation between those monitoring from the control room and those working the street. This leads to problems of system integration and makes a certain and immediate response to deviancy unlikely. With the current emphasis on creating centralized control rooms in order to carry out the monitoring functions for a number of spatially distanced and discrete systems, operators are further removed from the local cultural context, reducing the chance that they know, on the basis of face-to-face knowledge, the identity of those they watch. Thus, in the main, those who pass under the camera's lens remain anonymous, as there are few linkages to a named individual's record, which can then be used for the purposes of codification and classification.

In short, the rapid expansion of CCTV may clearly represent a massive quantitative increase in surveillance capacity, but only in a very partial sense can it be said to represent the panopticanization of urban space. However, this is about to change. The next generation of CCTV systems in Britain will be digital and this has profound implications for the nature of surveillance. For when CCTV systems are digitized, the images can be subject to automated storage, processing, and retrieval by computers.

The future is digital

"The future is digital" is certainly the message contained in a recent issue of the CCTV industry's trade magazine, *CCTV Today* (July 2001). Of the six main articles in the journal, three dealt with different aspects of the coming digital technologies. Already, according to Petrook, there has been an "explosion" in the digital recording market; the number of companies manufacturing Digital Video Recorders has increased from a handful five years ago to in excess of 80 today (Petrook 2001: 25). At the industry level, a Digital Forum was created in May 2000 to set up a common digital recording standard for systems interfacing with the criminal justice agencies. The draft guidelines were published in September 2001 (Constant 2001: 25). According to Greene, a number of fully digital systems have been introduced to surveille British streets, and at a recent CCTV users' group workshop half of the delegates reported that they were considering whether to switch to digital systems (Greene 2001: 16).

Similarly, in traffic management applications (see Bennett, Raab and Regan in this volume), the benefits of moving to digital systems are also being lauded. Traditionally, intelligent traffic management systems have relied on sensor technology with video pictures merely being used to provide visual confirmation of events. With digital video detection systems the video picture itself becomes the information source. If this can be automatically extracted through computer vision software technologies it represents a significant multi-functional advance on the information generated from traffic sensors. As Abernethy has recently noted:

> As every traffic engineer knows, the surveillance video image provides information on approximate speed, congestion, road conditions, debris in the road, status of road construction, weather, general visibility and impact on road conditions, verification of DMS messages, surveillance security for roadside jurisdictional equipment and perhaps most important – verification of and incident and assessment of its seriousness. Because CCTV provides a significant amount of information, it is in demand with just about every stakeholder associated with ITS [Intelligent Transportation Systems].
>
> (2001: 26)

Once images are digitized and algorithmic processing is enabled, the potential of linkages with existing databases are dramatically enhanced. In the case of vehicle traffic this is already regularly achieved. In the City of London, which installed one of the first digital systems in the country, the cameras comprising the so-called "Ring of Steel" are used to extract license plate details from every vehicle that enters the square mile of the city of London. This information is then automatically checked against a number of databases containing the registration numbers of vehicles linked to suspected criminals and terrorists. In Northampton, the city council has upgraded its town-center system to include an automatic number plate recognition system as part of a Home Office pilot scheme to evaluate the technology's effectiveness in contributing to the government's Crime Reduction Programme. The scheme uses the existing CCTV camera network to perform high-volume ANPR to detected wanted or stolen vehicles

> by comparing the number plates picked up on cameras with entries on the Police National Computer database. The system is also capable of checking against other databases, such as the DVLC's. A team of eight

police officers in cars and on motorbikes has been formed to respond to ANPR "hits". In just one month of operation, the system has captured 250,000 number plates and led to 50 arrests.

(*CCTV Today*, May 2001: 6)

The coupling of information extracted from CCTV images to database information containing identity exponentially increases its panoptic power. By being able to link a vehicle, and by association its occupants, to a database of named individuals, subjects no longer remain anonymous. Moreover, everyone who passes under this digitized surveillance gaze can be classified as "lawbreaker/law-abiding," "suspected/unsuspected," "wanted/not wanted," and so forth. Classification no longer relies on face-to-face knowledge; it is inscribed in the database.

While number plate recognition systems have now been perfected and offer highly reliable identification rates even in adverse environmental conditions and when vehicles are traveling at high speeds, this is of little help in identifying foot traffic in a city-center space. But a number of commercial systems now claim that they can accurately spot a face in a crowd. Most notably, the London Borough of Newham has installed Visionics *FaceIt* facial recognition system linked to a police database of known and suspected offenders. However, it appears that the success of this system has had less to do with its technological capacity than with the perception, encouraged by the police, that the system is far more effective than it really is. All offenders are encouraged to believe that they are being automatically monitored on the streets. Given that the database only contains the faces of 100 or so suspects, and the system has not resulted in a single arrest in three years of operation, it seems likely that its abilities in tracking and identifying have been significantly over-estimated (Rosen 2001).

But what are the prospects for facial recognition technology? Norris *et al.* wrote in 1996, after reviewing the technical problems associated with face recognition systems, "The prospect of being able to match a face from a city centre surveillance scene with one held on a computerised data base is advancing but still a long way off" (1996: 17).

In the intervening five years, there has been considerable technological progress. Software engineers have developed new and more sophisticated algorithms, and by early 2000 there were at least twenty-four commercial companies selling video-based facial recognition products in the US (Blackburn *et al.* 2001: 2). However, in the main, these systems have been perfected for access control applications, which rely on the consent and compliance of the subject. In this context the conditions under which a photograph is taken can largely be standardized, allowing the lighting conditions, head position, head orientation and focal distance between the lens and the subject's face to be held constant. Equally as important, the comparison picture in the database needs to be kept current (see Blackburn *et al.* 2001 for a description of the Facial Recognition Vendors Test, FRVT and evaluation). Under these conditions systems have been shown to perform reasonably well, at least well enough for one American company to be selling systems to the US prison authorities for the purposes of access control (Visionics 2001).

However, the ability to routinely match a face in a crowd is still elusive. First, given that the person walking the street is not necessarily going to be a cooperative or consenting subject, the chances of getting a full-frontal facial image is greatly reduced. Second, the system has to automatically locate the head and face in a sequence of video frames and because of differences in orientation, expression, and focal distance between the image on the database and the target image this is technically very difficult to achieve at an acceptable level of reliability (Norris *et al.* 1998: 266). Moreover, in a crowd setting there is a strong possibility the face will be partially obscured by other pedestrians. Third, in street scenes lighting conditions vary enormously between times of the day and at different times of the year. Finally, on the evidence of the FRVT evaluations, unless the database picture is relatively recent and taken under the same lighting conditions as the suspect image, the chances of recognition are significantly decreased.

With these limitations in mind commercial companies have concentrated on developing systems in relatively controlled environments such as banks, immigration desks, shop floors, and access points, which enable the crucial variables of lighting, distance, and face position to be held constant.

Digital systems and the transcendence of space and time

With the prospect of accurate facial recognition capabilities the loss in functionality caused by spatial distanciation becomes much less significant. Identification, which previously required face-to-face knowledge, can now be performed at a distance. By matching an image to a database, a person's movements can potentially be logged through space as cameras located in different parts of the system capture their image. Furthermore, when "known offenders" come into a field of view the algorithmic software can automatically display their image on the screen and alert the guard to the person's deviant status. In this way distanciation becomes far less important.

With analog tape-based technologies the distribution of the video image is severely limited; generally it reaches only the control room and a few peripheral video monitors, such as a dedicated link to police control room. With digital systems, it is possible to utilize the Internet as the platform by which the images can be distributed between the cameras and the control room monitors, allowing images to be viewed simultaneously from any point on the Internet. Any centralized authority may potentially have real-time access to any images from any system simply by connecting to the Internet. Therefore, MI6 operatives in London can view a "Stop the War" demonstration in Glasgow and simultaneously route the image to their CIA counterparts in Washington and Paris.

If digital systems help overcome the limitations in spatial distancing they also help to overcome the temporal limitations of retrospective searching. Digitally stored images significantly enhance the potential for retrospective automated searching. Digital imaging has the potential to capture and record far more information than current multiplex technologies. Rather than recording twenty-five frames of images from one camera continuously onto tape, a multiplex system records the frames from different cameras sequentially. Thus the frame from camera one is recorded followed by the frame from camera two followed by the frame from camera three, and so on. Each frame is given a camera code so that when play-back is required the multiplex recorder only selects the frames associated with the particular camera. In a five-camera system the picture from each camera will be updated every 0.2 seconds. Each of the images from each camera is recoded at only five frames per second as opposed to the twenty-five frames associated with normal video recording. What this effectively means is that 80 percent of the information available from each camera is lost (Constant and Turnbull 1994: 133–4). As it is not unusual to have the images of up to sixteen cameras stored on one multiplexed tape, the loss of information is even greater.

With the next generation of digital recorders that take full advantage of the MPEG standards for encoding and compression of video signals, the prospect of being able to capture images at twelve or even twenty-four frames a second is increasingly possible. This means that the archival record will be much more complete, greatly enhancing the ability to spot incidents and identify suspects retrospectively. Put simply, the crucial frame which captured the deft hand movement involved in an street drug transaction or provided a full-frontal facial shot is far more likely to be stored on the "tape." But most importantly, the digital medium greatly facilitates automated searching procedures. Thus, for instance, the same algorithms used to scan real-time images to match faces from a database image can also be used to retrospectively search the "tapes" for the presence of an individual across a variety of locations. As one currently marketed system claims:

> The FaceSnap recorder allows officials to document the movement of suspects automatically or manually – linking individuals to a crime or significant event. An advanced search function and activity monitoring graphic can cut the time needs to evaluate a 24 hour time lapse

observation video to less than one hour. Facial images can be compared against existing databases and images can be imported and exported in all common formats or printed out on a standard PC printer.

(FaceSnap 2001)

Digitized systems not only facilitate making the past visible, but the future too. As Bogard argues in his book *The Simulation of Surveillance* (1996), digitized information is increasingly integrated into simulated models of reality. Rather than just passively watching and recording, these software models seeks to extrapolate the future from the present and immediate past; they seek to predict the future. Thus, for example, the new Traffic Control Centre, which will open in 2003, will receive digitized information from the entire camera network overseeing Britain's roads. It is said to be developing a predictive computer model that will forecast congestion points:

> If, for example, a camera detects a collision the information will be fed into the computer which will predict the likely congestion levels that may arise at that and other points in the vicinity as a result of traffic back-up.
>
> (Hook 2000: 10)

It is not just traffic behavior that is subject to predictive modeling. Researchers at King's College London have developed a software package to automatically monitor crowd flows, congestion rates, and abnormal behavior which has been piloted on the London Underground. One of their algorithms models the behavior of suicidal commuters and uses it to predict if someone is a potential suicide risk and about to throw him- or herself under a train. The software's

> ability to spot people contemplating suicide stems from the finding made in analysing previous cases, that these individuals behave in a charac-teristic way. They tend to wait for at least ten minutes on the platform, missing trains, before taking their last few tragic steps. Velastin's deceptively simple solution is to identify patches of pixels that are not present on the empty platform and which stay unchanged between trains, once travellers alighting at the station have left. "If we know that there is a blob on the screen and it remains stationary for more than a few minutes then we raise an alarm".
>
> (Graham-Rowe 1999: 25)

Just as the past and the future become potentially more visible with the coupling of digital images to algorithmic software, so too does the here and now. Even with small systems with only twenty or so cameras it was never possible for the CCTV operatives to monitor the images from all the cameras simultaneously. They could only manage to concentrate their attention on a few areas at a time and, of course, as soon as they focus in on one event, then all the other images remain unmonitored. Algorithmic monitoring allows the prospect of always monitoring key events. For instance, for the night-time monitoring of a town center when there are few people about, the software could be programmed to analyze the images from all the cameras automatically and only display on the monitors those that record the presence of people. At present there are few algorithms of limited capacity to accurately identify deviant behavior or predict its occurrence. But computer vision scientists are actively trying to develop such algorithms. The European Commission, under its Information Society Programme, is currently sponsoring a "Face and Gesture Recognition Working Group" comprising vision scientists from six European countries "to encourage technology development in the area of face and gesture recognition" (EU-IST 2000). So we may expect that over the next ten years software engineers will try to develop algorithms that will automatically identify criminal events and suspicious behavior. Whether these algorithms will be any more successful than their human counterparts is uncertain. What is more certain, especially after the events of 11 September 2001, is that there will be increased investment in a whole raft of biometric surveillance technologies, and that the ability to identify a face and track an individual though space will be increasingly perfected.

Suspicion and social control in the digital age

As we argued earlier, the panoptic principle that observed acts of deviancy should be instantaneously responded to has not been achieved through the use of conventional CCTV systems, which are constrained by spatial and cultural distancing and the resulting loss of system integration. However, with digital systems there is the potential to transform radically the nature of decision-making that can both bypass the need for human mediation of the cameras and significantly reduce the need for human intervention at all. Potentially, digital systems facilitate not only automated facial and behavioral recognition but also automated enforcement. While the image of "Robocop" automatically intervening in a brawl outside a public house is best confined to the pages of science fiction writers, in much subtler, less visible ways, the potential of algorithmic surveillance is already being integrated in to Automated Social-Technical Systems for enforcement purposes.

Digital speed cameras, linked to a vehicle registration index and coupled to an automated billing system, are already in use. Given the speed of processing decisions, it is possible in real time to identify a vehicle exceeding the speed limit, extract the details of the number plate from the moving image, and match it against a database of registered owners. Within minutes a citation for a traffic violation can be printed and dispatched, demanding the payment of a fine if guilty or attendance at court to contest the charges.

It seems unlikely, but not impossible, that disorderly conduct at pub closing time will also meet with such an automated response, not least because the "objective" measurement of speed is very different from the subjective assessment of disorder. Furthermore, the ensuing legal disputes about the classificatory ability of the algorithms would provide a highly profitable arena for the legal profession. However, we already live in a world that utilizes automated enforcement systems. The bankcard with its PIN number, the automatic ticket barrier at the metro station, and the automated turnstile at the library entrance which is only activated when your staff card is scanned, are all enforcement systems. That we do not generally recognize them as such is because we see them as facilitative, allowing us access to our money, the train station, or the books we need for studying. However, as anyone who has incurred an unauthorized overdraft, held on to the library's books too long or tried to use an expired ticket on the railway knows, facilitation can immediately be transformed to exclusion as the cash card is gobbled by the machine or the access barrier refuses to open.

It is within the context of such access control systems that digitized CCTV systems can be expected to flourish. In any area where access can be regulated – the entrance to shopping malls, shops, metro systems, airports, leisure complexes, and so forth – CCTV systems can be integrated with automated access control systems. For instance, at a leisure center a digital database of those that have paid their subscriptions can be linked to the cameras monitoring the turnstile so that facial recognition software can determine whether the person is entitled to access. Similar technology on the metro could ensure that passengers convicted of assaulting members of staff are identified and barred from passing through the automated gates.

This represents a remarkable break with social control based on face-to-face interaction or CCTV-mediated control with a separation of monitoring and intervention functions. First, if such systems are reliable, the potential for full enforcement is significantly enhanced. Second, however, such systems dispense with the negotiated element of social control. For Lianos and Douglas (2000), this represents "a transformation of culture so radical that it amounts to denial." For them,

> Negotiation is the prime constituent of culture. The cultural process involves essentially the mutual understanding of communication and the development of mental skills that promote it. . . . But negotiating with an ASTE [Automated Socio-Technical Environment] is by definition

impossible. The limits of interaction are set in advance and the whole existence of the user is condensed into specific legitimising signals which are the only meaningful elements of the system. *ASTEs radically transform the cultural register of the societies in which they operate by introducing non-negotiable contexts of interaction.*

(2000: 106–7; emphasis in original)

In effect, such systems are profoundly reductive; they utilize no other logic than whatever is programmed into their software, and the end point of such processing is the creation of a binary system of classification: access is either accepted or denied; identity is either confirmed or rejected; behavior is either legitimate or illegitimate. This has fundamental implications for the normative basis of social control. Face-to-face control is negotiated, not absolute. It is based on a complex moral assessment of character which assesses demeanor, identity, appearance and behavior through the lens of context-specific relevancies. But most importantly it is negotiated and, as Lianos and Douglas argue, this negotiation has a crucial moral and educative function. For it is through negotiation, and the approval and disapproval it entails, that social values are learnt and reinforced, since the ASTE's binary classification is not based on nuanced and multi-faceted moral evaluation but

> on the single element of mediation that system recognises. In other words, there are no good and bad, honest and dishonest – or for that matter, poor or less poor – individuals. There are simply holders or non-holders of valid tokens for each predetermined level of access.
>
> (Lianos and Douglas 2000: 107)

As we have argued, face-to-face enforcement is inherently discretionary and therefore subject to very real accusations of discrimination, and the limitations of human-mediated CCTV monitoring inevitably results in the disproportionate targeting of already marginalized social groups. For a number of writers (cf. Marx 1995; Lianos and Douglas 2000) the prospect of digital enforcement brings with it the possibility of the end of discriminatory enforcement. As Lianos and Douglas write:

> It is the first time in history that we have the opportunity to experience forms of control that do not take into account any category of social division. Age, sex, race, beauty and attire are irrelevant and, what is equally important, guaranteed to be so. . . . The point is not that automated environments abolish other vehicles of class . . . but they

cannot discriminate among users on other grounds than their quality as users.

(2000: 108)

At one level these observations are certainly true. For instance, in the case of a camera-based speed enforcement system, it is now possible to implement a system in which every vehicle that violates the speed limit will trigger enforcement. The discretionary power of the traffic cop to waive a citation on the basis of demeanor, attractiveness, contriteness or any other reason is removed. However, the extent to which such systems are truly non-discriminatory depends centrally on the premise that everyone is equally subject to the same surveillance regime. For a system to be fair, every person must have an equal chance of being subject to the regime. But in the context of law enforcement what will be created is a set of discrete localized databases. For instance, a shopping mall might have a database of known or suspected shoplifters, the police a database of those under court-ordered curfews, and the security services a database of animal rights activists. These can then be used for the purposes of identification, tracking, and intervention. But entry into such databases will be based on previous discretionary decisions that are already the result of selective law enforcement which prioritize some kinds of crime as opposed to others.

If systems are not universal in their application, then there is a real danger that they will be deployed on a discretionary basis. In such a case particular communities are subject to intensive and extensive punishment-centered monitoring while others are subject to enabling surveillance. It is perhaps significant that the first and only street-based facial recognition system operating in Britain is also in the one of the poorest constituencies in the country and is used to track known offenders. Meanwhile US airports are preparing to deploy the same system to facilitate the rapid boarding of frequent flyers.

We noted in our introduction that commentators have highlighted the disciplinary potential of CCTV, with its inclusionary strategies of control Ironically, however, in operation it is the exclusionary potential of CCTV-mediated control that has become dominant in the semi-public spaces of the shopping mall and leisure center. This is of profound importance as this privatized space increasingly contains the amenities previously located in the public or civic realm such as shops, banks, pharmacists, and cinemas. But in this privatized space there is little commitment to democratic ideals of public access and assembly; the commitment is to commercial success. If people and their associated behaviors, whether legal or not, disrupt this entrepreneurial mission, they are to be excluded. In Britain at least, as Wakefield (2000) has shown, they can do so with impunity.

Moreover, as Jones has argued, identity – not behavior – is likely to be emphasized with the deployment of digital algorithmic systems for exclusionary purposes:

> Even future generations of CCTV systems, featuring computerised facial recognition systems . . . are likely to be used for this purpose: such systems are not designed to recognize "theft", for example, but rather a known shop-lifter. The system might be used to prompt shop security staff to focus their surveillance on that individual in the hope of catching the individual "in action", but a managerially more prudent (if from a civil liberties point of view, more disturbing) response would be to simply escort that individual from the premises and inform them they were not welcome to return.
>
> (Jones 2000: 18)

In conclusion, it is the computer – not the camera – that heralds the panopticonization of urban space. Anonymous bodies can be transformed into digital subjects, identified and linked to their digital personae residing in electronic databases. Enforcement can become more certain. The automated algorithmic scanning of digital images can alert the guardians to potential acts of deviance and those classified as "deviant" on the database are automatically excluded. But it is not the inclusionary project envisaged in Bentham's panopticon that will become operationalized by the spread of digitalized enforcement, but exclusion. Ironically then, it is in the treatment of the leper, rather than the plague victim, that we find the parallel with digital enforcement.

Bibliography

Abernethy, B. (2001) "Mass Market Appeal," *Traffic Technology International*, Oct/Nov 2001: 26–33.

Bannister, J., Fyfe, N., and Kearns, A. (1998) "Closed Circuit Television and the City," in C. Norris, J. Moran and G. Armstrong (eds) *Surveillance, Closed Circuit Television, and Social Control*, Aldershot: Ashgate.

Blackburn, D., Bone, M., and Phillips, P. (2001) *Facial Recognition Vendor Test: Evaluation Report*. Online. Available HTTP: http: //www.dodcounterdrug. com/facialrecognition/DLs/FRVT_2000.pdf (accessed 28 January 2002).

Bogard, W. (1996) *The Simulation of Surveillance: Hypercontrol in Telematic Societies*, Cambridge: Cambridge University Press.

Bulos, M. and Sarno, C. (1996) *Codes of Practice and Public Closed Circuit Television Systems*, London: Local Government Information Unit.

Clarke, R. and Hough, M. (1984) *Crime and Police Effectiveness*, London: Home Office.

Constant, M. (2001) "Digital Transfers" *CCTV Today*, 8(5): 25–8.

Constant, M. and Turnbull, P. (1994) *The Principles and Practice of CCTV*, Hertfordshire: Paramount Publishing.

Davis, M. (1990) *City of Quartz*, London: Vintage Press.

Ditton, J. and Short, E. (1999) "Yes, It Works, No, It Doesn't: Comparing the Effects of Open CCTV in Two Adjacent Scottish Town Centres" in K. Painter and N. Tilley (eds) *Crime Prevention Studies*, 10: 201–24.

Dixon, D., Bottomley, A. K., Coleman, C., Gill, M., and Wall, D. (1989) "Reality and Rules in the Construction and Regulation of Police Suspicion," *International Journal of the Sociology of Law*, 17.

Drury, I. (1997) "Safety First," *CCTV Today*, 4(4): 23.

—— (2001a) "Bus Lane Super-Highway," *CCTV Today*, 8(5): 50–1.

—— (2001b) "More Peaks to Scale as UK Market Reaches Plateau," *CCTV Today*, 8(6): 6.

Ericson, R. (1982) *Reproducing Order: A Study of Police Patrol Work*, Toronto: University of Toronto Press.

EU-IST (2000) "CVMT: Projects: FG-NET." Online. Available HTTP: <http://www.cvmt.dk/projects/fgnet/> (accessed 19 February 2002).

Evans, G. (1998) "Searching for Growth," *CCTV Today*, 5(1): 20–1.

FaceSnap (2001) "C-VIS: Computer Vision und Automation GmbH." Online. Available HTTP: <http://www.facesnap.de> (accessed 15 January 2002).

Fassbender, J. (2000) "When Image Is Everything," *CCTV Today*, 7(5): 34–5.

Foucault, M. (1977) *Discipline and Punish: The Birth of the Prison*, New York: Vintage.

Fyfe, N. R. and Bannister, J. (1996) "City Watching: Closed Circuit Television Surveillance in Public Spaces," *Area*, 28(1): 37–46.

Goffman, E. (1972) *Behaviour in Public Places*, Harmondsworth: Pelican.

Graham, S. (1998a) "Towards the Fifth Utility? On the Extension and Normalisation of Public CCTV" in C. Norris, J. Moran, and G. Armstrong (eds) *Surveillance, Closed Circuit Television, and Social Control*, Aldershot: Ashgate.

—— (1998b) "Spaces of Surveillant Simulation: New Technologies, Digital Representations, and Material Geographies," *Environment and Planning D: Society and Space*, 6: 483–504.

Graham-Rowe, D. (1999) "Warning! Strange Behaviour," *New Scientist*, 2216 (11 December): 25–8.

Greene, C. (2001) "User Options," *CCTV Today*, 8(6): 18–19.

Home Office (1990) *Digest of CCTV Schemes*, London: Home Office.

—— (1994) *CCTV: Looking Out For You*, London: Home Office.

—— (1996) *Closed Circuit Television Challenge Competition 1996/7 Successful Bids*, London: Home Office.

—— (2002) "Crime Reduction: CCTV Initiative: Round 2 Successful Bids." Online. Available HTTP: <http://www.crimereduction.gov.uk/cctv21.htm> (accessed 19 February 2002).

Hook, P. (1997) "Silent Witness" *CCTV Today*, 4(6): 10–11.

—— (2000) "Traffic Trauma," *CCTV Today*, 7(5): 10–12.

Hoyle, C. (1998) *Negotiating Domestic Violence: Police, Criminal Justice and Victims*, Oxford: Clarendon Press.

Jacobs, J. (1961) *The Death and Life of Great American Cities*, London: Jonathan Cape.

Jones, R. (2000) "Digital Rule: Punishment, Control and Technology," *Punishment and Society*, 2(1): 23–39.

Kemp, C., Fielding, N., and Norris, C. (1992) *Negotiating Nothing: Police Decision-Making in Disputes*, Aldershot: Avebury.

Lianos, M. and Douglas, M. (2000) "Dangerization and the End of Deviance: The Institutional Environment," in R. Sparks and D. Garland (eds) *Criminology and Social Theory*, Oxford: Oxford University Press.

Lofland, J. (1971) *Analyzing Social Settings*, California: Wadsworth.

Lofland, L. H. (1973) *A World of Strangers: Order and Action in Urban Public Space*, New York: Basic Books.

Lyon, D. (1993) "An Electronic Panopticon? A Sociological Critique of Surveillance Theory," *Sociological Review*, 41(4): 653–78.

McCahill, M. (1998) "Beyond Foucault: Towards a Contemporary Theory of Surveillance," in C. Norris, J. Moran, and G. Armstrong (eds) *Surveillance, Closed Circuit Television, and Social Control*, Aldershot: Ashgate.

—— (1999) "The Surveillance Web: The Rise and Extent of Visual Surveillance in a Northern City," unpublished PhD. thesis, Hull: University of Hull.

Marx, G. (1992) "The Engineering of Social Control: The Search for the Silver Bullet," in J. Hagan and R. Peterson (eds) *Crime and Inequality*, California: Stanford University Press.

Norris, C. and Armstrong, G. (1999a) "CCTV and the Social Structuring of Surveillance," in K. Painter and N. Tilley (eds) *Crime Prevention Studies*, 10: 157–78.

—— (1999b) *The Maximum Surveillance Society: The Rise of CCTV*, Oxford: Berg.

Norris, C., Moran, J., and Armstrong G. (1996) "Algorithmic Surveillance," paper presented at CCTV and Social Control Conference, Hull, July 1996.

—— (1998) "Algorithmic Surveillance: The Future of Automated Visual Surveillance," in C. Norris, J. Moran, and G. Armstrong (eds) *Surveillance, Closed Circuit Television, and Social Control*, Aldershot: Ashgate.

Orwell, G. (1949) *Nineteen Eighty-Four*, London: Secker and Warburg.

Petrook, D. (2001) "Digital Myths Explored," *CCTV Today*, 8(4): 25–7.

Poster, M. (1996) "Database as Discourse; or, Electronic Interpellations," in D. Lyon and E. Zureik (eds) *Computers, Surveillance and Privacy*, Minneapolis: University of Minnesota Press.

Reeve, A. (1998) "The Panopticisation of Shopping: CCTV and Leisure Consumption," in C. Norris, J. Moran, and G. Armstrong (eds) *Surveillance, Closed Circuit Television, and Social Control*, Aldershot: Ashgate.

Reiner, R. (1992) *The Politics of the Police*, London: Harvester Wheatsheaf.

Rosen, J. (2001) "A Cautionary Tale for a New Age of Surveillance," *New York Times*, 7 October.

Sacks, H. (1978) "Notes on Police Assessment of Moral Character," in J. van Maanen and P. Manning, (eds) *Policing: A View From the Street*, New York: Random House.

Simpson, L. (1995) *Technology, Time and the Conversations of Modernity*, London: Routledge.

Visionics (2001) "VISIONICS Corp. – Empowering Identification." Online. Available HTTP: <http://www.visionics.com> (accessed 15 January 2002).

Von Hirsch, A. and Shearing, C. (2000) "Exclusion from Public Space," in A. von Hirsch, D. Garland, and A. Wakefield (eds) *Ethical and Social Perspectives on Situational Crime Prevention*, Oxford: Hart Publishing.

Wade, G. (2000) "Funding CCTV: The Story so Far," *CCTV Today*, 7(2): 28–33.

Wakefield, A. (2000) "Situational Crime Prevention in Mass Private Property," in A von Hirsch, D, Garland, and A. Wakefield (eds) *Ethical and Social Perspectives on Situational Crime Prevention*, Oxford: Hart Publishing.

Webster, W. (1998) "Surveying the Scene: Geographic and Spatial Aspects of the Closed Circuit Television Surveillance Revolution in the UK," paper presented to the XII Meeting of the Permanent Study Group on Informatization in Public Administration, European Group of Public Administration Annual Conference, Paris, September.

Wright, S. (1998) *An Appraisal of Technologies of Political Control*, European Parliament, Scientific and Technological Options Assessments working document (consultation version), Luxembourg: European Parliament, Director General for Research, Directorate B, the STOA Programme.

Index

durhosz

506-236-306